Biosensors and Aptamers

Shriyansh Srivastava • Sachin Kumar
Sathvik Belagodu Sridhar
Malakapogu Ravindra Babu
Shaik Abdul Rahaman
Editors

Biosensors and Aptamers

A New Era in Cancer Diagnosis and Treatment

Springer

Editors
Shriyansh Srivastava
Department of Pharmacy
School of Medical and Allied Sciences
Galgotias University
Greater Noida, Uttar Pradesh, India

Sathvik Belagodu Sridhar
RAK College of Pharmacy
RAK Medical & Health Sciences University
Ras al Khaimah, United Arab Emirates

Shaik Abdul Rahaman
Department of Pharmacy
School of Medical and Allied Sciences
Galgotias University
Greater Noida, Uttar Pradesh, India

Sachin Kumar
Department of Pharmacology, Delhi
Institute of Pharmaceutical Sciences
and Research (DIPSAR)
Delhi Pharmaceutical Sciences
and Research University (DPSRU)
New Delhi, India

Malakapogu Ravindra Babu
Department of Pharmacy
School of Medical and Allied Sciences
Galgotias University
Greater Noida, Uttar Pradesh, India

ISBN 978-981-96-8386-4 ISBN 978-981-96-8387-1 (eBook)
https://doi.org/10.1007/978-981-96-8387-1

This Springer imprint is published by the registered company Springer Nature Singapore Pte Ltd.
The registered company address is: 152 Beach Road, #21-01/04 Gateway East, Singapore 189721, Singapore

I dedicate this book to my greatest inspiration, my father, ***Sanjay Srivastav****, and my most substantial support, my mother,* ***Pushpa Srivastava****, who always believed in me. They sowed the seeds of knowledge in my mind and nurtured them with unwavering love and care. I also dedicate this work to my younger brother,* ***Romil Srivastav****, and my beloved sister,* ***Soumya Srivastava****, whose presence brings me constant joy and motivation. Finally, I express heartfelt gratitude to all the teachers who teach passionately and patiently, shaping minds and igniting dreams.*

Shriyansh Srivastava

Foreword

Medical Science advances at an extraordinary pace, and with it, the fight against Cancer enters a bold new chapter. This book entitled *Biosensors and Aptamers: A New Era in Cancer Diagnosis and Treatment* edited by **Shriyansh Srivastava, Dr. Sachin Kumar, Dr. Sathvik Belagodu Sridhar, Dr. Malakapogu Ravindra Babu, and Dr. Shaik Abdul Rahaman** delivered a scientifically rich and forward-looking volume that actively engages with two of the most transformative technologies in modern oncology.

The authors dissect the power of biosensors with clarity and precision, demonstrating how these devices accelerate diagnosis by offering rapid, accurate, and minimally invasive detection of Cancer. Readers experience, firsthand, how biosensors shift the diagnostic paradigm from reactive to proactive, enabling earlier and more reliable detection.

Equally compelling is the focus on aptamers, small, synthetic molecules that redefine targeted therapy. The authors showcase how aptamers home in on tumor cells with molecular accuracy, delivering treatment with minimal collateral damage. They highlight how this approach significantly reduces side effects while maximizing therapeutic efficacy, paving the way for personalized, patient-centric care.

Throughout this book, the editors curate a wealth of case studies, real-world applications, and cutting-edge research that exemplify the impact of biosensors and aptamers. They present these advancements not as distant possibilities but as tangible solutions already shaping clinical outcomes. Their work reflects a deliberate and compassionate mission: to transform cancer diagnosis and treatment into processes that are not only more effective but also more humane.

This book invites readers to enter a new scientific frontier where biology and technology converge to redefine cancer care. It challenges scientists, clinicians, and innovators to embrace a future built on precision, innovation, and empathy. With its active voice, rigorous insight, and visionary outlook, this volume stands as both a roadmap and a rallying cry for all those committed to conquering cancer. This book guides your journey into the next cancer diagnosis and treatment era.

Emeritus Scientist, ICMR
Former DG (LS), DRDO & Director NIPER
Hyderabad, Telangana, India

Shashi Bala Singh
PhD, DSc, FNASc, FAMS, FIAN

Preface

In *Biosensors and Aptamers: A New Era in Cancer Diagnosis and Treatment*, we invite you on a transformative journey through the latest advancements in medical science. This book captures the groundbreaking innovations that scientists and innovators harness to unveil biosensors and aptamers' potential in the battle against cancer.

You will discover how these cutting-edge technologies are revolutionizing cancer diagnosis, providing unprecedented accuracy and facilitating early detection, which is crucial for effective treatment. As you delve deeper, you will explore the remarkable progress in targeted therapies, where aptamers deliver personalized treatments with precision that minimizes side effects while maximizing efficacy.

Through compelling narratives, we highlight real-world applications and success stories that illustrate the impact of these technologies on patient care. This book showcases the relentless pursuit of a future where cancer diagnosis and treatment become more effective and embrace a more humane approach.

Join the pioneers at the forefront of medical science as they usher in this new era in the war against cancer. Together, we can redefine the oncology landscape and work toward a brighter future for patients worldwide.

Greater Noida, Uttar Pradesh, India — Shriyansh Srivastava
New Delhi, Delhi, India — Sachin Kumar
Ras al Khaimah, United Arab Emirates — Sathvik Belagodu Sridhar
Greater Noida, Uttar Pradesh, India — Malakapogu Ravindra Babu
Greater Noida, Uttar Pradesh, India — Shaik Abdul Rahaman

Acknowledgments

I gratefully acknowledge Galgotias University for providing a supportive environment that enabled me to work on this book. I also sincerely thank our CEO, **Dr. Dhruv Galgotia**, for his visionary leadership and encouragement throughout this journey.

About the Book

In this book *Biosensors and Aptamers: A New Era in Cancer Diagnosis and Treatment*, readers explore the latest Medical and Life Sciences advancements. Scientists and innovators unveil the transformative potential of biosensors and aptamers in the fight against cancer. These cutting-edge technologies revolutionize diagnosis by enabling unprecedented accuracy and early detection. The book examines breakthroughs in targeted therapy, where aptamers deliver personalized treatments with remarkable precision, reducing side effects and enhancing efficacy. It highlights real-world applications and the pursuit of more effective and humane cancer diagnosis and treatment approaches. Join the pioneers in charge of medical science and help shape a new era in combating cancer.

Contents

Introduction to Biosensors and Aptamers: A New Era in Cancer Diagnosis and Treatment

1

Shriyansh Srivastava, Dheeraj Sharma, Sachin Kumar, Malakapogu Ravindra Babu, and Shaik Abdul Rahaman

1.1 Overview of Cancer Diagnostics and Treatment

The early detection of cancer is one of the best strategies for bettering the outcomes of the patient and reducing mortality. Treatment of the patient is more effective and less invasive when cancer is diagnosed in its initial stages, often with lower costs. For instance, survival rates for stage I colorectal cancer patients treated with localized surgery are greater than 90%. In contrast, survival rates for patients with stage IV colorectal cancer, where the disease has metastasized, drop to less than 15%. Likewise, cervical cancer screening programs through early detection have reduced incidence and mortality in countries that have well-organized screening efforts [1, 2]. Survival statistics aside, the benefits of early detection go much further. It reduces physical and psychological burdens that come with aggressive treatments like chemotherapy or surgeries needed for advanced cancers [3]. In addition, healthcare costs can be greatly reduced by avoiding complicated and lengthy treatment plans. Taking an example, the cost of managing early-stage breast cancer will be much lower than expensive metastatic breast cancer treatment because many

S. Srivastava (✉) · D. Sharma · M. Ravindra Babu · S. A. Rahaman
Department of Pharmacy, School of Medical and Allied Sciences, Galgotias University, Greater Noida, Uttar Pradesh, India

S. Kumar
Department of Pharmacology, Delhi Institute of Pharmaceutical Sciences and Research (DIPSAR), Delhi Pharmaceutical Sciences and Research University (DPSRU), New Delhi, India

S. Srivastava et al. (eds.), *Biosensors and Aptamers*,
https://doi.org/10.1007/978-981-96-8387-1_1

modalities are involved in the latter [4]. Despite its benefits, it remains a challenge worldwide as it is hampered by differences in access to screening programs, lack of awareness, and the limitations of current diagnostic technologies. Conventional methods usually fail to detect small, asymptomatic tumors, especially cancers like ovarian and pancreatic cancers, which are usually vaguely symptomatic at later stages [5]. The gaps that emerging technologies, including biosensors and aptamer-based diagnostics, are aiming to bridge would be an improvement in sensitivity and specificity for the detection of ultralow concentrations of cancer biomarkers. Introducing these tools into routine clinical practice will enable early and more reliable detection of cancer, thus offering better results for patients around the world. Traditional methods of cancer diagnostics, though foundational in oncology, are severely limited in effectiveness, especially at the early stages of the disease. Imaging techniques like computed tomography (CT), magnetic resonance imaging (MRI), and ultrasound are quite commonly used for tumor localization and disease progression. But these modalities are often incapable of detecting micrometastases or very small tumors. For instance, CT scans are very effective for staging lung cancer but have poor sensitivity for early-stage disease, where tumor sizes may be below detection thresholds [6]. The histopathological examination, being the gold standard in diagnosing cancer, mandates a biopsy a procedure that can be invasive, painful, and often not feasible in patients whose tumors are inaccessible. The process is time-consuming and requires the skills of pathologists; some may be subject to interobserver variability, thus delaying treatment decisions. For the low-resource setting, it becomes a multiple-problem scenario [7]. Tumor marker assays, such as prostate-specific antigen (PSA) for prostate cancer and carcinoembryonic antigen (CEA) for colorectal cancer, are noninvasive diagnostic options but have the disadvantages of low specificity and sensitivity. For example, an elevated PSA level is caused by benign prostatic hyperplasia rather than malignancy, which leads to inappropriate biopsies and increased patient anxiety. Similarly, CEA levels may rise due to inflammatory conditions that are unrelated to cancer [8]. These limitations highlight the need for new diagnostic tools that are more sensitive, specific, and accessible. Biosensors and aptamer-based technologies represent promising alternatives, allowing for rapid, noninvasive detection of biomarkers even at ultralow concentrations, addressing critical gaps left by traditional methods. Biosensors and aptamers have made their mark as revolutionary diagnostic tools for cancer, dealing with several critical disadvantages of conventional methods. A biosensor is an analytical device that incorporates a biological recognition element, such as an aptamer, coupled with a transducer to convert biomolecular interactions into measurable signals. The provided devices are outstanding for the fast, highly sensitive, and specific detection of cancer biomarkers, thus ideal for early diagnosis [9]. Aptamers, which are synthetic oligonucleotides or peptides, mimic the function of an antibody: high affinity toward a specific target. However, unlike the case of an antibody, an aptamer is synthesized chemically; hence, it presents the following major advantages, among others: much higher stability, cost-effectiveness, and ease of scalability, as well as versatility small molecules, proteins, and whole cells may be targeted [10]. For example, such aptamer-based biosensors for the HER2 marker in breast cancer have

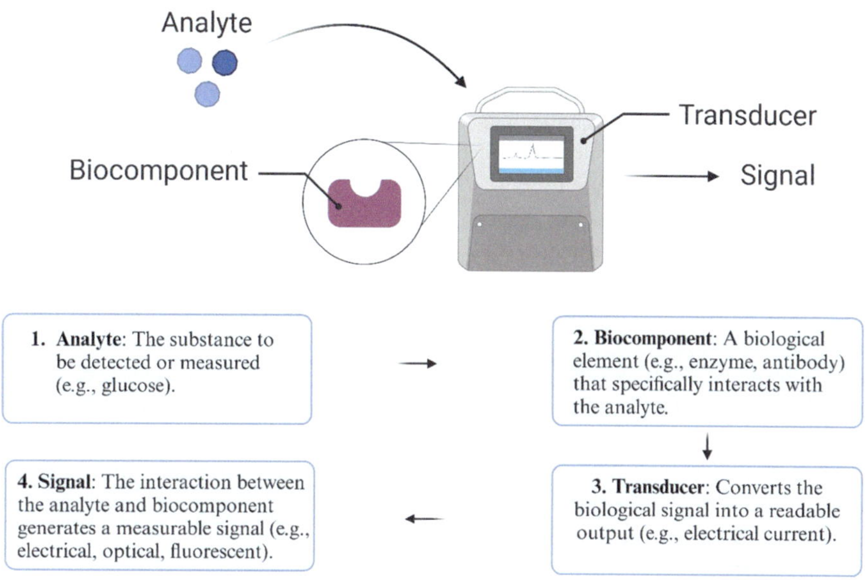

Fig. 1.1 Components of a biosensor

reported sensitivities with which their biomarkers are detectable at femtomolar concentration levels, undetectable by conventional means [11]. The integration of biosensors into diagnostic workflows is particularly valuable in resource-limited settings. These devices are portable and require minimal infrastructure, making them accessible for point-of-care testing. Moreover, biosensors reduce the time and cost associated with traditional diagnostics by enabling real-time detection and eliminating the need for extensive laboratory procedures [12]. As research continues, developments in nanotechnology and microfluidics are improving biosensors' and aptamers' capabilities further. These technologies pave the way for personalized medicine through early and precise cancer diagnosis and are trying to address global health inequalities in access [13] (Fig. 1.1).

1.2 Fundamentals of Biosensors

1.2.1 Definition and Components of Biosensors

Biosensors are analytical devices designed to sense specific biological molecules by translating molecular interactions into measurable signals. The fundamental building blocks include a biological recognition element, a transducer, and a signal processor. This biological recognition element specifically recognizes the target analyte for which the interaction initiates the detection event. Enzymes, antibodies, and aptamers are general types of recognition elements, with aptamers being beneficial in many areas because of their stability, specificity, and adaptability [14]. The transducer is between the biosensor and biological interaction or between the interaction and generation of a measurable signal, where the molecular recognition event is being converted into an electrical output [15]. Different biosensors result in varying types of changes through mechanisms involving electrical, optical, and mechanical methods. Electrochemical biosensors work in an electroactive process wherein, upon binding by the analyte to its recognition element, electrons are transferred to create a current relative to the amount of concentration [16]. The signal processor amplifies and interprets the transduced signal, thus allowing quantification and visualization of results. This is necessary for the accurate detection of biomarkers, especially in low concentrations [17]. Biosensors are engineered with high sensitivity, sometimes operating at the picomolar or femtomolar levels in terms of analyte concentrations. They are compact in design, and response times are very fast, allowing real-time analysis in cases of cancer diagnosis. Performance is further increased through the incorporation of innovations such as nanomaterials and microfluidics for the detection of multiple biomarkers within complex biological samples. Their use is now being assimilated into clinical workflows as biosensors contribute to diagnostic solutions that are precise, efficient, and accessible [18].

1.2.2 Types of Biosensors Used in Cancer Diagnostics

Biosensors can be classified based on the transduction mechanism used. The most widely used types in cancer diagnostics are electrochemical, optical, and piezoelectric biosensors, with different advantages and applications. The basic function of biosensors is that they transduce biomolecular interactions into measurable signals, and the choice of transducer will determine this process. Each electrochemical, optical, and piezoelectric biosensor relies on a different mechanism for signal transduction in order to achieve this.

1.2.2.1 Electrochemical Biosensors

Electrochemical biosensors are one of the most extensively used because of their ease, cost-effectiveness, and high sensitivity. These are designed to sense electrical variations like current, voltage, or impedance while detecting the interaction of the analyte and recognition element [19]. For example, an electrochemical HER2 biosensor used for detecting HER2 receptors in breast cancer has recorded detection limits as low as a few femtomolar units, and its early diagnostics and subsequent therapeutic response are monitored at that stage. These biosensors are portable and can be integrated into point-of-care platforms, which makes them very useful in decentralized healthcare settings [20]. Electrochemical biosensors operate by electron transfer events between the analyte and the electrode of the sensor. They produce electrical properties, for example, changes in current, voltage, or impedance values, directly proportional to analyte concentrations. Techniques applied include cyclic voltammetry and impedance spectroscopy to elevate the resolution and sensitivity in these sensors. For example, electrochemical aptamer-based biosensors

Table 1.1 Comparison of different types of biosensors in cancer diagnostics

Biosensor type	Principle	Advantages	Limitations	Example application	References
Electrochemical	Measures electrical changes (e.g., current, voltage, and impedance) generated by biomolecular interactions	High sensitivity, cost-effective, compact, and suitable for point-of-care diagnostics	Requires electrode surface modification; sensitivity affected by biological matrix interference	HER2 detection for breast cancer with femtomolar sensitivity	[19–21]
Optical	Utilizes light-based phenomena (e.g., fluorescence, absorbance, and refractive index changes)	High specificity, real-time and label-free detection, multiplexing capabilities.	Sophisticated instrumentation required, expensive for resource-limited settings.	CA125 detection in ovarian cancer using surface plasmon resonance (SPR)	[22, 23]
Piezoelectric	Detects mass-induced frequency shifts due to analyte binding on the sensor surface.	Rapid response, label-free detection, and effective for large analytes like circulating tumor cells.	Sensitivity dependent on surface functionalization,; prone to environmental vibrations.	Circulating tumor cell (CTC) detection in liquid biopsy for metastatic cancers	[24]

can measure the levels of PSA at femtomolar levels of detection, which reveals the exactness of its detection [21] (Table 1.1).

1.2.2.2 Optical Biosensors

Optical biosensors exploit light-related phenomena, such as fluorescence, absorbance, or refractive index changes, to monitor the interaction of biomolecules. Fluorescence-based sensors, for instance, employ labeled aptamers that emit light when binding occurs to their target molecules. This allows for the simultaneous qualitative and quantitative detection of the analyte [23]. SPR is one of the most popular optical techniques, allowing for real-time and label-free detection of cancer biomarkers, such as CA125, which is often associated with ovarian cancer. SPR biosensors have very high specificity and accuracy in giving information about the concentration of biomarkers. However, their dependence on complex instrumentation may make them inaccessible in resource-poor settings. High-throughput applications are very useful in fluorescent optical biosensors, which are based on aptamer-based labels and are both sensitive and multiplexed [22] (Table 1.1).

1.2.2.3 Piezoelectric Biosensors

Piezoelectric biosensors work by detecting a mechanical change, such as mass-induced frequency shifts of the surface of the sensor, by binding the analyte onto the surface. For liquid biopsies, these have been particularly suited for determining circulating tumor cells and even extracellular vesicles (EVs), and their responses are the fastest, in addition to being the most sensitive devices for sensing cancer metastasis and the progression level. Such mechanisms especially provide high sensitivity, as expected when detecting CTCs or extracellular vesicles. Each type of biosensor in cancer diagnostics plays an innovative role, and hence, efforts are on to put those technologies into compact, multifunctional platforms. These advancements will significantly elevate their utility in a clinic by combining the strengths of many different transduction mechanisms. Advances in materials science, for instance, have been very successful in incorporating nanomaterials into biosensors to enhance signal amplification. Gold nanoparticles and carbon nanotubes can improve the sensitivity and stability of the devices and thus allow ultralow biomarker concentrations in complex biological samples to be detected [24] (Table 1.1).

1.3 Introduction to Aptamers

1.3.1 Definition and Characteristics of Aptamers

Aptamers are short oligonucleotides containing DNA or RNA, peptides, or a combination of both, which fold into unique three-dimensional structures that can bind in a highly specific and selective manner to specific targets ranging from small molecules and ions to large proteins and even cells. Aptamers are often called "chemical antibodies" because they can mimic the binding properties of antibodies, but they give several advantages over other recognition elements based on antibodies [25]. One of the most prominent features of aptamers is their chemical stability. Unlike antibodies, which are sensitive to temperature and pH variations, aptamers can function under extreme conditions and are thus suitable for various diagnostic and therapeutic applications [26]. They are small in size, approximately 15–60 nucleotides, which enables them to bind to unique epitopes inaccessible to larger biomolecules. Aptamers are chemically synthesized, thus ensuring a consistent batch-to-batch preparation, scalability, and cost-effectiveness compared to antibodies, whose production requires biological systems [27]. Aptamers have a high degree of flexibility to be chemically modified. For example, fluorophores or nanoparticles can be attached to aptamers to improve the detection method in biosensor systems. In addition, their binding nature is reversible, thereby allowing them to be reused for certain diagnostic applications, further lowering the costs [28]. These characteristics make aptamers ideal candidates for applications in diagnostics related to cancer, where sensitivity, specificity, and stability are critical. Aptamers have been used successfully to detect biomarkers such as vascular endothelial growth factor (VEGF), an angiogenesis indicator, and HER2, a marker for breast cancer [29].

1.3.2 Comparison of Aptamers with Antibodies

Aptamers and antibodies are high-specificity recognition elements that can be used in diagnostics and therapeutics, but they differ significantly in their general properties and production methods. Antibodies are proteins that the immune system produces, which are usually generated using living organisms or cell culture systems. On the contrary, aptamers are totally synthetic substances [30]. They are synthesized through a chemical synthesis process, for instance, Systematic Evolution of Ligands by Exponential Enrichment (SELEX). This synthetic nature makes aptamers less expensive and considerably more reproducible compared with the rest of the antibody products [31]. Another important difference is stability. At extreme pH or high temperature, antibodies are easily denatured, whereas aptamers remain undamaged under the same conditions. This stability enables one to use aptamers where the environment might adversely affect the antibodies. Chemical modifications of aptamers further enhance binding affinity, add resistance to nuclease degradation, or attach functional groups suitable for targeted applications [26, 32]. Both show similarities between their binding specificity and affinity. However, the use of aptamers can easily be exploited when targeting small molecules or even non-immunogenic targets that are hard for antibodies to recognize. The aptamers, in particular, can bind highly accurately to ions, metabolites, and small ligands [33]. Despite these benefits, antibodies are still largely used because of their already established clinical acceptance and long history in biomedical applications. However, the scalability, stability, and adaptability of aptamers suggest that they may complement or even replace antibodies in certain applications, especially point-of-care diagnostics and personalized medicine.

1.3.3 Aptamer Selection Process (SELEX)

The Systematic Evolution of Ligands by Exponential Enrichment (SELEX) process, or aptamer selection, is a highly iterative process for isolating oligonucleotides with a high affinity and specificity for a given target. SELEX begins with a large, random library of oligonucleotide sequences, usually containing 10^13–10^15 unique variants. This library is exposed to the target molecule, allowing sequences that bind the target to form complexes. Unbound sequences are washed away, and the bound sequences are eluted and amplified by polymerase chain reaction (PCR) or reverse transcription polymerase chain reaction (RT-PCR) for RNA aptamers [34]. The amplified sequences are further submitted to additional rounds of binding and selection with increasing stringency to enrich for high-affinity sequences. Generally, this process requires 8–15 rounds; the enriched pool of aptamers is then sequenced to identify the best-performing candidates. The step has been further streamlined using high-throughput sequencing for the identification of aptamers with optimal binding characteristics [35]. Advances in SELEX methodology, including Cell-SELEX and in silico SELEX, have expanded its scope of targets and applications. By Cell-SELEX, aptamers that recognize a cell surface marker without prior information on the structure of their target can be selected particularly for cancer diagnostics. Using computational modeling to simulate in vitro binding interactions, the in silico SELEX method accelerates the pace of selection and reduces experiment costs [36, 37]. SELEX remains the gold standard for aptamer development, providing a robust and versatile framework for generating aptamers tailored to specific diagnostic or therapeutic needs.

1.4 Mechanisms of Aptamer-Based Biosensors

1.4.1 How Aptamers Function as Recognition Elements

Aptamers are very potent recognition elements in biosensors. This is due to the three-dimensional structural uniqueness of these elements and the exceptional specificity of their binding ability. Short, single-stranded oligonucleotides or peptides fold into complex conformations, which can enable interaction with the target by means of non-covalent forces such as hydrogen bonding, van der Waals forces, and electrostatic interactions. Aptamers thus differentiate between a target and its closest relative, thus providing the ability to select highly cancer biomarkers [38]. An advantage of aptamers is their adaptability to diverse targets, such as proteins, small molecules, and whole cells. This ability allows biosensors to sense a large range of cancer biomarkers, such as vascular endothelial growth factor (VEGF), the most critical molecule in the process of tumor angiogenesis, and prostate-specific antigen (PSA), the most frequent marker for prostate cancer. Aptamers also display reversible binding, which is an important feature in biosensors that are intended for real-time or repeated measurements. This is because they can release their targets under controlled conditions without losing functionality [39]. Besides these binding capabilities, aptamers are also stable at high temperatures and pH ranges, as well as resistant to denaturation. Chemically, aptamers can be modified to optimize their performance in biosensing. For instance, with fluorophores or nanoparticles embedded in the aptamer, signal detection and amplification are improved [40]. These features make aptamers superior substitutes for traditional recognition elements, such as antibodies, in cancer diagnostics. Since aptamers work as highly specific, stable, and adaptable recognition elements, biosensors can exhibit high sensitivity and specificity, even in complex biological samples such as blood or serum (Fig. 1.2).

1.4.2 Signal Transduction Mechanisms in Aptamer-Based Biosensors

Signal transduction of aptamer-based biosensors is the process of changing aptamer–target interactions into measurable signals. These signals can be electrical, optical, or colorimetric and are further processed for quantitative or qualitative information on the presence and concentration of cancer biomarkers. A signal transduction mechanism depends upon the design and application of a biosensor [41].

1.4.2.1 Electrochemical Detection

Electrochemical transduction is an extensively used mechanism in biosensors based on aptamers because of its simplicity, the sensitivity of the response, and cost-effectiveness. For example, when a particular target molecule binds to an aptamer adsorbed on an electrode, it induces changes within electrical properties, such as a change in current, voltage, or impedance. The changes measured are directly proportional to the

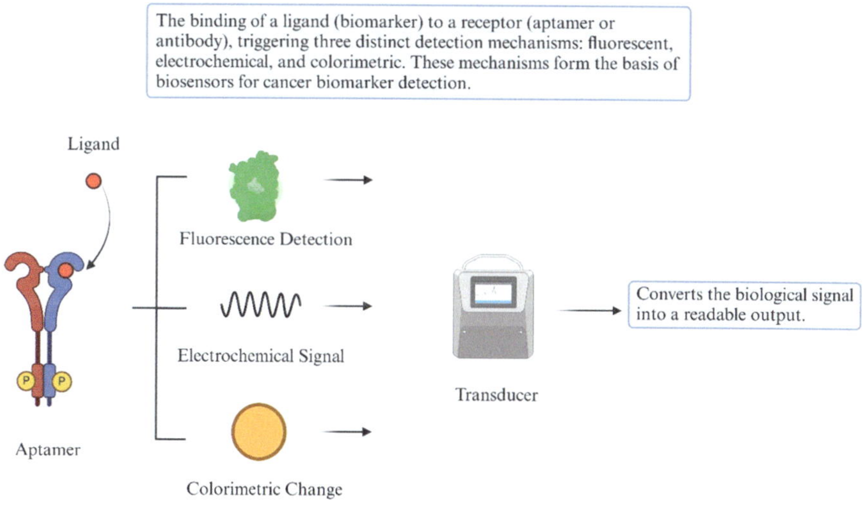

Fig. 1.2 Types of detection mechanisms in biosensors

concentration of the target, meaning that the biosensor responds quantitatively [42]. For instance, an electrochemical aptamer-based biosensor for HER2, a breast cancer biomarker, uses redox-active labels to amplify the detection signal. The binding of HER2 to the aptamer blocks the electron transfer between the label and the electrode, producing an electrochemical signal that can be measured. Cyclic voltammetry and electrochemical impedance spectroscopy are some of the techniques used to evaluate the signals, which have detection limits in the femtomolar range. This makes electrochemical aptamer-based biosensors very efficient for early cancer detection [43].

1.4.2.2 Fluorescent Detection

In the case of fluorescent detection, labeled aptamers release light on binding to the target molecules. Commonly attached fluorophores or quantum dots to the aptamers produce fluorescence signals, and fluorescence spectroscopy is applied for measurement. This is a preferred technique for low-abundance biomarkers because of the high sensitivity and specificity offered [44]. In terms of examples, an aptamer-based fluorescent biosensor applied for VEGF employs a fluorescence resonance energy transfer (FRET) mechanism, a conformational change process in the aptamer for binding to VEGF, bringing fluorophores and quencher molecules in close proximity to each other, where the generation of the fluorescent signal is according to the concentration of the VEGF. Fluorescent biosensors are utilized for high-throughput screenings that are also used for multiple reactions at the same time, wherein more than one biomarker can be detected in a single sample [29].

1.4.2.3 Colorimetric Detection

Colorimetric biosensors depend on visible color change for detecting the presence of a target molecule. Most colorimetric biosensors are based on nanoparticles, including gold nanoparticles (AuNPs), whose optical properties are sensitive to aggregation or dispersion. In a typical colorimetric aptamer-based biosensor, the aptamer will bind to the target biomarker and result in the aggregation or dispersion of gold nanoparticles, leading to a visible color change. A good example is the detection of thrombin using aptamer-functionalized AuNPs as a colorimetric biosensor. In this case, in the absence of thrombin, the color is red due to the dispersion of the nanoparticles. Upon binding of thrombin to the aptamer, the nanoparticles will aggregate, and the color will change to blue [45]. Colorimetric biosensors are simple and inexpensive, without the need for sophisticated instrumentation, which makes them particularly valuable for point-of-care applications. Nevertheless, their sensitivity is generally inferior to that of electrochemical or fluorescent biosensors and therefore less suited for the detection of biomarkers at ultralow concentrations [46]. This makes aptamer-based biosensors offer versatile platforms for the diagnostics of cancer through the mechanisms of diverse signal transduction methods employed. Their performance continuously gets enhanced with advancements in nanotechnology and materials science in detecting biomarkers sensitively and with unprecedented specificity.

1.5 Applications of Aptamer-Based Biosensors in Cancer Diagnosis

1.5.1 Detection of Cancer Biomarkers Using Aptamers

Detecting cancer biomarkers is currently an aspect of modern diagnostics, used to facilitate early diagnosis and prognosis, as well as to monitor the response to a treatment. Aptamer-based biosensors were introduced as powerful tools with great sensitivity and specificity, especially in detecting a vast number of cancer biomarkers such as proteins, nucleic acids, and small molecules. For instance, vascular endothelial growth factor, one of the most important mediators in tumor angiogenesis, is a widely investigated cancer biomarker. Biosensors based on aptamers targeting VEGF take advantage of the high affinity of the aptamer for the detection of VEGF in blood samples at the picomolar concentration level, allowing for early detection of colorectal and ovarian cancers, where VEGF has been known to significantly influence disease progression [47]. Similarly, HER2, which has become an important biomarker for breast cancer, can be monitored by electrochemical aptamer-based biosensors at femtomolar levels, while conventional immunoassays can hardly surpass such sensitivity to allow cancer to be detected earlier [39, 48]. Aptamer-based biosensors are also useful in the detection of circulating tumor cells (CTCs) and extracellular vesicles (EVs), which are important markers of metastasis. Piezoelectric biosensors functionalized with aptamers have been used to detect CTCs in blood samples, which is very informative about the progression of cancer and the possibility of recurrence [49]. The greatest strength of aptamer-based biosensors lies in their multiplexing capability, wherein a multiplicity of biomarkers can be detected within a single sample. Such an attribute is crucial for cancers having complex biomarker profiles, such as lung and pancreatic cancers. Multiplexed aptamer-based biosensors, therefore, improve the diagnostic accuracy and offer a complete view of the tumor microenvironment, thereby facilitating the planning of personalized treatment [50] (Table 1.2).

1.5.2 Case Studies of Aptamer-Based Biosensors in Clinical Settings

Several case studies reflect aptamer-based biosensors' successful clinical application in cancer diagnostics. For instance, an aptamer-functionalized electrochemical biosensor for alpha-fetoprotein, which is the liver cancer biomarker, has been developed for detection with a limit of detection of 0.1 ng/mL and has successfully helped in the early diagnosis of hepatocellular carcinoma, a silent-presenting disease in the early stages of its disease course. The device is relatively portable and cost-effective, making it suitable for point-of-care applications where advanced laboratory facilities are hard to come by [51]. Another notable application used aptamer-based fluorescent biosensors to detect prostate-specific antigen, a marker critical to identifying prostate cancer. In the case of this application, the biosensors employed FRET

Table 1.2 Applications of biosensors for specific cancer biomarkers

Cancer type	Biomarker	Biosensor type	Detection limit	Significance in diagnostics	References
Breast cancer	HER2	Electrochemical	Femtomolar range	Enables early detection and therapy monitoring for HER2-positive breast cancer.	[39, 48]
Liver cancer	Alpha-fetoprotein (AFP)	Electrochemical	0.1 ng/mL	Supports early diagnosis of hepatocellular carcinoma.	[51]
Prostate cancer	Prostate-specific antigen (PSA)	Fluorescent	0.05 ng/mL	Identifies prostate cancer at early stages with high specificity.	[52]
Ovarian cancer	CA125	Optical (SPR)	Nanomolar range	Aids in the diagnosis and monitoring of treatment response in ovarian cancer patients.	[53]
Colorectal cancer	Vascular endothelial growth factor (VEGF)	Colorimetric	Picomolar range	Facilitates early detection by identifying angiogenesis-associated biomarker levels.	[47]
Metastatic cancers	Circulating tumor cells (CTCs)	Piezoelectric	Single-cell detection	Tracks metastasis and recurrence, providing insights into disease progression.	[49]

mechanisms for highly rapid and specific detection down to 0.05 ng/mL. Quantum dots proved to be a further enhanced fluorescent probe, making it feasible to identify PSA in early-stage and recurring prostate cancers [52]. Aptamer-based surface plasmon resonance (SPR) biosensors have been successfully used in ovarian cancer diagnostics to measure the level of CA125. SPR biosensors offer label-free detection with high specificity, providing real-time insights into the dynamics of biomarkers. These tools are invaluable in monitoring treatment responses because changes in the levels of CA125 correlate with tumor burden and therapeutic efficacy [53]. Additionally, liquid biopsy approaches have been highly advantageous with aptamer-based biosensors. One of the good examples is the detection of circulating microRNAs (miRNAs), which are associated with cervical cancer. Biosensors have been made possible through the use of aptamers that specifically bind to sequences of miRNA. Noninvasive cancer diagnostics are made possible with biosensors, and such case studies underscore the versatility and clinical potential of aptamer-based biosensors in revolutionizing cancer diagnostics [54] (Table 1.2).

1.5.3 Advantages of Aptamer-Based Biosensors over Traditional Methods

Aptamer-based biosensors provide several benefits over traditional diagnostic techniques and help in overcoming the most critical shortcomings of current technologies. Probably, one of the biggest advantages is that these aptamer-based biosensors can be made to be very sensitive and specific. Conventional immunoassays, including enzyme-linked immunosorbent assay (ELISA), use antibodies for target recognition. Although these are successful assays, they suffer from poor sensitivity and have the disadvantage of cross-reactivity, causing false positives. In contrast, aptamers offer very high selective binding, allowing cancer biomarkers to be detected at ultralow concentrations that may be in the picomolar or femtomolar range. The second is stability. Aptamers are stable against changes in temperature and pH. The antibodies in conventional diagnostics require strict storage and handling procedures because of their sensitivity to changes in temperature and pH. The stability of aptamers also allows the use of aptamer-based biosensors in various settings, such as point-of-care and resource-limited environments [40, 55]. The ease and cost-effectiveness of the production of aptamers differentiate them from traditional methods. Antibody production involves complicated biological systems and may take months to develop. On the other hand, aptamers are synthesized chemically, ensuring batch-to-batch consistency and thus reducing production time and costs significantly. This makes the aptamer-based biosensor more accessible and scalable for widespread clinical use [56, 57]. What is more, aptamers can easily be adjusted in various ways to maximize their effectiveness. For example, nanoparticle or fluorophore conjugation increases the biosensor sensitivity as it augments signal transduction from the aptamers. Aptamers also have the advantage of multiplexing, the detection of different biomarkers simultaneously in the same assay, which poses a problem while using conventional methodologies [58, 59]. Finally, as a noninvasive modality with real-time detection capability, aptamer-based biosensors are very desirable in the monitoring of diseases and treatment response at any time. Such is not the case with classical techniques that cannot provide apt-level precision and accessibility compared to the use of this innovative method.

1.6 Therapeutic Applications of Aptamers in Cancer Treatment

1.6.1 Aptamer–Drug Conjugates for Targeted Therapy

Aptamer–drug conjugates (ADCs) are promising emerging drugs that integrate the specificity of aptamers with the cytotoxicity of chemotherapeutic agents, and these ADCs would be capable of reducing side effects and off-targeting while increasing therapeutic efficiency due to the targeted delivery to cancer cells. The mechanism of ADCs is based on the binding of the aptamer to a specific cancer biomarker that may be HER2, prostate-specific membrane antigen (PSMA), or any other cancer antigen. Once it is internalized by the cancerous cell, it releases the cytotoxic payload from its conjugated drug, significantly limiting systemic toxicity, a major challenge with traditional chemotherapy [60]. One of these examples involves aptamer–drug conjugates developed to directly target HER2-positive cancer cells using potent chemotherapeutic agents like doxorubicin. According to studies, these conjugates have the ability to slow down the growth of a tumor with relatively minimal toxicity against normal tissue [61]. Another interesting development has been aptamers targeting PSMA for prostate cancer treatment. PSMA-targeting aptamer conjugates can target chemotherapeutic agents selectively to the cancer cells expressing PSMA, thus avoiding noncancerous tissues and diminishing side effects. Similar strategies have been pursued to deliver siRNA and other agents, thereby significantly expanding the scope of therapeutics beyond simple drugs [62]. Because aptamers have a modular nature, the attachment of various payloads can be done, such as nanoparticles and imaging agents. This versatility enhances their use in combination therapies where, for example, an aptamer can deliver several agents to maximize the therapeutic outcome. As research advances, precision oncology is likely to see the use of aptamer–drug conjugates to create a highly effective and personalized approach toward treatment [63].

1.6.2 Use of Aptamers in Personalized Medicine

With their properties of adaptability and specificity, aptamers can tailor therapeutics for each individual based on their genetic and molecular profiles. They are so versatile; therefore, they could pinpoint targets specific to biomarkers or mutations expressed in patients' tumors. Perhaps the most important use of aptamers in personalized medicine has been in the creation of tumor-specific treatments. As such, aptamers designed to bind estimated glomerular filtration rate (EGFR) mutations in non-small-cell lung cancer have been utilized for the delivery of targeted therapies, improving treatment outcomes and reducing adverse effects [64]. Aptamers targeting VEGF have also been used to inhibit tumor angiogenesis on a patient-specific basis, taking into consideration the different vascularization profiles among cancers [65]. Aptamers are also combined with next-generation sequencing (NGS) technologies to identify new cancer biomarkers. With NGS data integration, researchers design aptamers that recognize patient-specific molecular targets, thereby making customized therapeutic solutions. This has been very effective in rare or refractory cancers, where conventional therapies are inadequate [66]. Another important role of aptamers is in the monitoring of treatment response and disease progression. Aptamer-based biosensors can even detect circulating biomarkers such as CTCs and miRNAs that give live information about the dynamics in tumor biology [67]. Such tools allow oncologists to adjust treatment regimens to an evolving patient's disease state for optimal therapeutic results. For instance, aptamers can play an important role in personalized medicine; their future promises to make even more targeted therapy possible with more effective treatment for cancer with fewer side effects so that it may perfectly match individual demands.

1.6.3 Challenges and Future Prospects in Therapeutic Applications

Although great promises have been made regarding the use of aptamers for therapeutic purposes, several challenges need to be overcome to utilize them as the most effective agents in cancer treatment. The most significant challenge of unmodified aptamers is nuclease degradation, which renders them liable to degradation and instability, limiting their bioavailability in vivo. Although chemical modifications, such as 2′-fluoro or 2′-O-methyl substitution, have made aptamers more stable, greater advances are required for better pharmacokinetic properties [68]. Another challenge is the potential for immunogenicity, although aptamers generally have lower immunogenic profiles than antibodies. However, their safety must be carefully tested in preclinical studies, especially if they are used in repeated dosing regimens or in combination therapies [69]. Scalability poses another logistical challenge: aptamer-based therapeutics. Aptamers are synthesized chemically, but large-scale production is optimized for consistency and lower cost. For clinical applications, stringent regulatory standards have to be met [70]. Despite these challenges, the future is bright for aptamer-based therapeutics. Recent advances in nanotechnology and drug delivery systems expand the possibilities of aptamer–drug conjugates and multifunctional aptamers. For example, nanoparticles that are functionalized with aptamers are designed for the co-delivery of drugs and imaging agents, thus combining therapy and diagnostics in one product, known as theranostics [71]. Further, aptamer engineering research in progress is providing new approaches that are enhancing affinity and specificity in binding. Designing next-generation aptamers with computer modeling and artificial intelligence (AI) to confront complex cancer targets is another big step forward. As these trends continue, the future of precision oncology becomes even more holistic, with aptamers as part of the cutting-edge and patient-centered solutions [72].

1.7 Current Trends and Innovations in Biosensing Technologies

1.7.1 Recent Advancements in Biosensor Technology

In the past few years, biosensor technology has gained great momentum in order to meet more sensitive, accurate, and versatile diagnostic needs. These advancements were focused on enhancing the fundamental building blocks of biosensors: the biological recognition elements, transducers, and signal processing systems. A new breakthrough is the incorporation of nanomaterials into biosensor platforms. In this aspect, nanoparticles, quantum dots, and carbon-based materials, such as graphene and carbon nanotubes, are used for improved sensitivity and specificity of biosensors. For example, gold nanoparticles have been applied for signal amplification in optical and electrochemical biosensors that have helped in detecting the biomarkers at femtomolar concentrations. The electrodes based on graphene have furthered the efficiency of electrochemical biosensors with improved electron transfer rates [73]. Miniaturization has also made tremendous strides with the advent of microfabrication and microfluidics. Devices are now produced for lab-on-a-chip technologies that provide multiplex diagnostic functionality on a small, self-contained platform with significant advantages for high-throughput analysis on very small samples. It can be useful at point-of-care sites, which require the ease of using rapidly portable diagnostic devices [74]. Advances in signal processing and data analysis enhance the biosensors further. AI, machine learning, and other computational algorithms are applied to interpret high-dimensional datasets, thus improving accuracy in diagnosis, predictive modeling, and more. For instance, AI-based biosensors have recently been applied in analyzing biomarker expression patterns and are being increasingly used for cancer detection at earlier stages and determining the treatment of cancer [75]. These developments indicate an increasing ability of biosensors to meet unmet needs in diagnostics, especially in complex diseases such as cancer.

1.7.2 Integration of Nanotechnology with Biosensors

The integration of nanotechnology into the design of biosensors has truly revolutionized its functionality, leading to ultrasensitive detection of biomarkers for cancers and improving diagnostics. Nanomaterials, due to their very unique physical and chemical properties, have become an essential entity in modern biosensors. AuNPs represent the most employed nanomaterial in biosensors. Their extremely high surface-to-volume ratio enhances efficient immobilization of biomolecules and improves performance characteristics of the recognition elements used in biosensors, such as aptamers. AuNPs also present optical properties including localized surface plasmon resonance that enhances optical and colorimetric biosensors through signal amplification. In particular, for the detection of prostate-specific antigen (PSA) in serum samples, a concentration sensitivity to picomolar was achieved through aptamer-functionalized AuNPs [76]. Graphene and carbon nanotubes have equally enabled the recent upgradation of electrochemical biosensors. Because of their high electrical conductivity, these compounds enable fast transfer of electrons, thus enhancing the sensitivity of biosensors for the detection of low-abundance cancer biomarkers. Another derivative called graphene oxide has also been used to enhance signal transduction due to its high biocompatibility [77]. Besides nanomaterials, nanoparticles and nanostructured surfaces for multiplex detection are under consideration. Such considerations are of exceptional value in many cancers with complex, multi-marker prognostic markers, including pancreatic and lung cancers. The synergy between nanotechnology and biosensors also continues to produce new innovation—precise, effective, and highly accessible diagnostics of diseases [78].

1.7.3 Future Directions in Biosensor Research for Cancer Diagnostics

Future biosensor research in cancer diagnostics is aimed at enhancing sensitivity, increasing multiplexing capability, and incorporating biosensors into holistic healthcare solutions. Given the heterogeneity of cancers, next-generation biosensors will have to address the challenge of providing a comprehensive profiling of multiple biomarkers to enhance the accuracy of diagnosis and guide the treatment. Advances in wearable biosensors for the continuous monitoring of cancer biomarkers hold much promise. Such devices, integrated into wearable patches or smartwatches, can offer real-time insights into tumor dynamics, achieving the possibility of early intervention and personally adjusted treatment. Flexible electronics and biocompatible materials are increasingly becoming a reality to allow for wearables in noninvasive, patient-centric diagnostics [79]. An additional crucial research area includes artificial intelligence (AI)– and machine learning–based applications for biosensor data interpretation. These can classify complex biomarker expression patterns against disease states with higher precision and accuracy, potentially improving the efficiency of cancer diagnosis. Additionally, AI-driven biosensors are currently being studied to be applied to predictive analytics that will allow clinicians to better anticipate the course of disease progression as well as the responses to therapy [80]. A theranostic biosensor is essentially a merging of diagnostic and therapeutic capabilities. This system combines aptamer-based detection with drug delivery mechanisms to diagnose cancer in a parallel manner to its treatment. For instance, an aptamer-functionalized nanoparticle can carry targeted drugs and also continuously monitor the levels of biomarkers for assessing therapeutic effectiveness [81]. Biosensors are to be integrated in the future with advances in research in precision oncology so that it will offer not only a diagnosis but also a predictive and therapeutic tool tailored for the patient's needs.

1.8 Conclusion

The integration of biosensors and aptamer-based technologies represents one of the biggest advances in the field of cancer diagnostics and therapeutics. Such tools address the many limitations associated with traditional approaches by providing sensitive, specific, and noninvasive means to detect cancer biomarkers. It has the potential to revolutionize early cancer detection by identifying low-abundance targets at the early stages of the disease. Aptamers are potent recognition elements in biosensors with outstanding specificity, stability, and flexibility for binding. Such elements have led to the establishment of diverse platforms that are useful for multiplexing and real-time diagnostics. The use of aptamers for conjugates in therapeutic drug applications and as personalized medicine approaches shows even wider possibilities for the role of aptamers in precision oncology. Nanotechnology, AI, and the microfluidic revolution have extended the capabilities of biosensors significantly, opening wide avenues for products such as a wearable device as well as creating theranostic platforms, which are capable not only of yielding improved diagnostic capability but also of permitting the monitoring of drug response and specific therapy delivery in the future. As biosensor and aptamer research continues to develop, the spotlight will be on scalability, affordability, and accessibility, ensuring these technologies reach all patients worldwide. Biosensors and aptamers are poised to make a transformative contribution to the future of cancer care by bridging the gap between diagnostics and therapy.

References

1. van den Bergh RCN, Loeb S, Roobol MJ. Impact of early diagnosis of prostate cancer on survival outcomes. Eur Urol Focus. 2015;1(2):137–46.
2. Ott JJ, Ullrich A, Miller AB. The importance of early symptom recognition in the context of early detection and cancer survival. Eur J Cancer. 2009;45(16):2743–8.
3. Girgis A, Lambert S, Johnson C, Waller A, Currow D. Physical, psychosocial, relationship, and economic burden of caring for people with cancer: a review. J Oncol Pract. 2013;9(4):197–202.
4. Kakushadze Z, Raghubanshi R, Yu W. Estimating cost savings from early cancer diagnosis. Data. 2017;2(3):30.
5. Lin K, Lin AN, Lin S, Lin T, Liu YX, Reddy M. A silent asymptomatic solid pancreas tumor in a nonsmoking athletic female: pancreatic ductal adenocarcinoma. Case Rep Gastroenterol. 2017;11(3):616–24.
6. Purandare NC, Rangarajan V. Imaging of lung cancer: implications on staging and management. Indian J Radiol Imaging. 2015;25(2):109–20.
7. Kimura M, Tsuda H, Morita D, Shinto E, Tanimoto T, Ichikura T, et al. Usefulness and limitation of multiple endoscopic biopsy sampling for epidermal growth factor receptor and c-erbB-2 testing in patients with gastric adenocarcinoma. Jpn J Clin Oncol. 2005;35(6):324–31.
8. Sturgeon CM, Lai LC, Duffy MJ. Serum tumour markers: how to order and interpret them. BMJ. 2009;339:b3527.
9. Coulet PR. What is a biosensor? In: Biosensor principles and applications. CRC Press; 1991.
10. Zhou W, Huang PJJ, Ding J, Liu J. Aptamer-based biosensors for biomedical diagnostics. Analyst. 2014;139(11):2627–40.
11. Şahin S, Caglayan MO, Üstündağ Z. Recent advances in aptamer-based sensors for breast cancer diagnosis: special cases for nanomaterial-based VEGF, HER2, and MUC1 aptasensors. Microchim Acta. 2020;187(10):549.
12. Ligler FS, Sapsford KE, Golden JP, Shriver-Lake LC, Taitt CR, Dyer MA, et al. The array biosensor: portable, automated systems. Anal Sci. 2007;23(1):5–10.
13. Fattahi Z, Hasanzadeh M. Nanotechnology-assisted microfluidic systems for chemical sensing, biosensing, and bioanalysis. TrAC Trends Anal Chem. 2022;152:116637.
14. Karunakaran C, Rajkumar R, Bhargava K. Introduction to biosensors. In: Biosensors and bioelectronics [Internet]. Elsevier; 2015 [cited 2025 Jan 1]. p. 1–68. Available from: https://www.sciencedirect.com/science/article/pii/B9780128031001000013
15. Polat EO, Cetin MM, Tabak AF, Bilget Güven E, Uysal BÖ, Arsan T, et al. Transducer technologies for biosensors and their wearable applications. Biosensors. 2022;12(6):385.
16. Ronkainen NJ, Halsall HB, Heineman WR. Electrochemical biosensors. Chem Soc Rev. 2010;39(5):1747–63.
17. Hassanzadeh P. New perspectives in biosensor technology. Gastroenterol Hepatol Bed Bench [Internet]. 2010 [cited 2025 Jan 1];3(3). Available from: http://ojs3.sbmu.ac.ir/ghfbb/index.php/ghfbb/article/download/94/78

18. Yoon J, Shin M, Lee T, Choi JW. Highly sensitive biosensors based on biomolecules and functional nanomaterials depending on the types of nanomaterials: a perspective review. Materials. 2020;13(2):299.
19. Pohanka M, Skládal P. Electrochemical biosensors–principles and applications. J Appl Biomed [Internet]. 2008 [cited 2025 Jan 1];6(2). Available from: https://www.researchgate.net/profile/Miroslav-Pohanka/publication/26585733_Electrochemical_Biosensors-Principles_and_Applications/links/0c96051a38bd2c4244000000/Electrochemical-Biosensors-Principles-and-Applications.pdf
20. Jarczewska M, Trojan A, Gągała M, Malinowska E. Studies on the affinity-based biosensors for electrochemical detection of HER2 cancer biomarker. Electroanalysis. 2019;31(6):1125–34.
21. Gutiérrez-Zúñiga GG, Hernández-López JL. Sensitivity improvement of a sandwich-type ELISA immunosensor for the detection of different prostate-specific antigen isoforms in human serum using electrochemical impedance spectroscopy and an ordered and hierarchically organized interfacial supramolecular architecture. Anal Chim Acta. 2016;902:97–106.
22. Valizadeh Shahbazlou S, Vandghanooni S, Dabirmanesh B, Eskandani M, Hasannia S. Biotinylated aptamer-based SPR biosensor for detection of CA125 antigen. Microchem J. 2023;194:109276.
23. Kaur B, Kumar S, Kaushik BK. Recent advancements in optical biosensors for cancer detection. Biosens Bioelectron. 2022;197:113805.
24. Recent uses of carbon nanotubes & gold nanoparticles in electrochemistry with application in biosensing: a review – ScienceDirect [Internet]. [cited 2025 Jan 3]. Available from: https://www.sciencedirect.com/science/article/abs/pii/S0956566318306432
25. Song S, Wang L, Li J, Fan C, Zhao J. Aptamer-based biosensors. TrAC Trends Anal Chem. 2008;27(2):108–17.
26. Figueroa-Miranda G, Feng L, Shiu SCC, Dirkzwager RM, Cheung YW, Tanner JA, et al. Aptamer-based electrochemical biosensor for highly sensitive and selective malaria detection with adjustable dynamic response range and reusability. Sens Actuators B Chem. 2018;255:235–43.
27. Zhou J, Battig MR, Wang Y. Aptamer-based molecular recognition for biosensor development. Anal Bioanal Chem. 2010;398(6):2471–80.
28. Sassolas A, Blum LJ, Leca-Bouvier BD. Optical detection systems using immobilized aptamers. Biosens Bioelectron. 2011;26(9):3725–36.
29. Dehghani S, Nosrati R, Yousefi M, Nezami A, Soltani F, Taghdisi SM, et al. Aptamer-based biosensors and nanosensors for the detection of vascular endothelial growth factor (VEGF): a review. Biosens Bioelectron. 2018;110:23–37.
30. Hidding J. A therapeutic battle: antibodies vs. aptamers. Nanosci Master Progr. 2017;109:1–20.
31. Wu YX, Kwon YJ. Aptamers: the "evolution" of SELEX. Methods. 2016;106:21–8.
32. Bauer M, Strom M, Hammond DS, Shigdar S. Anything you can do, i can do better: can aptamers replace antibodies in clinical diagnostic applications? Molecules. 2019;24(23):4377.
33. Nezlin R. Aptamers in immunological research. Immunol Lett. 2014;162(2 Part B):252–5.
34. Gopinath SCB. Methods developed for SELEX. Anal Bioanal Chem. 2007;387(1):171–82.
35. Zimmermann B, Gesell T, Chen D, Lorenz C, Schroeder R. Monitoring genomic sequences during SELEX using high-throughput sequencing: neutral SELEX. PLoS One. 2010;5(2):e9169.
36. Guo KT, Paul A, Schichor C, Ziemer G, Wendel HP. CELL-SELEX: novel perspectives of aptamer-based therapeutics. Int J Mol Sci. 2008;9(4):668–78.
37. Wondergem JAJ, Schiessel H, Tompitak M. Performing SELEX experiments in silico. J Chem Phys [Internet]. 2017 [cited 2025 Jan 3];147(17). Available from: https://pubs.aip.org/aip/jcp/article/147/17/174101/195017
38. Chen Z, Luo H, Gubu A, Yu S, Zhang H, Dai H, et al. Chemically modified aptamers for improving binding affinity to the target proteins via enhanced non-covalent bonding. Front Cell Dev Biol [Internet]. 2023 [cited 2025 Jan 5];11. Available from: https://www.frontiersin.org/journals/cell-and-developmental-biology/articles/10.3389/fcell.2023.1091809/full

39. Ahirwar R, Khan N, Kumar S. Aptamer-based sensing of breast cancer biomarkers: a comprehensive review of analytical figures of merit. Expert Rev Mol Diagn. 2021;21(7):703–21.
40. Belleperche M, DeRosa MC. pH-control in aptamer-based diagnostics, therapeutics, and analytical applications. Pharmaceuticals. 2018;11(3):80.
41. Mo T, Liu X, Luo Y, Zhong L, Zhang Z, Li T, et al. Aptamer-based biosensors and application in tumor theranostics. Cancer Sci. 2022;113(1):7–16.
42. Radi AE. Electrochemical aptamer-based biosensors: recent advances and perspectives. Int J Electrochem. 2011;2011(1):863196.
43. Jayaswal N, Srivastava S, Kumar S, Sridhar SB, Khalid A, Najmi A, Zoghebi K, Alhazmi HA, Mohan S, Tambuwala MM. Precision arrows: Navigating breast cancer with nanotechnology siRNA. International Journal of Pharmaceutics. 2024:124403.
44. Kalkal A, Pradhan R, Kadian S, Manik G, Packirisamy G. Biofunctionalized graphene quantum dots based fluorescent biosensor toward efficient detection of small cell lung cancer. ACS Appl Bio Mater. 2020;3(8):4922–32.
45. Wang H, Wu T, Li M, Tao Y. Recent advances in nanomaterials for colorimetric cancer detection. J Mater Chem B. 2021;9(4):921–38.
46. Krishnan S, Syed Z, ul Q. Colorimetric visual sensors for point-of-needs testing. Sens Actuators Rep. 2022;4:100078.
47. Srivastava S, Bagang N, Yadav S, Rajput S, Sharma D, Dahiya A, Bhardwaj L, Deshmukh K, Joshi JC, Singh G. Evolution of β-catenin-independent Wnt–GSK3–mTOR signalling in regulation of energy metabolism in isoproterenol-induced cardiotoxicity model. Inflammation Research. 2021;70(7):743–7.
48. Li Z, Xue G, Mei Y. Applications of electrochemical analytical techniques in HER2 detection for breast cancer. Int J Electrochem Sci. 2024;19(10):100813.
49. Puranik N, Kumar P, Paliwal P, Yadav SK, Song M. Nanobiosensor based rapid detection of circulating biomarkers of cancer. In: Nano biosensors for non-invasive diagnosis of cancer [Internet]. Bristol: IOP Publishing; 2024 [cited 2025 Jan 5]. p. 12–1. Available from: https://iopscience.iop.org/book/edit/978-0-7503-6234-4/chapter/bk978-0-7503-6234-4ch12
50. Liang L, Su M, Li L, Lan F, Yang G, Ge S, et al. Aptamer-based fluorescent and visual biosensor for multiplexed monitoring of cancer cells in microfluidic paper-based analytical devices. Sens Actuators B Chem. 2016;229:347–54.
51. Tran Ngoc Huy D, Iswanto AH, Catalan Opulencia MJ, Al-Saikhan F, Timoshin A, Abed AM, et al. Optical and electrochemical aptasensors developed for the detection of alpha-fetoprotein. Crit Rev Anal Chem. 2024;54(4):857–71.
52. Yao H, Wang L, Guo J, Liu W, Li J, Wang Y, et al. Genetically encoded FRET biosensor detects the enzymatic activity of prostate-specific antigen. Mol Cell Biomech. 2020;17(3):101.
53. Valerievich Yumashev A, Rudiansyah M, Chupradit S, Kadhim MM, Turki Jalil A, Abdelbasset WK, et al. Optical-based biosensor for detection of oncomarker CA 125, recent progress and current status. Anal Biochem. 2022;655:114750.
54. Tamaian R. Aptamer-based biosensor design for simultaneous detection of cervical cancer-related MicroRNAs. Eng Proc. 2023;58(1):88.
55. Yoo H, Jo H, Soo OS. Detection and beyond: challenges and advances in aptamer-based biosensors. Mater Adv. 2020;1(8):2663–87.
56. Chen K, Zhou J, Shao Z, Liu J, Song J, Wang R, et al. Aptamers as versatile molecular tools for antibody production monitoring and quality control. J Am Chem Soc. 2020;142(28):12079–86.
57. Birch JR, Racher AJ. Antibody production. Adv Drug Deliv Rev. 2006;58(5–6):671–85.
58. Sargazi S, Simge ER, Mobashar A, Gelen SS, Rahdar A, Ebrahimi N, et al. Aptamer-conjugated carbon-based nanomaterials for cancer and bacteria theranostics: a review. Chem Biol Interact. 2022;361:109964.
59. Grabowska I, Hepel M, Kurzątkowska-Adaszyńska K. Advances in design strategies of multiplex electrochemical aptasensors. Sensors. 2021;22(1):161.
60. Chen K, Liu B, Yu B, Zhong W, Lu Y, Zhang J, et al. Advances in the development of aptamer drug conjugates for targeted drug delivery. WIREs Nanomed Nanobiotechnol. 2017;9(3):e1438.

61. Kim DH, Seo JM, Shin KJ, Yang SG. Design and clinical developments of aptamer-drug conjugates for targeted cancer therapy. Biomater Res. 2021;25(1):42.
62. Ye Y, Zhang L, Dai Y, Wang Z, Li C, Peng Y, et al. PSMA-targeting reduction-cleavable hyperbranched polyamide-amine gene delivery system to treat the bone metastases of prostate cancer. Int J Nanomedicine. 2020;15:7173–84.
63. Porciani D, Cardwell LN, Tawiah KD, Alam KK, Lange MJ, Daniels MA, et al. Modular cell-internalizing aptamer nanostructure enables targeted delivery of large functional RNAs in cancer cell lines. Nat Commun. 2018;9(1):2283.
64. Srivastava S, Jayaswal N, Kumar S, Sharma PK, Behl T, Khalid A, Mohan S, Najmi A, Zoghebi K, Alhazmi HA. Unveiling the potential of proteomic and genetic signatures for precision therapeutics in lung cancer management. Cellular Signalling. 2024;113:110932.
65. Riccardi C, Napolitano E, Platella C, Musumeci D, Melone MAB, Montesarchio D. Anti-VEGF DNA-based aptamers in cancer therapeutics and diagnostics. Med Res Rev. 2021;41(1):464–506.
66. Dickey DD, Giangrande PH. Oligonucleotide aptamers: a next-generation technology for the capture and detection of circulating tumor cells. Methods. 2016;97:94–103.
67. Wu L, Wang Y, Xu X, Liu Y, Lin B, Zhang M, et al. Aptamer-based detection of circulating targets for precision medicine. Chem Rev. 2021;121(19):12035–105.
68. Nuzzo S, Roscigno G, Affinito A, Ingenito F, Quintavalle C, Condorelli G. Potential and challenges of aptamers as specific carriers of therapeutic oligonucleotides for precision medicine in cancer. Cancers. 2019;11(10):1521.
69. Zhou J, Rossi J. Aptamers as targeted therapeutics: current potential and challenges. Nat Rev Drug Discov. 2017;16(3):181–202.
70. Jiang W, Jones JC, Shankavaram U, Sproull M, Camphausen K, Krauze AV. Analytical considerations of large-scale aptamer-based datasets for translational applications. Cancers. 2022;14(9):2227.
71. Zhang L, Radovic-Moreno AF, Alexis F, Gu FX, Basto PA, Bagalkot V, et al. Co-delivery of hydrophobic and hydrophilic drugs from nanoparticle–aptamer bioconjugates. ChemMedChem. 2007;2(9):1268–71.
72. Fallah A, Havaei SA, Sedighian H, Kachuei R, Fooladi AAI. Prediction of aptamer affinity using an artificial intelligence approach. J Mater Chem B. 2024;12(36):8825–42.
73. Rostamabadi PF, Heydari-Bafrooei E. Impedimetric aptasensing of the breast cancer biomarker HER2 using a glassy carbon electrode modified with gold nanoparticles in a composite consisting of electrochemically reduced graphene oxide and single-walled carbon nanotubes. Microchim Acta. 2019;186(8):495.
74. Khan NI, Song E. Lab-on-a-chip systems for aptamer-based biosensing. Micromachines. 2020;11(2):220.
75. Cui F, Yue Y, Zhang Y, Zhang Z, Zhou HS. Advancing biosensors with machine learning. ACS Sens. 2020;5(11):3346–64.
76. Atapour A, Khajehzadeh H, Shafie M, Abbasi M, Mosleh-Shirazi S, Kasaee SR, et al. Gold nanoparticle-based aptasensors: a promising perspective for early-stage detection of cancer biomarkers. Mater Today Commun. 2022;30:103181.
77. Yang Y, Yang X, Yang Y, Yuan Q. Aptamer-functionalized carbon nanomaterials electrochemical sensors for detecting cancer relevant biomolecules. Carbon. 2018;129:380–95.
78. Synergizing Functional Nanomaterials with Aptamers Based on Electrochemical Strategies for Pesticide Detection: Current Status and Perspectives: Critical Reviews in Analytical Chemistry: Vol 52, No 8 [Internet]. [cited 2025 Jan 6]. Available from: https://www.tandfonline.com/doi/abs/10.1080/10408347.2021.1919987
79. Rabiee N, Rabiee M. Wearable aptasensors. Anal Chem. 2024;96(49):19160–82.
80. Futane A, Jadhav P, Mustafa AH, Srinivasan A, Narayanamurthy V. Aptamer-functionalized MOFs and AI-driven strategies for early cancer diagnosis and therapeutics. Biotechnol Lett. 2024;46(1):1–17.
81. Liu B, Zhang J, Liao J, Liu J, Chen K, Tong G, et al. Aptamer-functionalized nanoparticles for drug delivery. J Biomed Nanotechnol. 2014;10(11):3189–203.

The Biology of Cancer: Understanding the Disease and Its Challenges

2

Garla Venkateswarlu, Sachin Kumar, Suddikattu Bhargavi, and Ramesh Bodla

2.1 Introduction

Cancer is categorized by uncontrolled cell evolution and spread, driven by genetic mutations and changes in cellular signaling pathways [1]. Cancer research has made significant strides over the past century, leading to major advances in our understanding of the disease and how to treat it. From the identification of cancer's genetic and molecular foundations to the improvement of targeted therapies and immunotherapies, many milestones have shaped modern oncology [2]. Despite these advances, many challenges remain in our quest to improve the quality of life of cancer patients because cancer is a complex genetic/molecular disease, and more effective therapies are needed. A comprehensive understanding of the biological mechanisms of cancer will provide new opportunities for the development of more effective diagnostic and therapeutic modalities, so cancer research should continue to be a major focus of medical research (Fig. 2.1).

G. Venkateswarlu · R. Bodla
Department of Pharmaceutical Chemistry, Delhi Institute of Pharmaceutical Sciences and Research (DIPSAR), Delhi Pharmaceutical Sciences and Research University, New Delhi, India

S. Kumar (✉)
Department of Pharmacology, Delhi Institute of Pharmaceutical Sciences and Research (DIPSAR), Delhi Pharmaceutical Sciences and Research University (DPSRU), New Delhi, India

S. Bhargavi
Department of Pharmaceutics, Delhi Institute of Pharmaceutical Sciences and Research (DIPSAR), Delhi Pharmaceutical Sciences and Research University, New Delhi, India

S. Srivastava et al. (eds.), *Biosensors and Aptamers*,
https://doi.org/10.1007/978-981-96-8387-1_2

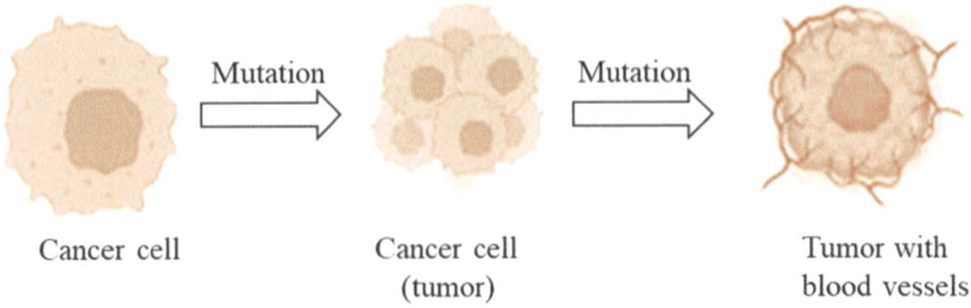

Fig. 2.1 Development of cancer

2.1.1 Cancer at the Cellular Level

2.1.1.1 Cell Cycle Dysregulation and Uncontrolled Proliferation

The cell cycle is tightly regulated to maintain controlled cell division and tissue homeostasis. In cancer, these regulatory mechanisms become disrupted, resulting in uncontrolled cell proliferation. Mutations in key regulatory genes, particularly cyclin-dependent kinases (CDKs) and their inhibitors, play a critical role in bypassing cell cycle checkpoints. CDKs function as master regulators of the cell cycle, controlling transitions between different phases and coordinating DNA damage responses. When CDKs become dysregulated, genomic instability and tumorigenesis can occur. CDKs work in conjunction with cyclins to regulate cell cycle progression and DNA damage repair, thereby maintaining genomic integrity. Certain CDKs have specialized functions in the DNA damage response pathway. CDK7, CDK9, and CDK12/13 are particularly important in modulating responses to DNA damage and replication stress [3]. CDK inhibitors serve as essential regulators of the cell cycle by binding to and inhibiting cyclin–CDK complexes, thus preventing uncontrolled cell proliferation. When these inhibitors become inactivated or mutated, cells can divide without proper regulation, which is a hallmark characteristic of cancer. Specific CDK inhibitors such as p21 and p27 play crucial roles in maintaining cell cycle checkpoints by inhibiting cyclin–CDK complexes, particularly at the G1 to S phase transition point in the cell cycle [4]. This dysregulation permits cancer cells to divide continuously, contributing to tumor growth.

2.1.1.2 Loss of Contact Inhibition and Programmed Cell Death

Normal cells cease proliferation upon interaction with neighboring cells, a phenomenon well-known as contact inhibition. Cancer cells lose this property, enabling them to develop uncontrollably, even in crowded environments [5]. Additionally, cancer cells evade programmed cell death (apoptosis), a critical mechanism that eliminates damaged or abnormal cells (Fig. 2.2). Mutations in proapoptotic genes (e.g., *BAX* and *BAK*) and the overexpression of antiapoptotic proteins (e.g., BCL-2) allow cancer cells to survive and proliferate despite cellular stress or damage [6, 7].

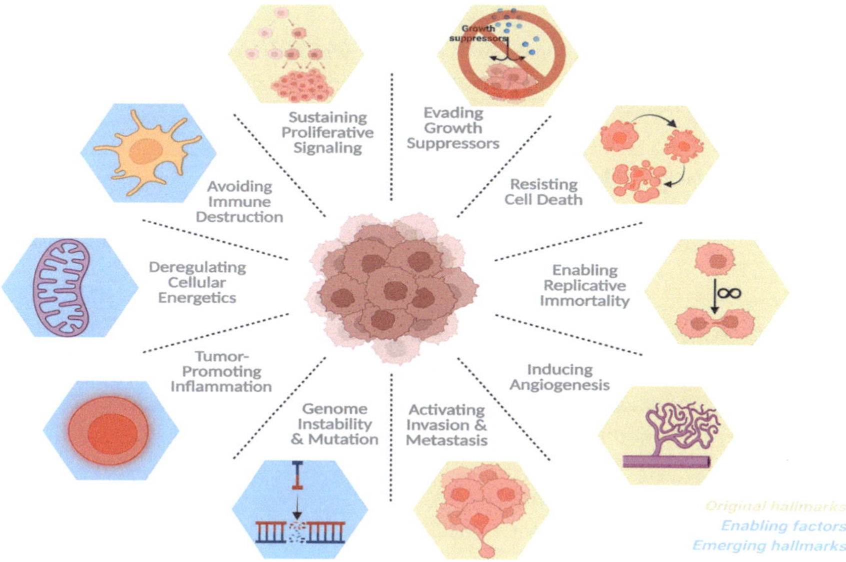

Fig. 2.2 Hallmarks of cancer

2.1.1.3 Cellular Immortalization and Telomerase Activation

Cellular immortalization is a critical process in cancer biology, enabling cells to bypass senescence and proliferate indefinitely. Normally, cells undergo a finite number of divisions due to progressive telomere shortening—a natural process associated with DNA replication. Telomeres, repetitive nucleotide sequences at the ends of chromosomes, act as protective caps, preventing damage to essential genetic information. However, when telomeres become critically short, cells enter senescence or apoptosis to maintain genomic stability [8]. Cancer cells overcome this limitation by activating telomerase, an enzyme that elongates telomeres, thereby achieving cellular immortality. This capability is a hallmark of many cancers and enables the sustained growth of tumors [9].

2.1.2 The Hallmarks of Cancer

The hallmarks of cancer, first described by Hanahan and Weinberg, outline the biological traits that enable cancer development and progression. Hanahan and Weinberg first described the hallmarks of cancer, which define the biological characteristics that drive the development and progression of cancer (Fig. 2.2).

2.1.2.1 Sustaining Proliferative Signaling

Cancer cells continuously activate growth-promoting pathways, often through mutations in oncogenes such as *RAS* and *MYC* [10]. This allows them to bypass normal growth controls and maintain unchecked proliferation.

2.1.2.2 Evading Growth Suppressors

Tumor suppressor genes (TSGs), such as *TP53* and *RB1*, act as natural brakes on cell division [11]. Mutations or deletions in these genes remove these growth-inhibitory signals, facilitating tumor progression.

2.1.2.3 Resisting Cell Death

Apoptosis, a programmed cell death process, is evaded by cancer cells through mutations in proapoptotic genes or the overexpression of antiapoptotic proteins like BCL-2.

2.1.2.4 Enabling Replicative Immortality

Normal cells have a restricted division capacity due to telomere shortening. Cancer cells reactivate telomerase, an enzyme that extends telomeres, granting them the ability to divide indefinitely [12].

2.1.2.5 Inducing Angiogenesis

To support rapid growth, tumors stimulate the formation of new blood vessels (angiogenesis), ensuring an adequate supply of oxygen and nutrients. This process is often driven by factors such as vascular endothelial growth factor (VEGF) [13].

2.1.2.6 Activating Invasion and Metastasis

Cancer cells invade nearby tissues and spread to distant organs via the bloodstream or lymphatic system, causing metastasis. This process involves altered cell adhesion molecules (e.g., E-cadherin) and the activation of enzymes that break down the extracellular matrix (ECM) [14].

2.1.2.7 Emerging Hallmarks: Metabolic Reprogramming and Immune Evasion

Cancer cells reprogram their metabolism to support rapid growth, often favoring glycolysis even in the presence of oxygen (the Warburg effect) [15]. Additionally, they evade immune surveillance by modulating immune checkpoints and creating an immunosuppressive microenvironment [15, 16].

2.2 Molecular Basis of Cancer

The molecular basis of cancer stems from genetic and epigenetic changes that drive malignant transformation. These alterations disrupt normal cellular functions, causing uncontrolled growth, evasion of cell death, and other cancer hallmarks.

2.2.1 Genetic Alterations

2.2.1.1 Oncogenes and Tumor Suppressor Genes

Oncogenes, derived from mutated proto-oncogenes, drive uncontrolled cell growth and division, whereas tumor suppressor genes (TSGs) inhibit cell proliferation and stimulate apoptosis. The interplay of these genetic alterations underpins the development of cancer through mechanisms such as mutations, copy number changes, and epigenetic modifications [17]. Mutations in proto-oncogenes like *RAS* and *MYC* are particularly significant. Mutant RAS proteins remain in an active guanosine triphosphate (GTP)-bound state, persistently signaling for cell proliferation and survival while inhibiting apoptosis [18]. Overexpression of MYC drives hallmark cancer traits, including enhanced DNA replication, transcription, and protein synthesis, alongside altered metabolism [19]. Conversely, tumor suppressor genes such as *TP53, RB1, and BRCA1/2* act as genomic safeguards. Their inactivation through mutations or deletions removes growth-inhibitory signals, facilitating tumor progression [20, 21].

2.2.1.2 Chromosomal Abnormalities

Chromosomal instability (CIN), encompassing structural and numerical abnormalities, is a hallmark of cancer. CIN involves either whole-chromosome instability (W-CIN) or structural chromosomal instability (S-CIN), leading to aneuploidy—an abnormal number of chromosomes—frequently observed in cancer cells [22]. Aneuploidy arises from chromosome segregation errors during cell division, resulting in gains or losses of chromosomes. For example, trisomies are common in cancers such as Ewing's sarcoma and renal adenocarcinoma, while monosomies are associated with meningiomas and ovarian adenocarcinomas [23].

Chromosomal translocations, such as the Philadelphia chromosome (t (9;22)), create fusion proteins like BCR-ABL, which drive malignancies like chronic myeloid leukemia [24]. Other abnormalities, such as deletions, duplications, inversions, and amplifications, also contribute to cancer progression. For instance, *MYCN* amplification, often seen in neuroblastoma, involves complex structural rearrangements [25].

2.2.1.3 DNA Repair Mechanisms and Their Failure

DNA repair pathways are critical for maintaining genomic integrity by correcting replication errors and damage caused by environmental factors. The mismatch repair (MMR) and homologous recombination (HR) pathways are particularly significant. Mutations in genes like *MLH1, MSH2, BRCA1, and BRCA2* are associated with increased risks of cancers such as breast and ovarian cancers [26–28].

The MMR system repairs replication errors, including base mismatches and insertion–deletion loops. Defects in MLH1 and MSH2 disrupt protein stability and function, leading to mutation accumulation. Similarly, the HR pathway repairs double-strand breaks in DNA using a homologous sequence as a template. Mutations in BRCA1/2 impair HR, resulting in genomic instability, characterized by deletions and chromosomal rearrangements, increasing cancer susceptibility [29]. The MMR system also interacts with other pathways, such as base excision repair (BER), to address oxidative DNA damage, with combined pathway failures amplifying mutagenesis and cancer risk [30].

2.2.1.4 Epigenetic Modifications in Cancer

Epigenetic changes, comprising DNA methylation, histone modifications, and noncoding RNA (ncRNA) regulation, are crucial in cancer biology. DNA methylation characteristically silences gene expression, particularly in Cytosine-phosphate-Guanine (CpG) islands within gene promoters. Aberrant methylation in cancer results in the silencing of tumor suppressor genes and global hypomethylation, which destabilizes the genome and activates oncogenes [31, 32].

Histone modifications, such as methylation and acetylation, regulate chromatin structure and transcription. Dysregulated histone-modifying enzymes contribute to inappropriate gene expression patterns in cancer [33, 34]. DNA methylation and histone modifications are interdependent, with methylation recruiting histone-modifying enzymes to reinforce chromatin changes and gene silencing [35].

Noncoding RNAs (ncRNAs) further influence gene regulation. Long noncoding RNAs (lncRNAs) serve as scaffolds for protein complexes that modify chromatin states. They interact with Polycomb repressive complexes and mixed-lineage leukemia (MLL) complexes to regulate gene expression [36]. Additionally, ncRNAs modulate epigenetic modifications, such as the ncRNA/DNMT3B axis in DNA methylation, and influence pathways like Wnt/β-catenin and cyclin-dependent kinase (CDK), which are essential for cancer cell survival and metastasis [37].

2.2.2 Key Signaling Pathways

2.2.2.1 Growth Factor Signaling Pathways

Growth factor signaling pathways play a critical role in cancer development and progression. The epidermal growth factor receptor (EGFR) and vascular endothelial growth factor (VEGF) pathways are frequently dysregulated in cancer, contributing to tumor growth and metastasis. These pathways operate through receptor tyrosine kinases (RTKs) that activate intracellular signaling cascades, promoting key cancer hallmarks, including sustained proliferation, evasion of apoptosis, and angiogenesis. When EGFR becomes activated, it triggers several downstream pathways, including MAPK, PI3K/AKT, and JAK/STAT, which are crucial for cell proliferation and survival. Beyond these direct signaling effects, EGFR also interacts with adhesion molecules like integrins and cadherins, enhancing cell adhesion and motility and facilitating epithelial–mesenchymal transition (EMT) [38].

The platelet-derived growth factor (PDGF) pathway significantly influences the tumor microenvironment (TME). It promotes angiogenesis and recruits pericytes to blood vessels, which helps maintain vascular integrity and supports tumor vascularization [39]. Additionally, PDGF affects stromal cells by enhancing their proliferation and survival, which creates a supportive environment for tumor growth and metastasis [40]. VEGF serves as a primary driver of angiogenesis, facilitating the formation of new blood vessels that supply tumors with essential nutrients and oxygen. This process is vital for tumor progression and metastasis. Specifically, the VEGF-A isoform promotes lymphangiogenesis, which enables cancer cells to spread through the lymphatic system [41].

2.2.2.2 Cell Survival Pathways

The PI3K/AKT/mTOR pathway plays a fundamental role in cellular regulation, controlling processes essential for cell survival and function. This signaling cascade governs cell growth, metabolic activities, and programmed cell death (apoptosis). Mutations in *PI3K* or loss of Phosphatase and TENsin homolog deleted on chromosome 10 (*PTEN*) leads to the hyperactivation of this pathway, promoting cancer cell survival. The pathway drives protein synthesis and cell cycle progression through mTOR activation, which phosphorylates targets like S6 kinase and 4E-BP1 [42]. AKT, a central player, inhibits apoptosis by inactivating proapoptotic factors such as caspase-9 and BAD, enabling cancer cells to survive under stress. Additionally, this pathway enhances glucose uptake and glycolysis while influencing lipid and protein synthesis, ensuring that the metabolic demands of rapidly proliferating cancer cells are met [43].

2.2.2.3 Cell Death Pathways

Cancer cells evade apoptosis by disrupting the balance between proapoptotic and antiapoptotic factors. Overexpression of antiapoptotic proteins like BCL-2 and BCL-xL prevents the release of cytochrome c from mitochondria, blocking the intrinsic apoptotic pathway. Upregulation of inhibitors such as cIAP2 and FLIP further suppresses apoptosis, as seen in esophageal adenocarcinoma. Additionally, reduced expression of proapoptotic proteins such as BAX and BAK, along with mutations or inactivation of p53, diminishes apoptosis and enhances cancer cell survival. NF-κB activation contributes to this process by upregulating survival genes and inhibiting apoptotic pathways, promoting cancer progression and therapy resistance [44].

2.2.2.4 Metabolic Pathways

Cancer cells undergo metabolic reprogramming to meet their high energy and biosynthetic demands. One prominent feature is the Warburg effect, where cancer cells depend on glycolysis, followed by lactic acid fermentation, even in the presence of oxygen. This shift supports rapid ATP production and supplies intermediates for biosynthetic pathways. *MYC* oncogene and *TP53* tumor suppressor gene play important roles in regulating glycolytic enzymes, enhancing glycolysis, and supporting cellular proliferation. Under hypoxic conditions within tumors, hypoxia-inducible factor 1 (HIF-1) becomes a critical regulator, upregulating glycolytic enzymes and glucose transporters to maintain energy production [45].

Beyond glucose metabolism, cancer cells also reprogram lipid metabolism to support membrane biosynthesis, energy storage, and signaling pathways. This includes increased de novo fatty acid synthesis and lipid oxidation processes, which are regulated by transcription factors such as FOXM1. Additionally, many cancer cells exhibit glutamine addiction, using this amino acid as a source of carbon and nitrogen for nucleotide synthesis and maintaining redox balance. HIF-1 further influences amino acid metabolism by optimizing their uptake and utilization under hypoxic conditions [46].

The growing understanding of cancer signaling pathways has significantly influenced biosensor technology development. These advances have enabled early detection, diagnosis, and monitoring of cancer through various biosensor platforms. Biosensors designed to detect specific cancer biomarkers—including DNA, RNA, and enzymes—provide rapid and sensitive diagnostic capabilities. For example, YbTixOy electrolyte-insulator-semiconductor (EIS) biosensors can detect KRAS mutations in colorectal cancer, while other biosensors measuring VEGF and BCL-2 protein levels provide insights into tumor angiogenesis and apoptosis resistance [47]. Epigenetic biosensors represent another promising area, detecting changes such as DNA methylation for noninvasive cancer diagnostics. These technologies enable real-time monitoring of cancer progression and treatment efficacy. The integration of molecular insights into biosensor development demonstrates significant potential for improving cancer management strategies [48].

2.3 Cancer Progression and Heterogeneity

Cancer progression involves a complex series of events where normal cells transform into malignant cells that can invade surrounding tissues and spread to distant sites. This process is influenced by multiple factors working in concert: epigenetic modifications that alter gene expression without changing the DNA sequence, genetic mutations that directly affect cellular function, and dynamic interactions with the surrounding tumor microenvironment. This diversity presents significant challenges for cancer management [49].

2.3.1 Stages of Cancer Development

2.3.1.1 Initiation

This first stage involves genetic damage to cells, often affecting proto-oncogenes, tumor suppressor genes, or DNA repair genes. The damage is typically caused by carcinogens (chemicals, radiation, and viruses) and creates permanent genetic alterations that make cells susceptible to further mutations [50].

2.3.1.2 Promotion

During this stage, initiated cells proliferate to form benign neoplasms or preneoplastic lesions [51]. The tumor microenvironment supports cancer cell survival through growth factors and cytokines. Unlike initiation, promotion can potentially be reversed through interventions like dietary changes or fasting [52].

2.3.1.3 Progression

This stage involves the accumulation of additional mutations, leading to increased genetic diversity within the tumor. Characteristics include changes in cell morphology (dysplasia), development of carcinoma in situ, and angiogenesis (formation of new blood vessels) that supports invasive growth [53].

2.3.1.4 Metastasis

The final stage involves cancer cells spreading to distant organs via the blood or lymphatic systems. Metastatic cells must survive detachment, circulation, and colonization in new environments. This stage typically carries a poor prognosis and presents significant treatment challenges [54].

2.3.2 Tumor Microenvironment

2.3.2.1 Cellular Components

The tumor microenvironment (TME) comprises diverse cellular elements that critically influence cancer progression. Cancer-associated fibroblasts (CAFs) represent a predominant TME component that facilitates tumor development through multiple mechanisms: They restructure the extracellular matrix (ECM), stimulate angiogenesis, and support immune evasion strategies. CAFs produce essential growth factors and cytokines—notably transforming growth factor-beta (TGF-β) and vascular endothelial growth factor (VEGF)—that drive tumor proliferation and metastasis. These specialized fibroblasts also enhance cancer cells' invasive properties, thereby promoting metastatic dissemination [55].

The TME contains various immune cells, including T cells, macrophages, and dendritic cells, that exhibit dual roles in cancer progression. While certain immune populations attempt to eliminate malignant cells, others, such as tumor-associated macrophages (TAMs), develop immunosuppressive characteristics that shield tumors from immune surveillance and accelerate metastasis. Contemporary immunotherapeutic approaches, particularly immune checkpoint inhibitors and CAR-T cell therapies, have demonstrated significant potential by specifically targeting these immune components within the TME.

Endothelial cells within the TME orchestrate tumor angiogenesis—a vital process that supplies growing tumors with nutrients and oxygen. VEGF signaling constitutes the primary pathway through which endothelial cells promote vascularization, thereby sustaining tumor growth and facilitating metastatic spread. Additional stromal elements, including mesenchymal stem cells and tumor-associated adipocytes, contribute to tumor metabolism, disease progression, and therapeutic resistance by modulating immune responses and altering the tumor microenvironment [56].

2.3.2.2 Extracellular Matrix

The ECM serves as a structural scaffold for tumor cells, influencing their survival and proliferation through embedded biochemical signals such as cytokines and growth factors. Proteolytic enzymes, particularly metalloproteinases, degrade ECM components, facilitating tumor invasion and metastasis. Dysregulation of these enzymes often leads to enhanced tumor progression by modifying the ECM's biochemical and physical properties [57].

Increased ECM stiffness, frequently resulting from collagen cross-linking, activates mechanotransduction pathways that promote cancer cell proliferation and metastasis. This mechanical stress can also induce hypoxia, further exacerbating the invasive potential of cancer cells. Beyond the primary tumor site, ECM remodeling plays a crucial role in preparing distant organs for metastatic colonization by creating pre-metastatic niches. Through complex interactions with resident stromal cells, tumor-derived factors systematically modify the ECM at potential metastatic sites. These modifications establish favorable microenvironments that support the survival and growth of disseminated tumor cells. The remodeled matrix simultaneously promotes new blood vessel formation and creates immunosuppressive conditions that shield metastatic cells from immune surveillance [58].

2.3.2.3 Signaling Molecules

The TME contains a rich array of signaling molecules—cytokines, growth factors, and chemokines—that orchestrate tumor progression through multiple mechanisms. TGF-β signaling emerges as a central regulator of epithelial–mesenchymal transition (EMT), fundamentally enhancing cancer cell invasiveness and metastatic potential. Concurrently, VEGF signaling drives angiogenesis, establishing the vascular infrastructure necessary for tumor growth and dissemination.

Pro-inflammatory cytokines, particularly interleukins IL-1β, IL-15, and IL-18, show consistent upregulation within tumors, creating immunosuppressive conditions while promoting cancer proliferation. These cytokines additionally maintain cancer stem cell–like properties, contributing to therapeutic resistance and tumor recurrence. Chemokine–G protein-coupled receptors (GPCR) signaling pathways further support EMT processes while regulating both cancer cell migration and immune cell recruitment to the tumor site. The Wnt signaling cascade complements these mechanisms by stimulating cancer cell proliferation and enhancing migratory behavior. Together, these molecular signals shape the tumor microenvironment's immunological landscape and metastatic capabilities [59].

2.3.2.4 Metabolic Characteristics

The metabolic profile of the TME is characterized by two predominant features—hypoxia and acidosis—both significantly influencing cancer progression and treatment resistance. Rapid tumor growth, coupled with inadequate vascularization, creates oxygen-deprived regions that stabilize hypoxia-inducible factors (HIFs). These transcription factors regulate genes controlling metabolism, angiogenesis, and cellular survival mechanisms. HIF activation promotes EMT processes while maintaining cancer stem–like cell populations through pathways involving HSP90, a chaperone protein that stabilizes HIF complexes [60].

Under hypoxic conditions, cancer cells undergo a metabolic shift from oxidative phosphorylation to glycolysis, resulting in lactate accumulation and environmental acidification. This acidosis facilitates extracellular matrix remodeling, creating pathways for tumor invasion and metastasis. Acidic conditions additionally enhance cancer cells' capacity for vasculogenic mimicry—the formation of vessel-like structures that support tumor vascularization, independent of conventional angiogenesis. Cancer cells maintain intracellular pH homeostasis through specialized enzymes like carbonic anhydrase IX (CA IX), preserving optimal conditions for glycolysis-driven proliferation.

A comprehensive understanding of the TME enables the development of advanced biosensors capable of detecting tumor-specific markers and environmental parameters, such as hypoxia and cytokine fluctuations. These biosensing technologies offer promising approaches for early cancer detection and real-time therapeutic response monitoring. Hypoxia-targeting biosensors can identify therapy-resistant tumor regions, while cytokine-detecting biosensors provide critical insights into tumors' immunological status, particularly valuable for monitoring immunotherapy efficacy. Emerging exosome-based biosensors detect tumor-derived biomarkers that indicate disease progression and treatment response. The integration of these biosensing technologies into clinical practice represents a significant advancement toward personalized cancer management strategies with improved diagnostic accuracy and treatment optimization [61].

2.3.3 Tumor Heterogeneity

2.3.3.1 Intratumor Heterogeneity

Intratumor heterogeneity (ITH) represents a defining characteristic of cancer, characterized by the simultaneous existence of diverse cancer cell subpopulations within individual tumors. This cellular diversity emerges through multiple mechanisms, including genetic mutations, epigenetic alterations, and microenvironmental influences, collectively enhancing cancer's adaptability and therapeutic resistance. The molecular underpinnings of ITH involve complex signaling networks, dynamic gene expression patterns, and evolutionary processes that collectively drive cancer progression and treatment challenges. Cancer cell plasticity significantly amplifies ITH by enabling malignant cells to modify their phenotypic identity in response to both genetic signals and environmental conditions. Critical cellular programs, particularly epithelial-to-mesenchymal transition (EMT) and metabolic reprogramming, function as central mechanisms in this adaptive process. These pathways allow cancer cells to transition between different functional states, further increasing tumor heterogeneity and complicating therapeutic targeting.

The cancer cell secretome—the collection of proteins and molecules secreted by tumor cells—plays a substantial role in maintaining heterogeneity, especially in colorectal cancer. Research demonstrates that these secreted factors enhance chemotherapy resistance by selectively protecting specific cancer cell subpopulations while simultaneously promoting invasive characteristics. This secretome-mediated protection creates additional layers of functional diversity within tumors.

Expression noise—defined as the variability in gene expression among genetically identical cells—is another significant contributor to ITH. This nongenetic source of heterogeneity has been directly linked to cancer progression and treatment resistance. In lung adenocarcinoma, specific genes demonstrate progressively increased expression variability as the disease advances from early to late stages, creating functional diversity even among genetically similar cancer cells [62].

2.3.3.2 Intertumor Heterogeneity

Intertumor heterogeneity refers to the molecular and genetic differences observed among tumors of the same type across different individuals. This variability significantly influences cancer progression and treatment outcomes, as tumors originating from the same tissue type can exhibit distinct molecular behaviors and therapeutic responses. Intertumor heterogeneity is exemplified by variations in molecular markers such as HER2, dMMR, and PD-L1 in gastric cancer, where discrepancies between primary tumors and metastatic sites can complicate treatment strategies. Similarly, in breast cancer, distinct molecular and genetic signatures among patients contribute to differences in disease progression and response to therapy. The presence of intertumor heterogeneity poses challenges for developing universal treatment protocols, as therapeutic approaches effective in one patient may not yield similar results in another due to these underlying molecular differences [63].

2.3.3.3 Impact on Diagnosis and Treatment

Tumor heterogeneity presents significant obstacles in cancer diagnosis and treatment. Standard diagnostic techniques may fail to detect rare subclonal populations, leading to incomplete disease characterization. Variations in biomarker expression, influenced by factors such as blood supply and hypoxia, further complicate accurate diagnosis, as seen in breast cancer, where these factors affect tumor growth and biomarker distribution. Spatial heterogeneity within tumors can diminish the prognostic reliability of biomarkers, as averaging expression levels across a tumor may obscure critical variations. Furthermore, targeted therapies designed to address specific genetic mutations often demonstrate limited clinical efficacy against heterogeneous or evolving cancer cell populations, as treatment-resistant subclones can rapidly emerge and dominate the tumor landscape [64].

2.3.3.4 Challenges for Biosensor Development

Addressing tumor heterogeneity requires biosensors capable of capturing comprehensive molecular profiles across diverse cancer cell populations. Recent innovations include biomimetic biosensors employing dual-targeting multivalent aptamer-regulated 3D DNA walkers, specifically designed to enhance the detection of heterogeneous circulating tumor cells (CTCs). This advanced technology significantly improves detection efficiency by minimizing leukocyte interference while facilitating the capture of viable CTCs for subsequent molecular analysis. Multiplexed biosensors, capable of detecting multiple biomarkers simultaneously, provide a more holistic view of tumor heterogeneity, aiding in personalized treatment strategies. Advances in next-generation sequencing and multi-omics technologies have further refined biosensor capabilities, enabling high-resolution analysis of genetic, transcriptomic, and proteomic variations within tumors. These innovations offer deeper insights into tumor biology and support the development of more effective, targeted therapies [65].

2.4 Current Diagnostic Approaches and Their Limitations

Cancer diagnosis is a critical step in managing and treating the disease. Accurate and timely diagnosis enables clinicians to determine the tumor's stage, subtype, and molecular characteristics, guiding therapeutic decisions. However, current diagnostic approaches have inherent limitations that pose challenges to achieving optimal outcomes [66].

2.4.1 Traditional Diagnostic Methods

2.4.1.1 Imaging Techniques

Imaging techniques are fundamental tools for detecting and monitoring cancer, offering noninvasive visualization of tumors. Common modalities include computed tomography (CT), magnetic resonance imaging (MRI), positron emission tomography (PET), X-rays, and ultrasound. Advanced applications, such as the integration of functional imaging with CT, enable adaptive treatment strategies by adjusting radiation fields based on tumor response during therapy [67].

Molecular imaging, particularly PET, excels in characterizing tumors at the molecular level, while optical imaging provides real-time visualization of molecular events. MRI is particularly effective for detecting occult diseases and assessing tumor extent, especially in dense breast tissues and high-risk individuals, making it crucial for accurate staging and treatment planning. Innovations in ultrasound, including elastography, contrast-enhanced imaging, and 3D techniques, have improved sensitivity for detecting nonpalpable carcinomas, supporting more conservative surgical approaches and better treatment outcomes. X-rays remain instrumental for detecting lung nodules, assessing tumor size, and determining cancer stages [68].

2.4.1.2 Tissue Biopsy and Histopathological Analysis

Tissue biopsy is the gold standard for cancer diagnosis, involving the extraction of tissue samples from suspected tumor sites for histological analysis. Methods such as excisional, incisional, and needle biopsies are used to obtain material for cytological and histological examination, each with distinct advantages and limitations [69].

Histopathological analysis involves microscopic examination of tissue samples to identify cellular abnormalities indicative of cancer. It plays a vital role in determining malignancy, tumor grading, staging, and detecting biomarkers that influence treatment decisions. Techniques like immunohistochemistry (IHC) enable detailed characterization of molecular markers, aiding in tumor classification and staging [70].

2.4.1.3 Limitations of Current Approaches

While imaging and biopsy techniques are pivotal in cancer diagnosis, they face inherent limitations that affect their diagnostic accuracy and clinical utility.

Imaging Techniques

The use of ionizing radiation poses a risk of secondary malignancies, especially in pediatric patients. Contrast agents can cause allergic reactions or nephropathy, limiting their use in patients with renal impairment.

Contraindications include metallic implants or foreign bodies, and the enclosed nature of MRI machines can induce claustrophobia. Artifacts may degrade image quality, complicating interpretation. High costs of PET scans restrict accessibility and routine use in some healthcare settings. X-rays provide limited contrast for soft tissues, making it challenging to detect certain types of tumors. Like CT, X-rays involve ionizing radiation, which carries a cancer risk. The effectiveness of ultrasound diminishes in obese patients or those with bloating, and operator skill significantly impacts diagnostic accuracy [66].

Tissue Biopsy and Histopathology

Biopsies are invasive and carry risks such as bleeding and infection, limiting their feasibility in certain patients. Tumor heterogeneity may lead to sampling errors, particularly in cancers like hepatocellular carcinoma, where characteristics vary within a single lesion. Traditional histology provides a two-dimensional view, potentially missing critical aspects of tumor invasiveness and micro-infiltrations, leading to under-staging or false negatives. Lack of consensus on evaluating key histopathological features, such as differentiation in hepatocellular carcinoma, can affect diagnostic consistency [71].

To address these limitations, noninvasive diagnostic tools, molecular diagnostic techniques, and advanced imaging technologies are being developed. These innovations aim to enhance diagnostic precision, minimize risks, and improve patient care, paving the way for more accurate and comprehensive cancer diagnosis [72].

2.4.2 Molecular Diagnostic Techniques

2.4.2.1 PCR-Based Methods

Polymerase chain reaction (PCR)-based diagnostic technologies serve as essential tools in cancer detection and monitoring, providing exceptional sensitivity and specificity for identifying cancer-associated genetic alterations and nucleic acids. When integrated with liquid biopsy approaches, these techniques offer minimally invasive methods for tracking disease progression and evaluating treatment efficacy. Ongoing technological developments focus on enhancing detection sensitivity, expanding the range of identifiable mutations, and combining PCR with complementary genomic technologies to achieve comprehensive cancer profiling [73].

Advanced PCR methodologies such as droplet digital PCR (ddPCR) enable the detection of rare mutant DNA molecules within circulating tumor DNA (ctDNA) obtained from simple blood draws, facilitating earlier cancer detection when treatment interventions are most effective [73]. Primer exchange reaction (PER)-based signal amplification strategies further enhance sensitivity by allowing detection of cancer-specific mutations, even when vastly outnumbered by wild-type DNA sequences—a critical capability for early-stage cancer diagnosis [74]. These PCR-based approaches significantly advance personalized medicine by identifying specific genetic markers that guide therapeutic decision-making. For example, the detection of EGFR mutations in lung cancer patients helps identify candidates for tyrosine kinase inhibitor therapy, improving treatment outcomes through targeted approaches [75]. Additionally, these technologies enable precise monitoring of minimal residual disease and therapeutic response, allowing clinicians to anticipate potential tumor recurrence and adjust treatment strategies proactively [76].

2.4.2.2 Next-Generation Sequencing (NGS)

Next-generation sequencing (NGS) technologies have revolutionized cancer diagnostics by enabling comprehensive genetic profiling that identifies markers indicative of early-stage malignancy, supporting timely intervention and improved patient outcomes [77]. Powerful approaches including whole-genome sequencing (WGS) and whole-exome sequencing (WES) provide unprecedented insights into cancer's genetic landscape, facilitating earlier and more accurate diagnosis [78].

By systematically identifying driver mutations and clinically actionable genetic alterations, NGS enables the development of personalized treatment strategies with enhanced efficacy and reduced side effects [79, 80]. Integration with sophisticated bioinformatics tools further improves the prediction of therapeutic responses and management of treatment resistance mechanisms. NGS technologies provide a comprehensive analysis of tumor heterogeneity, clonal evolution patterns, and resistance mechanisms—critical insights for tailoring individualized treatment plans [81]. The high-throughput capabilities of NGS platforms support large-scale genomic studies that continue to advance the understanding of cancer biology while informing clinical applications [82].

2.4.2.3 Protein-Based Assays

Protein-based diagnostic assays leverage advances in proteomics to enhance cancer detection sensitivity and specificity, offering promising alternatives to traditional diagnostic approaches. These assays detect cancer-associated proteins at early stages, enabling timely intervention and improving patient outcomes.

A multidimensional serum proteomic strategy integrates various proteomic techniques, achieving comprehensive serum proteome coverage and demonstrating 87.5% localization accuracy for multiple cancers, including breast, lung, and liver cancers. Recent advancements in plasma proteomics have enabled the development of multi-cancer screening tests. For instance, a proximity extension assay identified the proteins capable of detecting early-stage cancers with high accuracy (Area Under Curve (AUC): 0.98 for males and 0.983 for females) and determining the tissue of origin in over 80% of cases [83].

Extracellular vesicle (EV) protein-based tests utilize biomarkers in circulating EVs to detect early-stage cancers, demonstrating high specificity and sensitivity for stage I and II pancreatic, ovarian, and bladder cancers. Combining protein markers with other biomarker classes, such as DNA methylation, further enhances detection sensitivity. For example, integrating these markers improved overall sensitivity to

75% at 99% specificity, highlighting the potential of multi-biomarker approaches for early cancer detection [84].

2.4.2.4 Current Challenges and Limitations

Despite their potential, molecular diagnostic techniques face several challenges.

PCR-Based Methods

Variability in assay design, particularly for DNA methylation biomarkers, can hinder reproducibility and comparability across studies. Low concentrations and high fragmentation of cell-free DNA (cfDNA) in blood plasma complicate analysis, requiring sufficient DNA quantity and quality for accurate detection. Cancer heterogeneity results in variable biomarker expression, affecting diagnostic reliability. PCR methods are often limited to predefined mutation sets, restricting their ability to capture the full spectrum of genetic alterations [73].

NGS Technology

High costs of sequencing and bioinformatics analyses limit accessibility, especially in low- and middle-income countries. Infrastructure requirements, including computational resources and skilled personnel, remain expensive and complex. Interpreting vast data volumes requires sophisticated bioinformatics tools and specialized expertise, creating bottlenecks.

Targeted approaches, such as gene panels, often miss critical noncoding regions and structural variants [85]. Sample quality and preservation are crucial, as poor-quality samples can lead to inaccurate results [86].

Protein-Based Assays

The complexity of the human proteome, including posttranslational modifications, complicates biomarker identification and validation. Variability in biomarker expression and pre-analytical factors, such as blood collection and storage conditions, impact assay reliability. Innovations like Protein Plus BCT have been developed to stabilize blood cells and minimize proteome changes during storage, but these solutions are not yet widely adopted in clinical practice [87].

Emerging technologies, such as single-cell sequencing and long-read sequencing, hold promise for addressing these challenges. However, they introduce new complexities, including increased computational demands and the need for further technological development [88]. Continued advancements in molecular diagnostics are essential to overcome these limitations and improve cancer detection and management.

2.5 Biomarkers in Cancer

Biomarkers are essential tools in cancer detection, diagnosis, prognosis, and treatment monitoring. These measurable biological molecules provide critical insights into tumor biology, enable patient stratification for targeted therapies, and enhance the precision of clinical decision-making.

2.5.1 Types of Cancer Biomarkers

2.5.1.1 Genetic Biomarkers

Genetic biomarkers encompass mutations, deletions, amplifications, and translocations in DNA sequences associated with cancer. These biomarkers illuminate the molecular mechanisms underlying cancer, facilitating accurate diagnosis, prognosis, and personalized treatment strategies. Mutations in oncogenes (e.g., *KRAS* and *BRAF*) and tumor suppressor genes (e.g., *TP53* and *BRCA1/2*) are commonly used to assess disease risk and guide therapy [89]. For instance, EGFR mutations in non-small cell lung cancer (NSCLC) predict the responsiveness to tyrosine kinase inhibitors [90].

2.5.1.2 Protein Biomarkers

Protein biomarkers include proteins that are overexpressed, underexpressed, or aberrantly modified in cancer cells or the tumor microenvironment. Advances in proteomics have identified numerous protein biomarker candidates across various cancers (https://doi.org/10.1002/qub2.35). Examples include prostate-specific antigen (PSA) for prostate cancer and human epidermal growth factor receptor 2 (HER2) for breast cancer [91]. These biomarkers are critical for cancer subtyping, such as in breast cancer, where they guide therapy selection for both primary and recurrent tumors [92].

2.5.1.3 Metabolic Biomarkers

Metabolic biomarkers arise from alterations in cellular metabolism characteristic of cancer cells. Metabolomics—the study of metabolites—has become a key approach to identifying biochemical markers indicative of cancer presence and progression. These biomarkers, such as those associated with the Warburg effect (increased glucose uptake and lactate production), aid in early cancer diagnosis. Additionally, tumor-associated metabolites play roles in cancer progression, including promoting angiogenesis and invasion, offering new therapeutic targets [93].

2.5.1.4 Circulating Tumor Cells

CTCs, which detach from primary tumors and enter the bloodstream, are key contributors to metastasis and are increasingly utilized in liquid biopsies for cancer detection and management. CTCs also provide insights into immunological checkpoints, aiding cancer immunotherapy, particularly in patients undergoing chemotherapy and targeted therapies. The development of CTC-derived organoids

(CTCDOs) offers promising tools for studying tumor heterogeneity and metastasis, advancing precision oncology [94].

2.5.1.5 Cell-Free DNA (CfDNA)

CfDNA consists of small DNA fragments released into the bloodstream by apoptotic or necrotic tumor cells. Analyzing cfDNA fragmentation patterns, integrity indices, and tumor fraction scores provides insights into tumor presence and burden. These patterns, particularly those linked to nucleosome positioning, enable the enrichment of tumor-derived cfDNA for sensitive cancer diagnosis. CfDNA is also valuable for real-time monitoring of treatment efficacy and predicting relapse, offering a noninvasive method for tracking disease progression [95].

2.5.2 Challenges in Biomarker Detection

Despite their potential, biomarker detection faces several challenges that limit their clinical utility.

2.5.2.1 Sensitivity and Specificity Issues

Many biomarkers lack cancer specificity and may also be elevated in benign conditions, leading to false positives. Conversely, low biomarker levels in early-stage cancers can result in false negatives. Variability in biomarker concentrations between patients and over time complicates detection [96].

2.5.2.2 Sample Preparation and Handling

The isolation of biomarkers, such as cell-free nucleic acids, is labor-intensive and requires large sample volumes, hindering rapid clinical application. Pre-analytical and analytical factors, including sample collection, storage, and processing, significantly affect biomarker measurement validity, leading to potential misinterpretations [97].

2.5.2.3 Cost and Accessibility

High costs associated with biomarker detection technologies, coupled with the need for advanced equipment and trained personnel, limit widespread accessibility. The financial burden is further exacerbated by the high failure rate in biomarker development and the stringent requirements for validation and regulation [98].

2.5.2.4 Time to Results

Traditional diagnostic methods often involve delays due to process complexity, hindering timely clinical decisions. Rapid detection technologies, such as point-of-care testing (POCT), are essential to minimize delays and improve outcomes [99].

2.5.2.5 Need for Point-of-Care Diagnostics

Point-of-care testing (POCT) offers immediate results at the patient's location, but developing reliable platforms with high sensitivity and specificity remains challenging. Innovations like noninvasive skin patches for biomarker detection show promise, offering advantages such as ease of use and reduced infection risks [96, 100].

2.6 Future Challenges and Opportunities

The field of cancer diagnostics is rapidly evolving, driven by advances in technology and a growing understanding of tumor biology. However, significant challenges remain, particularly in achieving early detection, improving treatment monitoring, and addressing disparities in access to diagnostic tools.

2.6.1 Current Challenges in Cancer Diagnosis

2.6.1.1 Early Detection

Detecting cancer at an early stage significantly improves patient outcomes. However, countless cancers, such as ovarian and pancreatic cancers, are often diagnosed late due to vague symptoms and the lack of effective screening tools [101]. Early detection biomarkers are often present in very low concentrations, making them problematic to identify with existing methods.

2.6.1.2 Monitoring Treatment Response

Assessing how a patient responds to therapy is serious for optimizing treatment plans. Traditional methods, such as imaging and biopsy, are not always reliable or timely. These approaches may fail to capture real-time changes in tumor biology or drug resistance, leading to suboptimal treatment decisions [102].

2.6.1.3 Predicting Recurrence

Cancer recurrence remains a significant concern, even after successful initial treatment. The identification of biomarkers capable of predicting recurrence is particularly compelling, given the inherent tumor heterogeneity and the dynamic nature of cancer progression [103]. Current methods often rely on periodic imaging and clinical evaluations, which may miss early signs of relapse.

2.6.1.4 Personalized Medicine Approaches

While personalized medicine has transformed cancer care, its implementation is hampered by the complexity of tumor biology and the need for comprehensive biomarker profiling. The lack of standardized protocols and high costs further limit its widespread adoption [104].

2.6.2 Opportunities for Biosensor Development

2.6.2.1 Point-of-Care Testing

Biosensors offer a promising solution for decentralized, rapid cancer diagnostics. Portable and user-friendly devices can enable point-of-care testing, reducing the need for centralized laboratories [105]. These technologies can facilitate early detection, particularly in low-resource settings, where access to advanced diagnostics is limited.

2.6.2.2 Real-Time Monitoring

Biosensors can provide real-time data on biomarkers, enabling dynamic monitoring of treatment response and disease progression. For example, wearable biosensors could continuously measure specific biomarkers in bodily fluids, offering immediate insights into therapeutic efficacy [106].

2.6.2.3 Multiplexed Detection

Multiplexed detection capabilities represent a significant advantage of modern biosensor technologies in cancer management. Rather than relying on individual biomarkers that may not reflect the complete disease profile, multiplexed biosensors generate integrated datasets that better characterize cancer's biological complexity [107]. This approach is particularly valuable for addressing tumor heterogeneity.

2.6.2.4 Integration with Existing Technologies

Biosensor technologies demonstrate remarkable compatibility with established diagnostic modalities, creating powerful synergies that enhance overall clinical utility. Integration with conventional imaging techniques and molecular profiling methods creates complementary diagnostic systems that leverage the strengths of each approach [108]. The combination of biosensors with artificial intelligence algorithms supports more precise clinical decision-making and truly personalized cancer management.

2.6.2.5 Cost-Effective Solutions

Developing economically accessible biosensor technologies represents a critical priority for democratizing advanced cancer diagnostics globally. Affordable and scalable biosensor platforms can significantly reduce disparities between high-resource and low-resource healthcare settings, ensuring that cutting-edge diagnostic capabilities reach diverse patient populations worldwide [109].

Despite persistent challenges in early cancer detection, treatment monitoring, and personalized medicine implementation, these areas present substantial opportunities for biosensor innovation. With their potential for rapid, sensitive, and cost-effective biomarker detection, biosensor technologies are uniquely positioned to address many current limitations in cancer diagnostics. By leveraging interdisciplinary advances in materials science, microfluidics, and artificial intelligence, biosensors continue to transform the cancer diagnostic landscape, making sophisticated molecular analysis more accessible and effective for patients across diverse healthcare environments.

2.7 Conclusion

Cancer represents one of medicine's most complex challenges, characterized by multidimensional cellular and molecular alterations. These include dysregulated cell cycle control mechanisms, apoptosis evasion strategies, disrupted signaling pathways, and metabolic reprogramming that allows cancer cells to thrive in otherwise hostile environments. The heterogeneity of tumors presents a particularly formidable obstacle. This variability exists not only between different cancer types (inter-tumoral heterogeneity) but also within individual tumors (intra-tumoral heterogeneity). Such diversity complicates both accurate diagnosis and effective treatment planning. Traditional diagnostic approaches, while valuable, face significant limitations. These include insufficient sensitivity for early-stage detection, limited specificity leading to false positives, and accessibility barriers that prevent equitable cancer care globally. Emerging biosensor technologies offer potential solutions to these diagnostic challenges. These innovative approaches may enable early detection of biomarkers, real-time monitoring of disease progression and treatment response, personalized treatment, and point-of-care testing capabilities. By integrating our expanding knowledge of cancer biology with advances in biosensor development, one can envision a future where cancer diagnosis becomes more precise, accessible, and actionable. This integration could transform clinical practice across diverse healthcare settings globally, ultimately improving outcomes for cancer patients through earlier intervention and more targeted therapeutic approaches.

References

1. Hassanpour SH, Dehghani M. Review of cancer from perspective of molecular. J Cancer Res Pract. 2017;4(4):127–9.
2. Orzetti S, Tommasi F, Bertola A, Bortolin G, Caccin E, Cecco S, et al. Genetic therapy and molecular targeted therapy in oncology: safety, pharmacovigilance, and perspectives for research and clinical practice. Int J Mol Sci. 2022;23(6)
3. Ben-Salem S, Venkadakrishnan VB, Heemers HV. Novel insights in cell cycle dysregulation during prostate cancer progression. Endocr Relat Cancer. 2021;28(6):R141–R55.
4. Besson A, Dowdy SF, Roberts JM. CDK inhibitors: cell cycle regulators and beyond. Dev Cell. 2008;14(2):159–69.
5. Jorgensen I, Rayamajhi M, Miao EA. Programmed cell death as a defence against infection. Nat Rev Immunol. 2017;17(3):151–64.
6. Hartman ML, Czyz M. BCL-w: apoptotic and non-apoptotic role in health and disease. Cell Death Dis. 2020;11(4):260.
7. Mustafa M, Ahmad R, Tantry IQ, Ahmad W, Siddiqui S, Alam M, et al. Apoptosis: a comprehensive overview of signaling pathways, morphological changes, and physiological significance and therapeutic implications. Cells. 2024;13(22):1838.
8. Dolcetti R, Giunco S, Dal Col J, Celeghin A, Mastorci K, De Rossi A. Epstein-Barr virus and telomerase: from cell immortalization to therapy. Infect Agents Cancer. 2014;9:1–7.

9. Saretzki G. Telomeres, telomerase and ageing. Biochem Cell Biol Ageing Part I Biomed Sci. 2018;90:221–308.
10. Ciccarone F, Ciriolo MR. Hallmark of cancer: sustained proliferative signalling. Frontiers Media SA; 2023. p. 1328827.
11. Nicolini A, Ferrari P, Rossi G, Carpi A. Tumour growth and immune evasion as targets for a new strategy in advanced cancer. Endocr Relat Cancer. 2018;25(11):R577–604.
12. Wani AK, Akhtar N, Sharma A, El-Zahaby SA. Fighting carcinogenesis with plant metabolites by weakening proliferative signaling and disabling replicative immortality networks of rapidly dividing and invading cancerous cells. Curr Drug Deliv. 2023;20(4):371–86.
13. Saman H, Raza SS, Uddin S, Rasul K. Inducing angiogenesis, a key step in cancer vascularization, and treatment approaches. Cancers. 2020;12(5):1172.
14. Jiang WG, Sanders AJ, Katoh M, Ungefroren H, Gieseler F, Prince M, et al. Tissue invasion and metastasis: molecular, biological and clinical perspectives. Semin Cancer Biol. 2015;35:S244–75.
15. Zhang H, Li S, Wang D, Liu S, Xiao T, Gu W, et al. Metabolic reprogramming and immune evasion: the interplay in the tumor microenvironment. Biomark Res. 2024;12(1):96.
16. Huang H, Li S, Tang Q, Zhu G. Metabolic reprogramming and immune evasion in nasopharyngeal carcinoma. Front Immunol. 2021;12:680955.
17. Zhu K, Liu Q, Zhou Y, Tao C, Zhao Z, Sun J, et al. Oncogenes and tumor suppressor genes: comparative genomics and network perspectives. BMC Genomics. 2015;16:1–11.
18. Grzes M, Oron M, Staszczak Z, Jaiswar A, Nowak-Niezgoda M, Walerych D. A driver never works alone—interplay networks of mutant p53, MYC, RAS, and other universal oncogenic drivers in human cancer. Cancers. 2020;12(6):1532.
19. Casacuberta-Serra S, González-Larreategui Í, Capitán-Leo D, Soucek L. MYC and KRAS cooperation: from historical challenges to therapeutic opportunities in cancer. Signal Transduct Target Ther. 2024;9(1):205.
20. Rosen EM, Pishvaian MJ. Targeting the BRCA1/2 tumor suppressors. Curr Drug Targets. 2014;15(1):17–31.
21. Siles MP. Translational readthrough of nonsense mutant TP53, RB1 and PTEN tumor suppressor genes as a strategy for novel cancer therapy. Karolinska Institutet (Sweden); 2023.
22. Dhital B, Rodriguez-Bravo V. Mechanisms of chromosomal instability (CIN) tolerance in aggressive tumors: surviving the genomic chaos. Chromosom Res. 2023;31(2):15.
23. Potapova T, Gorbsky GJ. The consequences of chromosome segregation errors in mitosis and meiosis. Biology. 2017;6(1):12.
24. Peiris MN, Li F, Donoghue DJ. BCR: a promiscuous fusion partner in hematopoietic disorders. Oncotarget. 2019;10(28):2738.
25. Bartolucci D, Montemurro L, Raieli S, Lampis S, Pession A, Hrelia P, et al. MYCN impact on high-risk neuroblastoma: from diagnosis and prognosis to targeted treatment. Cancers. 2022;14(18):4421.
26. Incorvaia L, Bazan Russo TD, Gristina V, Perez A, Brando C, Mujacic C, et al. The intersection of homologous recombination (HR) and mismatch repair (MMR) pathways in DNA repair-defective tumors. NPJ Precis Oncol. 2024;8(1):190.
27. Sajjadi E, Venetis K, Piciotti R, Invernizzi M, Guerini-Rocco E, Haricharan S, et al. Mismatch repair-deficient hormone receptor-positive breast cancers: biology and pathological characterization. Cancer Cell Int. 2021;21:1–10.
28. Kim J, Jeong K, Jun H, Kim K, Bae JM, Song MG, et al. Mutations of TP53 and genes related to homologous recombination repair in breast cancer with germline BRCA1/2 mutations. Hum Genomics. 2023;17(1):2.
29. Cilona M, Locatello LG, Novelli L, Gallo O. The mismatch repair system (MMR) in head and neck carcinogenesis and its role in modulating the response to immunotherapy: a critical review. Cancers. 2020;12(10):3006.
30. Stratigopoulou M, van Dam TP, Guikema JE. Base excision repair in the immune system: small DNA lesions with big consequences. Front Immunol. 2020;11:1084.

31. Lujambio A, Portela A, Liz J, Melo S, Rossi S, Spizzo R, et al. CpG Island hypermethylation-associated silencing of non-coding RNAs transcribed from ultraconserved regions in human cancer. Oncogene. 2010;29(48):6390–401.
32. Bure IV, Nemtsova MV, Kuznetsova EB. Histone modifications and non-coding RNAs: mutual epigenetic regulation and role in pathogenesis. Int J Mol Sci. 2022;23(10):5801.
33. Qin J, Wen B, Liang Y, Yu W, Li H. Histone modifications and their role in colorectal cancer. Pathol Oncol Res. 2020;26:2023–33.
34. Szczepanek J, Tretyn A. MicroRNA-mediated regulation of histone-modifying enzymes in cancer: mechanisms and therapeutic implications. Biomol Ther. 2023;13(11):1590.
35. Vaissière T, Sawan C, Herceg Z. Epigenetic interplay between histone modifications and DNA methylation in gene silencing. Mutat Res Rev Mutat Res. 2008;659(1–2):40–8.
36. Taylor DH, Chu ETJ, Spektor R, Soloway PD. Long non-coding RNA regulation of reproduction and development. Mol Reprod Dev. 2015;82(12):932–56.
37. Huang C, Azizi P, Vazirzadeh M, Aghaei-Zarch SM, Aghaei-Zarch F, Ghanavi J, et al. Non-coding RNAs/DNMT3B axis in human cancers: from pathogenesis to clinical significance. J Transl Med. 2023;21(1):621.
38. Wee P, Wang Z. Epidermal growth factor receptor cell proliferation signaling pathways. Cancers. 2017;9(5):52.
39. Heldin CH, Lennartsson J, Westermark B. Involvement of platelet-derived growth factor ligands and receptors in tumorigenesis. J Intern Med. 2018;283(1):16–44.
40. Oncul S, Cho MS. Interactions between platelets and tumor microenvironment components in ovarian cancer and their implications for treatment and clinical outcomes. Cancers. 2023;15(4):1282.
41. Paduch R. The role of lymphangiogenesis and angiogenesis in tumor metastasis. Cell Oncol. 2016;39:397–410.
42. Maddika S, Ande SR, Panigrahi S, Paranjothy T, Weglarczyk K, Zuse A, et al. Cell survival, cell death and cell cycle pathways are interconnected: implications for cancer therapy. Drug Resist Updat. 2007;10(1–2):13–29.
43. Henson ES, Gibson SB. Surviving cell death through epidermal growth factor (EGF) signal transduction pathways: implications for cancer therapy. Cell Signal. 2006;18(12):2089–97.
44. Jin Z, El-Deiry WS. Overview of cell death signaling pathways. Cancer Biol Ther. 2005;4(2):147–71.
45. Hoxhaj G, Manning BD. The PI3K–AKT network at the interface of oncogenic signalling and cancer metabolism. Nat Rev Cancer. 2020;20(2):74–88.
46. Asl ER, Amini M, Najafi S, Mansoori B, Mokhtarzadeh A, Mohammadi A, et al. Interplay between MAPK/ERK signaling pathway and MicroRNAs: a crucial mechanism regulating cancer cell metabolism and tumor progression. Life Sci. 2021;278:119499.
47. Mayoral-Pena K, Gonzalez Pena OI, Orrantia Clark AM, Flores-Vallejo RC, Oza G, Sharma A, et al. Biorecognition engineering technologies for cancer diagnosis: a systematic literature review of non-conventional and plausible sensor development methods. Cancers. 2022;14(8):1867.
48. Zakari S, Niels NK, Olagunju GV, Nnaji PC, Ogunniyi O, Tebamifor M, et al. Emerging biomarkers for non-invasive diagnosis and treatment of cancer: a systematic review. Front Oncol. 2024;14:1405267.
49. Maishi N, Annan DA, Kikuchi H, Hida Y, Hida K. Tumor endothelial heterogeneity in cancer progression. Cancers. 2019;11(10):1511.
50. Deshmukh S, Saini S. Phenotypic heterogeneity in tumor progression, and its possible role in the onset of cancer. Front Genet. 2020;11:604528.
51. Hennings H, Glick AB, Greenhalgh DA, Morgan DL, Strickland JE, Tennenbaum T, et al. Critical aspects of initiation, promotion, and progression in multistage epidermal carcinogenesis. Proc Soc Exp Biol Med. 1993;202(1):1–8.
52. Pitot HC, Campbell HA, Maronpot R, Bawa N, Rizvi TA, Xu Y-H, et al. Critical parameters in the quantitation of the stages of initiation, promotion, and progression in one model of hepatocarcinogenesis in the rat. Toxicol Pathol. 1989;17(4_part_1):594–612.

53. Zhang KJ, Tan XL, Guo L. The long non-coding RNA DANCR regulates the inflammatory phenotype of breast cancer cells and promotes breast cancer progression via EZH2-dependent suppression of SOCS3 transcription. Mol Oncol. 2020;14(2):309–28.
54. Kim S, Karin M. Role of TLR2-dependent inflammation in metastatic progression. Ann N Y Acad Sci. 2011;1217(1):191–206.
55. Wei R, Liu S, Zhang S, Min L, Zhu S. Cellular and extracellular components in tumor microenvironment and their application in early diagnosis of cancers. Anal Cell Pathol. 2020;2020(1):6283796.
56. Kerkar SP, Restifo NP. Cellular constituents of immune escape within the tumor microenvironment. Cancer Res. 2012;72(13):3125–30.
57. Walker C, Mojares E, del Río Hernández A. Role of extracellular matrix in development and cancer progression. Int J Mol Sci. 2018;19(10):3028.
58. Huang J, Zhang L, Wan D, Zhou L, Zheng S, Lin S, et al. Extracellular matrix and its therapeutic potential for cancer treatment. Signal Transduct Target Ther. 2021;6(1):153.
59. Liu JY, Wellen KE. Advances into understanding metabolites as signaling molecules in cancer progression. Curr Opin Cell Biol. 2020;63:144–53.
60. Di Francesco AM, Toesca A, Cenciarelli C, Giordano A, Gasbarrini A, Puglisi MA. Metabolic modification in gastrointestinal cancer stem cells: characteristics and therapeutic approaches. J Cell Physiol. 2016;231(10):2081–7.
61. Zakian KL, Eberhardt S, Hricak H, Shukla-Dave A, Kleinman S, Muruganandham M, et al. Transition zone prostate cancer: metabolic characteristics at 1H MR spectroscopic imaging—initial results. Radiology. 2003;229(1):241–7.
62. Sun X-x, Yu Q. Intra-tumor heterogeneity of cancer cells and its implications for cancer treatment. Acta Pharmacol Sin. 2015;36(10):1219–27.
63. Turashvili G, Brogi E. Tumor heterogeneity in breast cancer. Front Med. 2017;4:227.
64. Williams K, Jackson SE, Beeken RJ, Steptoe A, Wardle J. The impact of a cancer diagnosis on health and well-being: a prospective, population-based study. Psycho-Oncology. 2016;25(6):626–32.
65. De La Franier B, Thompson M. Early stage detection and screening of ovarian cancer: a research opportunity and significant challenge for biosensor technology. Biosens Bioelectron. 2019;135:71–81.
66. Kowalik A, Kowalewska M, Góźdź S. Current approaches for avoiding the limitations of circulating tumor cells detection methods – implications for diagnosis and treatment of patients with solid tumors. Transl Res. 2017;185(58–84):e15.
67. Rai HM, Yoo J, Moqurrab SA, Dashkevych S. Advancements in traditional machine learning techniques for detection and diagnosis of fatal cancer types: comprehensive review of biomedical imaging datasets. Measurement. 2024;225:114059.
68. Hussain S, Mubeen I, Ullah N, Shah SSUD, Khan BA, Zahoor M, et al. Modern diagnostic imaging technique applications and risk factors in the medical field: a review. Biomed Res Int. 2022;2022(1):5164970.
69. Barocas D, Rohan S, Kao J, Gurevich R, Del Pizzo J, Vaughan E, et al. Diagnosis of renal tumors on needle biopsy specimens by histological and molecular analysis. J Urol. 2006;176(5):1957–62.
70. Brown MV, McDunn JE, Gunst PR, Smith EM, Milburn MV, Troyer DA, et al. Cancer detection and biopsy classification using concurrent histopathological and metabolomic analysis of core biopsies. Genome Med. 2012;4:1–12.
71. Berardi R, Morgese F, Rinaldi S, Torniai M, Mentrasti G, Scortichini L, et al. Benefits and limitations of a multidisciplinary approach in cancer patient management. Cancer Manag Res. 2020:9363–74.
72. Moreno-Sánchez R, Saavedra E, Gallardo-Pérez JC, Rumjanek FD, Rodríguez-Enríquez S. Understanding the cancer cell phenotype beyond the limitations of current omics analyses. FEBS J. 2016;283(1):54–73.
73. Bernard PS, Wittwer CT. Real-time PCR technology for cancer diagnostics. Clin Chem. 2002;48(8):1178–85.

74. Ahmad E, Ali A, Sharma AK, Ahmed F, Dar GM, Singh AM, et al. Molecular approaches in cancer. Clin Chim Acta. 2022;537:60–73.
75. Kalemkerian GP, Narula N, Kennedy EB, Biermann WA, Donington J, Leighl NB, et al. Molecular testing guideline for the selection of patients with lung cancer for treatment with targeted tyrosine kinase inhibitors: American Society of Clinical Oncology Endorsement of the College of American Pathologists/International Association for the Study of Lung Cancer/Association for Molecular Pathology Clinical Practice Guideline Update. J Clin Oncol. 2018;36(9):911–9.
76. Ghafoor Q, Baijal S, Taniere P, O'Sullivan B, Evans M, Middleton G. Epidermal growth factor receptor (EGFR) kinase inhibitors and non-small cell lung cancer (NSCLC)–advances in molecular diagnostic techniques to facilitate targeted therapy. Pathol Oncol Res. 2018;24:723–31.
77. Natrajan R, Reis-Filho JS. Next-generation sequencing applied to molecular diagnostics. Expert Rev Mol Diagn. 2011;11(4):425–44.
78. Shuai Y, Ma Z, Ju J, Wei T, Gao S, Kang Y, et al. Liquid-based biomarkers in breast cancer: looking beyond the blood. J Transl Med. 2023;21(1):809.
79. Zalli D, Mai Z, Ferati E, Ramaj A, Bregu R, Pranjol MZI. Advancing precision medicine: integrating next-generation sequencing and tumor markers for early cancer detection and personalized treatment. In: Handbook of cancer and immunology; 2023. p. 1–31.
80. Vashisht V, Vashisht A, Mondal AK, Woodall J, Kolhe R. From genomic exploration to personalized treatment: next-generation sequencing in oncology. Curr Issues Mol Biol. 2024;46(11):12527–49.
81. Morganti S, Tarantino P, Ferraro E, D'Amico P, Viale G, Trapani D, et al. Complexity of genome sequencing and reporting: next generation sequencing (NGS) technologies and implementation of precision medicine in real life. Crit Rev Oncol Hematol. 2019;133:171–82.
82. Kiran NS, Yashaswini C, Maheshwari R, Bhattacharya S, Prajapati BG. Advances in precision medicine approaches for colorectal cancer: from molecular profiling to targeted therapies. ACS Pharmacol Transl Sci. 2024;7(4):967–90.
83. Koga Y, Yamazaki N, Matsumura Y. New molecular diagnosis and screening methods for colorectal cancer using fecal protein, DNA and RNA. Expert Rev Mol Diagn. 2014;14(1):107–20.
84. Hinestrosa JP, Kurzrock R, Lewis JM, Schork NJ, Schroeder G, Kamat AM, et al. Early-stage multi-cancer detection using an extracellular vesicle protein-based blood test. Commun Med. 2022;2(1):29.
85. Rheinbay E, Nielsen MM, Abascal F, Wala JA, Shapira O, Tiao G, et al. Analyses of non-coding somatic drivers in 2,658 cancer whole genomes. Nature. 2020;578(7793):102–11.
86. Ellingford JM, Ahn JW, Bagnall RD, Baralle D, Barton S, Campbell C, et al. Recommendations for clinical interpretation of variants found in non-coding regions of the genome. Genome Med. 2022;14(1):73.
87. Sequist LV, Skates SJ, Haas W. A new era of protein-based assays for cancer early detection. J Thorac Oncol. 2021;16(2):191–3.
88. Peabody J, Paculdo D, Swagel E, Fugaro S, Tran M. Clinical utility of a blood-based protein assay to increase screening of elevated-risk patients for colorectal cancer in the primary care setting. J Cancer Res Clin Oncol. 2017;143:2301–7.
89. Carethers JM, Jung BH. Genetics and genetic biomarkers in sporadic colorectal cancer. Gastroenterology. 2015;149(5):1177–90. e3
90. John T, Liu G, Tsao M. Overview of molecular testing in non-small-cell lung cancer: mutational analysis, gene copy number, protein expression and other biomarkers of EGFR for the prediction of response to tyrosine kinase inhibitors. Oncogene. 2009;28(1):S14–23.
91. Zamay TN, Zamay GS, Kolovskaya OS, Zukov RA, Petrova MM, Gargaun A, et al. Current and prospective protein biomarkers of lung cancer. Cancers. 2017;9(11):155.
92. Shu X, Bao J, Wu L, Long J, Shu XO, Guo X, et al. Evaluation of associations between genetically predicted circulating protein biomarkers and breast cancer risk. Int J Cancer. 2020;146(8):2130–8.

93. Bi G, Bian Y, Liang J, Yin J, Li R, Zhao M, et al. Pan-cancer characterization of metabolism-related biomarkers identifies potential therapeutic targets. J Transl Med. 2021;19(1):219.
94. Alix-Panabières C, Schwarzenbach H, Pantel K. Circulating tumor cells and circulating tumor DNA. Annu Rev Med. 2012;63(1):199–215.
95. Salvi S, Gurioli G, De Giorgi U, Conteduca V, Tedaldi G, Calistri D, et al. Cell-free DNA as a diagnostic marker for cancer: current insights. Onco Targets Ther. 2016:6549–59.
96. Wu L, Qu X. Cancer biomarker detection: recent achievements and challenges. Chem Soc Rev. 2015;44(10):2963–97.
97. Tiberio P, Callari M, Angeloni V, Daidone MG, Appierto V. Challenges in using circulating miRNAs as cancer biomarkers. Biomed Res Int. 2015;2015(1):731479.
98. Taube SE, Clark GM, Dancey JE, McShane LM, Sigman CC, Gutman SI. A perspective on challenges and issues in biomarker development and drug and biomarker codevelopment. J Natl Cancer Inst. 2009;101(21):1453–63.
99. Mordente A, Meucci E, Martorana GE, Silvestrini A. Cancer biomarkers discovery and validation: state of the art, problems and future perspectives. In: Advances in cancer biomarkers: from biochemistry to clinic for a critical revision; 2015. p. 9–26.
100. Campuzano S, Pedrero M, Yáñez-Sedeño P, Pingarrón JM. New challenges in point of care electrochemical detection of clinical biomarkers. Sens Actuators B Chem. 2021;345:130349.
101. Zugazagoitia J, Guedes C, Ponce S, Ferrer I, Molina-Pinelo S, Paz-Ares L. Current challenges in cancer treatment. Clin Ther. 2016;38(7):1551–66.
102. Sanz-Garcia E, Zhao E, Bratman SV, Siu LL. Monitoring and adapting cancer treatment using circulating tumor DNA kinetics: current research, opportunities, and challenges. Sci Adv. 2022;8(4):eabi8618.
103. Tufail AB, Ma Y-K, Kaabar MK, Martínez F, Junejo A, Ullah I, et al. Deep learning in cancer diagnosis and prognosis prediction: a minireview on challenges, recent trends, and future directions. Comput Math Methods Med. 2021;2021(1):9025470.
104. Verma M. Personalized medicine and cancer. J Pers Med. 2012;2(1):1–14.
105. Soper SA, Brown K, Ellington A, Frazier B, Garcia-Manero G, Gau V, et al. Point-of-care biosensor systems for cancer diagnostics/prognostics. Biosens Bioelectron. 2006;21(10):1932–42.
106. Karimi F, Karimi-Maleh H, Rouhi J, Zare N, Karaman C, Baghayeri M, et al. Revolutionizing cancer monitoring with carbon-based electrochemical biosensors. Environ Res. 2023;117368
107. Rosa BG, Akingbade OE, Guo X, Gonzalez-Macia L, Crone MA, Cameron LP, et al. Multiplexed immunosensors for point-of-care diagnostic applications. Biosens Bioelectron. 2022;203:114050.
108. Sengupta J, Hussain CM. Early detection of cancer utilizing biosensors based on "green graphene": an innovative and sustainable methodology for advancing cancer diagnosis. TrAC Trends Anal Chem. 2023:117254.
109. Denny L, Prendiville W. Cancer of the cervix: early detection and cost-effective solutions. Int J Gynecol Obstet. 2015;131:S28–32.

Aptamers: A Novel Class of Targeted Therapeutics

3

Laxmi Yadav, Sachin Kumar, Shriyansh Srivastava, and Pougang Golmei

3.1 Introduction

Aptamers are 20–100-nucleotide-long, single-stranded DNA or RNA sequences. These are often called "chemical antibodies" as they serve as alternatives to antibodies in various biomedical applications. They can bind to diverse targets, including proteins, small molecules, and cells. Aptamers are structurally stable and, therefore, can be useful in harsh conditions like high temperatures. Aptamers cost less than antibodies because they are made through chemical synthesis. They are cheaper to produce, especially when needed in large quantities [1–3].

Two independent research teams led by Larry Gold and Jack W. Szostak defined aptamers for the first time in the early 1990s. Aptamers are produced using a process called Systematic Evolution of Ligands by Exponential Enrichment (SELEX). This method isolates aptamers from a combinatorial library through repeated cycles of selection and amplification. Since its inception, SELEX has undergone significant advancements, which have improved its efficiency and application and reduced costs [1, 2].

Aptamers offer several advantages over monoclonal antibodies. They are cheaper and easier to produce, smaller in size, and non-immunogenic and can bind to a wider range of molecules [2–4]. The year 2004 was an important milestone in the development of aptamers. The US Food and Drug Administration (FDA) approved Macugen (pegaptanib) for age-related macular degeneration (AMD) [5].

Aptamers are typically composed of nucleotides, though some aptamers are composed of peptides. They can form a variety of three-dimensional structures, including stem-loops, G-quadruplexes, and pseudoknots. These unique structures

L. Yadav · S. Kumar (✉) · S. Srivastava · P. Golmei
Department of Pharmacology, Delhi Institute of Pharmaceutical Sciences and Research (DIPSAR), Delhi Pharmaceutical Sciences and Research University (DPSRU), New Delhi, India

S. Srivastava et al. (eds.), *Biosensors and Aptamers*,
https://doi.org/10.1007/978-981-96-8387-1_3

create special pockets and surfaces that contribute to the binding of aptamers to a target [6]. Further, the formation of hydrogen bonds, Van der Waals forces, and electrostatic forces enhances the affinity of aptamers to their targets [7]. Aptamers can match or even surpass antibodies in their ability to identify closely related targets [8]. Aptamers with reversible binding affinities have been designed to allow controlled interactions with their targets. Aptamer sequences can also be modified to enhance their pharmacokinetic properties, stability, and binding affinity [9].

3.2 Selection and Evolution of Therapeutic Aptamers

The detection and refinement of aptamers depend on selection and evolution techniques. These procedures influence the binding characteristics and therapeutic efficacy of aptamers. Various methodologies have been used to identify and optimize aptamers with specific properties.

3.2.1 SELEX Technology

The SELEX technique is the cornerstone of aptamer development. This in vitro method systematically identifies nucleic acid sequences that specifically bind to targets. The process starts with a combinatorial library of oligonucleotides. These libraries contain about 10^{15} unique sequences of aptamers [10]. Each sequence in this large collection has a central random region surrounded by fixed segments. These constant regions help in primer attachment during amplification steps.

3.2.1.1 Key Steps of the SELEX Technique

The SELEX methodology is a combination of several essential steps, including library preparation, binding, partitioning, elution, amplification, and enrichment. Initially, a synthetic oligonucleotide library with millions to trillions of unique sequences is created. During the binding phase, the library is combined with target molecules under controlled conditions. The environment is kept similar to physiological settings to ensure optimized functioning of aptamers. Factors like temperature, pH, and salt concentrations significantly influence aptamers' affinity for the target. During partitioning, bound sequences are separated from unbound ones without disrupting legitimate interactions. Affinity chromatography or magnetic beads coated with target molecules could be used for this purpose. Following partitioning, the bound aptamers are eluted without damaging their structure. After that, the eluted aptamers are amplified by using different approaches. DNA aptamers undergo standard polymerase chain reaction (PCR), while RNA aptamers require reverse transcription before amplification. The enrichment phase involves repeating these steps with increasing stringency. Each cycle refines the pool, focusing on sequences with stronger binding properties. Typically, 8 to 15 rounds are performed before identifying candidate aptamers. This iterative process gradually transforms a random collection of sequences into highly specific molecular recognition elements (Fig. 3.1) [11–13].

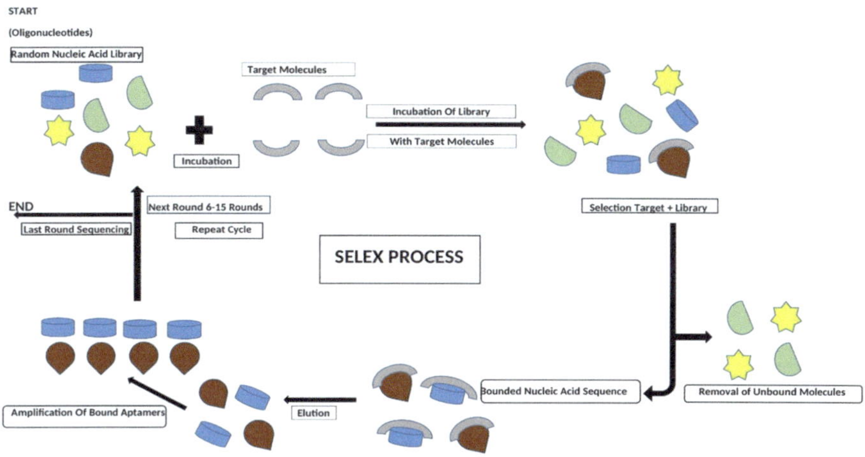

Fig. 3.1 Overview of the SELEX technique

The SELEX technique, despite its effectiveness, presents several practical challenges for researchers. Overcoming these challenges often requires significant resources and expertise. Traditional SELEX protocols can take weeks or even months to complete. Each selection round involves careful attention to detail and the precise execution of various procedures. One of the most challenging aspects of SELEX is optimization. The technique also struggles with certain target types. For example, membrane proteins are challenging because they need specific environments to maintain their natural structure. Similarly, small molecules with limited binding surfaces often result in aptamers with low affinity, even after multiple selection rounds. Another issue is due to PCR bias. Some sequences amplify more easily than others, notwithstanding their binding properties [14].

3.2.1.2 Modified SELEX Methods

The challenges of traditional SELEX are addressed by modified SELEX approaches. These modifications have made aptamer synthesis more efficient and accessible.

Cell-SELEX

In Cell-SELEX, whole intact cells are used as targets instead of isolated molecules. Aptamers bind to cell surface markers, which are present in their natural states. With Cell-SELEX, aptamers that differentiate between cell types can be created. This makes it a powerful tool for developing targeted therapies and diagnostic tests. The elimination of protein purification steps provides substantial practical advantages. Preparation time and resources could be significantly reduced as the target cells could be cultured according to standard protocols. This approach streamlines the selection process by eliminating the need for purified proteins [15]. This approach is particularly beneficial for cancer research, as aptamers that specifically recognize malignant cells could be developed [16].

Toggle-SELEX

In the Toggle-SELEX technique, different but related targets are exposed to the aptamer pool in successive selection rounds. This method recognizes shared structural features and accommodates target-specific variations. The resulting aptamers demonstrate cross-reactivity across a defined group of molecules or cells rather than exclusive binding to a single target. DNA aptamers capable of binding across multiple bacterial genera have been identified. These aptamers exhibit dissociation constants between 9.22 and 38.5 nM, which indicate significant binding interactions [17]. The selection of appropriate toggle targets significantly influences the resulting aptamer characteristics. Too much structural diversity between targets may yield aptamers with weak affinity to all targets, whereas insufficient diversity renders the toggle approach useless [18].

Capillary Electrophoresis–SELEX (CE-SELEX)

Capillary electrophoresis is used as the partitioning method in CE-SELEX. This method provides accurate separation of bound and unbound aptamer sequences on the basis of molecular size. Aptamers with dissociation constants of approximately 27.6 nM have been successfully isolated using CE-SELEX [19].

High-Throughput SELEX (HT-SELEX)

HT-SELEX utilizes high-throughput sequencing to improve aptamer development. Unlike traditional SELEX, HT-SELEX allows detailed tracking of individual sequences throughout the selection process. Millions of unique sequences could be analyzed at once [19]. With HT-SELEX, better aptamer candidates can be identified just after 3 to 4 selection rounds, compared to the 8 to 15 rounds needed with traditional methods. This helps in achieving efficiency, even if the initial aptamer count is low.

3.2.1.3 Advanced SELEX for Cancer

The SELEX methodology has undergone significant revisions, which were made keeping in view the challenges posed by tumor biology. These approaches help synthesize potential aptamer sequences for cancer therapeutics.

In Vivo SELEX

In vivo SELEX conducts selection directly within living organisms. It creates aptamers that are optimized for real physiological environments rather than laboratory conditions. This method naturally selects aptamers with beneficial pharmacokinetic traits. These traits include a suitable circulation duration, resistance to nuclease breakdown, and minimal nonspecific tissue buildup. The RNA aptamer RA16 validates the potential of in vivo SELEX for cancer treatments. RA16 was synthesized using mice with tumors. It shows very specific binding to non-small cell lung cancer cells. RA16 retains its targeting ability in both laboratory cell cultures and living organisms [20].

Hybrid-SELEX

The hybrid approach to aptamer development uses multiple selection techniques. It combines methods like capillary separation and cellular targeting to create aptamers with specific functions. This strategy has been used to develop aptamers that enter cells by interacting with the Trophoblast cell-surface antigen 2 (TROP2) surface marker [21]. The field has advanced further through the incorporation of microfluidic systems within these hybrid protocols. This technological enhancement substantially decreases both the temporal investment and manual effort traditionally required [22].

Negative Selection

Negative selection involves preliminary filtering steps that remove unwanted aptamers from the candidate pool. Lin et al. introduced an innovative selection protocol featuring alternating enrichment and elimination rounds with carefully limited enzymatic multiplication cycles. This strategic methodology yielded highly specific aptamers that recognize distinctive cancer-associated structures, including peptide fragments presented by major histocompatibility complex (MHC) complexes and the claudin-6 membrane component [23].

3.2.2 Post-SELEX Modifications

3.2.2.1 Chemical Modifications

Strategic chemical modification of the aptamer can improve the biostability and therapeutic potential of the aptamer.

Nucleotide Modifications

Researchers incorporate nonnatural nucleic acid structures (XNAs), add 2′-O-methyl groups, or integrate locked nucleic acids (LNAs) to create aptamers that resist breakdown by nucleases while maintaining or even enhancing their binding capabilities to targets [24, 25].

Backbone Modifications

Replacing oxygen atoms with sulfur (thiophosphate) or double sulfur (dithiophosphate) in the aptamer backbone significantly protects against enzymatic degradation. These modifications also slow kidney clearance, allowing aptamers to remain active longer in the body. In cancer research, such modifications have shown extended inhibition of targets like phospho-AXL, effectively widening the treatment time frame [26].

Terminal Protective Groups

Adding protective molecules to aptamer ends provides substantial stability benefits. For example, attaching naphthalene diimide and 3-hydroxypropylphosphate to the terminal regions of aptamers increases their thermal stability and resistance to nucleases. The modified N-TBA-p aptamer demonstrated a 14 °C improvement in

G-quadruplex stability and became ten times more resistant to nuclease degradation, resulting in better anticoagulant performance [27].

3.2.2.2 Conjugation Strategies

Nanomaterial Conjugation

Aptamers have been combined with carbon-based nanomaterials to create better treatment systems. These combinations have improved optical properties and work well with biological systems. The new systems serve two main purposes. First, they allow doctors to see inside the body without surgery. Second, they deliver cancer drugs like doxorubicin directly to tumors. These targeted delivery systems help medications reach cancer cells more effectively. The precision of these systems means better treatment outcomes for patients [28].

Circulation Enhancement

Aptamers have been modified with nanomaterials to prevent them from being quickly cleared from the body. This change greatly extends how long they stay in the bloodstream. Their improved pharmacokinetic behavior allows for longer-lasting treatment effects. Patients may benefit from more sustained therapy with these modified aptamers [28].

Stimuli-Responsive Systems

Aptamers with special linkers that react to specific environmental triggers have been created. These systems can sense unique conditions in tumor environments, like changes in acidity or the presence of certain enzymes. This ability ensures that medications are released exactly where and when they are needed. It enhances therapeutic effects while minimizing harm to healthy tissues [29].

Targeted Delivery

Aptamer conjugates are highly effective at identifying specific tumor markers, such as nucleolin and epidermal growth factor receptor (EGFR). This ability allows them to deliver therapeutic agents directly to cancer cells. As a result, healthy tissues are protected, and treatment side effects may be reduced [30].

3.2.2.3 Sequence Optimization

A step-by-step library approach is used to find and remove unnecessary parts of aptamer sequences. This creates smaller, more cost-effective aptamers that bind more strongly to their targets. This optimization process turns promising aptamer candidates into more practical treatments. The resulting minimized aptamers have greater potential for use in clinical settings [31].

3.2.2.4 Enhancing Therapeutic Efficacy

Sophisticated approaches such as structural and functional innovation in aptamer sequences have substantially elevated the therapeutic potential of aptamers.

Multivalent Aptamers

Advanced aptamers with multiple binding regions have been developed. These regions can bind to different targets at the same time or interact with multiple sites on a single target. This multipoint binding approach greatly strengthens the connection between the aptamer and its target. It also improves the precision of targeting, resulting in more effective therapeutic agents [32].

Aptamer–siRNA Chimeras

Hybrid molecules combine the precise targeting of aptamers with the gene-silencing ability of small interfering RNAs (siRNAs). The aptamer part of the molecule guides the siRNA to specific target cells. Once there, the siRNA suppresses the expression of genes related to the disease. In cancer research, these hybrid molecules have shown promising results. Tumor size is reduced by aptamer–siRNA conjugates by decreasing the expression of biomarkers such as Human Epidermal Growth Factor Receptor 2 (HER2) and Epithelial Cell Adhesion Molecule (EpCAM) [33, 34].

Switchable Aptamers

Smart aptamers have been designed to become active in the presence of specific triggers. This controlled activation minimizes side effects and toxicity risks. Switchable aptamers, which become active in disease-specific conditions, improve safety while ensuring efficacy as needed [35].

3.3 Advantages of Aptamers as Therapeutic Agents

Aptamer-based platforms have flexible applications due to the molecular characteristics of the aptamer. They are valuable alternatives to antibodies. Because of their small size, aptamers can reach targets that are not accessible to larger molecules. Aptamers also have minimal immunogenic potential.

3.3.1 Molecular Properties

3.3.1.1 Small Size and Enhanced Tissue Penetration

Aptamers have a small and compact structure, which permits swift movement through tissues. They can penetrate tissues, which makes aptamers suitable for drug delivery to specific locations in the body. This targeting ability gives them a major advantage, which is not possible with larger and bulkier treatment options [36].

3.3.1.2 Chemical Stability

Aptamers are more stable than protein molecules and, therefore, could be stored for long periods without losing their efficacy. Aptamers can also withstand environmental stresses better [37]. Aptamers' properties can be improved with chemical modifications. They can be made resistant to enzyme action, and modifications can also improve their pharmacokinetics, consequently increasing their stay in the body [38].

3.3.1.3 Low Immunogenicity Profile

Aptamers are usually less immunogenic compared to antibodies. This makes repeated administration of aptamers possible without toxicity during long-term treatment of chronic illnesses [39].

3.3.1.4 Controlled Production Process

The chemical synthesis of aptamers ensures high consistency with very little batch-to-batch variation. Unlike antibodies, aptamers are produced with precise control over their structure and composition [40]. This level of precision is essential for ensuring the predictability and safety of the therapy.

3.3.1.5 Cost-Effectiveness

Aptamers are cheaper to produce than antibodies due to the use of chemical synthesis methods. This cost difference is important at a commercial scale. For aptamer synthesis, solid-phase synthesis techniques are utilized because of their efficient scalability. Further, the quality and consistency remain high even when synthesizing in larger amounts. This approach offers major economic advantages throughout the drug development process. The cost savings extend from early research phases to final production [41].

3.3.2 Therapeutic Applications

3.3.2.1 Target Specificity

Aptamers can fold into complex 3D shapes. This allows them to recognize molecules with high precision. Their flexible structure helps them tell apart very similar targets accurately [42]. Chemical changes can make aptamers even more specific. These modifications can change how the molecules are arranged. They can strengthen the bonds between nucleic acids and proteins. New structural patterns can also be created to improve how aptamers bind to their targets [43].

3.3.2.2 Versatility in Target Recognition

Aptamers can target many different substances in the body. They can bind to proteins, peptides, small molecules, carbohydrates, whole cells, and cell parts. They even work on targets that antibodies struggle to attach to [43]. This flexibility has led to real-world success. The FDA has approved some aptamer-based treatments. Doctors are also using aptamers more often in medical tests as an alternative to antibody methods [44].

3.3.2.3 Multiplexing Capabilities

Multivalent aptamer designs can bind to multiple targets or different parts of the same target at once. This ability significantly improves their therapeutic effectiveness [32]. Advanced strategies like aptamer-based lysosome-targeting chimeras (AptLYTACs) use sophisticated structures for multivalent binding. This approach allows precise control over protein degradation therapies [45].

Aptamers offer several advantages for personalized medicine. They can be quickly selected to target specific molecules in a patient's body. This helps doctors treat the exact pathways causing the disease. Aptamers work well with genetic profiling. This makes it easier to find biomarkers that indicate specific diseases [46]. These molecules can also be combined with advanced delivery methods. For example, they can be attached to nanomedicines to improve treatment delivery [38].

3.4 Aptamers in Cancer Therapy

Aptamers have several advantages, such as small size, easy synthesis, possibilities of structural modifications, and non-immunogenicity. These properties are especially useful for designing targeted therapeutics for cancer. Aptamers can be effectively used in various treatments, including immune checkpoint inhibition, gene therapy, and drug delivery systems.

3.4.1 Cancer-Specific Targets

3.4.1.1 Cell Surface Receptors

The structure of aptamers allows precise binding to receptor tyrosine kinases (RTKs), such as Axl, epidermal growth factor receptor (EGFR), and platelet-derived growth factor receptor (PDGFR), often overexpressed in cancer cells. By inhibiting receptor dimerization and autophosphorylation of RTKs, aptamers have been shown to significantly slow tumor growth [38].

3.4.1.2 Protein Markers

Aptamers can selectively inhibit vascular endothelial growth factor (VEGF), which plays a significant role in angiogenesis. This antiangiogenic effect prevents the tumor's growth and metastasis [47]. Further, aptamers exhibit anticancer effects by additional mechanisms. For instance, certain c-Met-targeting aptamers induce proteasomal degradation of their target protein, leading to tumor suppression in mouse models [48].

3.4.1.3 Signaling Molecules

Aptamers can enhance chemotherapy efficacy, particularly in drug-resistant cancers, by selectively binding to key signaling molecules. When integrated into advanced delivery systems like DNA origami nanostructures, aptamers can facilitate the co-delivery of chemotherapeutic agents and antisense oligonucleotides, simultaneously targeting multiple resistance pathways such as Bcl2 and P-glycoprotein [49]. Additionally, aptamers targeting proteins involved in metastasis, such as filamin A, can inhibit cancer cell migration and invasion, effectively limiting tumor spread [50].

3.4.1.4 Metabolic Targets

Cancer cells often exhibit altered metabolism, providing unique targeting opportunities. Aptamers like SYL-6, which binds to prohibitin 2, have been successfully employed for both tumor imaging and targeted chemotherapy, enabling precise distinction between cancerous and normal tissues [51]. Innovative diagnostic applications include aptamer–cyclometalated iridium(III) complexes that produce strong fluorescence signals when bound to nucleolin, an overexpressed marker on cancer cells [52].

3.4.2 Therapeutic Strategies

3.4.2.1 Direct Inhibition of Cancer Pathways

Aptamers can directly inhibit oncogenic pathways by binding to specific proteins involved in cancer progression. For instance, a DNA aptamer targeting the c-Met receptor has been shown to induce its degradation via the proteasomal pathway, effectively inhibiting tumor growth in mouse models [53]. The Aptamer-Ribonuclease Targeting Chimera (RIBOTAC) strategy represents an innovative approach where the aptamer binds to oncogenic miRNAs like miR-210-3p and miR-155-5p and facilitates the recruitment of endogenous ribonucleases that degrade these miRNAs. By catalyzing the degradation of these oncogenic miRNAs within tumor cells, the Aptamer-RIBOTAC strategy effectively reduces their abundance and inhibits their cancer-promoting functions [54].

3.4.2.2 Drug Delivery Vehicles

Aptamer-based drug delivery systems enhance therapeutic specificity while minimizing systemic toxicity. These conjugates can transport conventional chemotherapeutic agents, therapeutic RNAs (siRNAs and miRNAs), and antisense oligonucleotides. For example, aptamers have successfully delivered siRNAs targeting osteopontin (OPN), a protein involved in tumor progression, resulting in significant tumor suppression across various cancer models [55, 56].

3.4.2.3 Immunotherapy Applications

By targeting checkpoint molecules such as CTLA-4, PD-1, and PD-L1, aptamers can effectively release the brakes on immune responses against tumors. The aptamer AYA22T-R2–13 interacts with both CTLA-4 and NKG2A simultaneously to improve the function of CD8+ T cells and NK cells and destroy tumor cells [57]. This dual targeting is better than the inhibition of either molecule alone. Another aptamer, Ap3-7c, simultaneously blocks both PD-1 and PD-L1 and improves immune checkpoint inhibition by preventing the effect of backup mechanisms that could reduce the efficiency of the checkpoint inhibition therapy [58]. Furthermore, aptamer-functionalized chimeric antigen receptor (CAR) T cell therapy, Apt-CAR, can reportedly activate T cells without genetic modifications and provide better flexibility and adjustability compared to traditional CAR T cell therapy [59]. Similarly, modified macrophages with the cholesterol-AS1411-M1 (CAM1) aptamer, which targets nucleolin, have better antitumor effects than unmodified ones [60].

3.4.2.4 Combination Therapy Approaches

The conjugation of aptamers with nanoparticles can be used as a target drug delivery system with remarkable tumor-targeting specificity. This approach substantially improves the biodistribution of drugs by increasing drug concentration within tumor tissues and reducing exposure to healthy cells. The therapeutic index of doxorubicin has been improved, which, otherwise, has a narrow therapeutic window [30, 61]. The Nb2C-PAA-DOX@Apt-M platform exemplifies this capability through its integration of photothermal therapy with chemotherapy [62].

3.5 Engineering Therapeutic Aptamers

Therapeutic aptamer engineering requires a comprehensive approach to optimize structure, stability, and pharmacokinetic properties for better efficacy and safety. Here is how researchers are advancing this field.

3.5.1 Design Considerations

3.5.1.1 Structure–Function Relationships

Researchers use computational modeling and biophysical analyses to understand aptamer conformations. Molecular dynamics simulations help identify binding sites in aptamers, like those targeting adenosine monophosphate [62, 63]. NMR, X-ray crystallography, and circular dichroism provide insights into structural changes when aptamers bind to targets [64]. Advanced techniques like replica exchange molecular dynamics further reveal RNA aptamer flexibility and how sequence affects structure [65].

3.5.1.2 Enhancing Stability

To combat the body's natural degradation of aptamers, scientists employ chemical modifications. Adding 2′-fluoro and 2′-O-methyl groups improves resistance to enzymes that would normally break down these molecules, as seen in HIV-1 reverse transcriptase studies [66]. Locked nucleic acid modifications make VEGF-targeting aptamers more thermally stable and resistant to degradation [67]. These modified aptamers show better retention in the bloodstream during animal studies [68].

3.5.1.3 Pharmacokinetic Optimization

PEGylation (attaching polyethylene glycol) shields aptamers from enzymes and extends their circulation time in the body [69]. Researchers also use truncation to remove unnecessary segments, which can dramatically improve binding affinity—one PDGF-BB-targeting aptamer showed 150 times better binding after truncation [70]. Combining truncation with chemical modifications further enhances stability and specificity [71].

3.5.1.4 Safety Considerations

Minimizing off-target effects is crucial for therapeutic aptamers. Techniques like the aptamer target chain reaction help ensure aptamers only interact with their intended targets [72]. When combined with nanoparticles, aptamers can improve biocompatibility by preventing unwanted immune recognition [73]. Aptamers generally trigger fewer immune responses than antibodies, making them potentially safer therapeutic options [74, 75].

3.5.2 Advanced Engineering Approaches

3.5.2.1 Multivalent Aptamers

Aptamers with multiple binding sites have increased binding strength because of avidity effects. This multivalent configuration improves retention on the target and enhances therapeutic effectiveness. Based on this concept, multivalent glycomimetic ligands have been developed for lectin receptors [76]. By adjusting structural parameters, such as size, number of binding sites, and spatial arrangement, interactions with the target could be regulated. By optimizing the structure of thrombin-binding aptamers, the binding affinity and therapeutic effectiveness of these aptamers have been improved [43].

3.5.2.2 Aptamer–Drug Conjugates

The combination of aptamers with therapeutic agents has created effective targeted delivery systems, particularly for cancer treatment. Several aptamer–drug conjugates have been designed to recognize specific tumor-associated biomarkers such as EpCAM. These conjugates can precisely deliver drugs to cancer cells [77]. The aptamer–drug conjugate interacts with its cellular target and promotes internalization of the entire therapeutic payload directly into the cancer cell [77].

3.5.2.3 Switchable Aptamers

Switchable aptamers are the most revolutionary developments in aptamer engineering. These switchable aptamers can detect changes in pH, temperature, or other stimuli, triggering controlled drug release or activating biosensing mechanisms [78, 79]. Their core mechanism involves structural transitions that selectively expose or hide functional domains, allowing precise control of molecular interactions. Recent advances in toehold exchange mechanisms have further enhanced the thermal stability and programmability of these aptamers, allowing researchers to fine-tune their response characteristics for specific analytical and therapeutic applications [79].

3.5.2.4 Smart Delivery Systems

The integration of aptamers with nanoparticles and liposomes has opened new frontiers in targeted therapeutics. These sophisticated delivery platforms leverage aptamer specificity to concentrate drugs at disease sites while minimizing systemic exposure and associated toxicities. Liposome-based aptamer therapies have shown promise in cancer treatment, demonstrating enhanced therapeutic indices [80, 81] Aptamer-functionalized nanocarriers designed to recognize specific cellular markers like nucleolin ensure that therapeutic agents reach their intended targets with unprecedented precision, potentially transforming treatment outcomes for patients with challenging malignancies [82, 83].

3.6 Clinical Applications and Case Studies

Aptamers have emerged as promising candidates for both diagnostic and therapeutic applications. Their exceptional specificity, remarkable stability, and cost-effective production make them particularly valuable for addressing various clinical challenges, from chronic and infectious diseases to cancer management.

3.6.1 FDA-Approved Aptamers

The 2004 FDA approval of Macugen (pegaptanib) marked a watershed moment in aptamer therapeutics. As the first aptamer-based drug to receive regulatory clearance, Macugen pioneered anti-VEGF therapy for neovascular age-related macular degeneration (AMD). This RNA aptamer works by selectively inhibiting VEGF165, a critical mediator of pathological blood vessel formation in AMD [84].

More recently, avacincaptad pegol (Izervay) received FDA approval for geographic atrophy, an advanced form of AMD. This innovative aptamer targets the complement system by binding to complement protein C5, thereby preventing membrane attack complex formation and reducing the oxidative damage and chronic inflammation characteristics of this condition [85].

Despite its groundbreaking status, Macugen eventually faced stiff competition from monoclonal antibody therapies like ranibizumab (Lucentis®) and bevacizumab (Avastin®). These antibody-based treatments demonstrated superior clinical outcomes in comparative trials, highlighting one of the challenges aptamers face in the therapeutic landscape [84, 86]. Nevertheless, Macugen's approval established aptamers as viable precision medicine tools, capable of highly selective targeting with minimal off-target effects.

3.6.2 Clinical Trials and Development

3.6.2.1 AS1411 (Anticancer Aptamer for Renal Cell Carcinoma)

AS1411, a guanosine-rich oligonucleotide aptamer, specifically targets nucleolin—a protein abundantly expressed in renal cell carcinoma and other tumor types. Upon binding to nucleolin, AS1411 induces S-phase cell cycle arrest and triggers apoptotic pathways in cancer cells while leaving normal cells unaffected. This selective cytotoxicity makes AS1411 particularly promising for targeted cancer therapy [87].

3.6.2.2 NOX-A12 (CXCL12-Binding Aptamer for Cancer Immunotherapy)

NOX-A12 (olaptesed pegol) represents an innovative approach to cancer immunotherapy. By binding to CXCL12, a chemokine that regulates the tumor microenvironment, NOX-A12 disrupts signaling pathways essential for tumor survival, migration, and immune evasion. This mechanism enhances immune cell infiltration into tumors, effectively breaking down the tumor's immune-privileged status and potentially improving responses to checkpoint inhibitor therapies [88].

3.6.2.3 Pegnivacogin (RNA Aptamer–Based Anticoagulant)

Pegnivacogin exemplifies aptamer versatility beyond oncology. This RNA aptamer provides highly selective anticoagulation by targeting factor IXa in the coagulation cascade. As part of the REG1 system, pegnivacogin works in tandem with its antidote, anivamersen, allowing for unprecedented control over anticoagulation effects. This precision makes it particularly valuable for patients with acute coronary syndrome undergoing cardiac catheterization, offering effective anticoagulation with reduced bleeding risk compared to conventional options [89, 90]. A list of aptamers in different phases of clinical trial is given in Table 3.1.

Table 3.1 Aptamers in different phases of clinical trials

S. No.	Aptamer	Study type	NCT number	Study title	Study status	Disease conditions	Clinical trial phase	Study URL
1	ARC1905 (Aanti-C5 aptamer)	Therapeutic	NCT00709527	ARC1905 (anti-C5 aptamer) given in combination with Lucentis® 0.5 mg/eye in subjects with neovascular age-related macular degeneration	Completed	Neovascular age-related macular degeneration	Phase 1	[91]
2	EYE001 (anti-VEGF pegylated aptamer)	Therapeutic	NCT00021736	Phase 2/3 study of anti-VEGF in neovascular AMD	Completed	Macular degeneration, choroidal neovascularization	Phase 2, phase 3	[92]
3	Tenofovir (TFV) aptamer–based biosensor (aptasensor)	Diagnostic	NCT04870671	Project ADHERE: Clinical proof-of-concept of a tenofovir (TFV) aptamer–based biosensor	Completed	HIV/AIDS, adherence, medication, drug use	Early-phase 1	[93]

(continued)

Table 3.1 (continued)

S. No.	Aptamer	Study type	NCT number	Study title	Study status	Disease conditions	Clinical trial phase	Study URL
4	Electrophage and colorimetric aptamers	Diagnostic	NCT02957370	Molecular biosensors for the detection of bladder cancer	Unknown	Urinary bladder neoplasms		[94]
5	REG1aptamer-RNA target to factor IXa	Diagnostic	NCT00113997	Safety and dosing evaluation of REG1 anticoagulation system	Completed	Healthy	Phase 1	[95]
6	ARC1905 (anti-C5 aptamer)	Therapeutic	NCT00950638	A study of ARC1905 (anti-C5 aptamer) in subjects with dry age-related macular degeneration	Completed	Dry age-related macular degeneration	Phase 1	[96]
7	E10030 (anti-PDGF pegylated aptamer)	Therapeutic	NCT01089517	A safety and efficacy study of E10030 (anti-PDGF pegylated aptamer) plus Lucentis for neovascular age-related macular degeneration	Completed	Age-related macular degeneration	Phase 2	[97]

8	EYE001 (anti-VEGF pegylated aptamer)	Therapeutic	NCT00056199	EYE001 to treat retinal tumors in patients with Von Hippel–Lindau syndrome	Completed	Hippel–Lindau disease	Phase 1	[98]
9	Zimura® (anti-C5 aptamer) in combination with anti-VEGF therapy	Therapeutic	NCT02397954	A study to establish the safety and tolerability of Zimura® (anti-C5 aptamer) in combination with anti-VEGF therapy in subjects with idiopathic polypoidal choroidal vasculopathy (IPCV)	Completed	Idiopathic polypoidal choroidal vasculopathy	Phase 2	[99]

(continued)

Table 3.1 (continued)

S. No.	Aptamer	Study type	NCT number	Study title	Study status	Disease conditions	Clinical trial phase	Study URL
10	E10030 (anti-PDGF pegylated aptamer)	Therapeutic	NCT00569140	A phase 1, safety, tolerability, and pharmacokinetic profile of intravitreous injections of E10030 (anti-PDGF pegylated aptamer) in subjects with neovascular age-related macular degeneration	Completed	Age-related macular degeneration	Phase 1	[100]
11	AS1411 combined with cytarabine	Therapeutic	NCT01034410	A study of AS1411 combined with cytarabine in the treatment of patients with primary refractory or relapsed acute myeloid leukemia	Terminated	Acute myeloid leukemia	Phase 2	[101]

12	Zimura™ (anti-C5 aptamer)	Therapeutic	NCT02686658	Zimura® in participants with geographic atrophy secondary to dry age-related macular degeneration	Completed	Geographic atrophy, macular degeneration	Phase 2, phase 3	[102]
13	Fovista® (anti-PDGF-BB pegylated aptamer) regiment administered in combination with Avastin®, Eylea®, or Lucentis®	Therapeutic	NCT02214628	Phase 2A open-label safety study of Fovista® (anti-PDGF BB) regimen administered in combination with anti-VEGF therapy to study subretinal fibrosis in neovascular AMD	Terminated	Age-related macular degeneration	Phase 2	[103]

(continued)

Table 3.1 (continued)

S. No.	Aptamer	Study type	NCT number	Study title	Study status	Disease conditions	Clinical trial phase	Study URL
14	Fovista® administered in combination with anti-VEGF therapy	Therapeutic	NCT02387957	A 24-month phase 2A open-label, randomized study of Avastin®, Lucentis®, or Eylea® (anti-VEGF therapy) administered in combination with Fovista® (anti-PDGF-BB pegylated aptamer)	Terminated	Age-related macular degeneration	Phase 2	[104]
15	Fovista® (anti-PDGF-BB pegylated aptamer) administered in combination with Lucentis®	Therapeutic	NCT01944839	A phase 3 safety and efficacy study of Fovista® (E10030) intravitreous administration in combination with Lucentis® compared to Lucentis® monotherapy	Terminated	Age-related macular degeneration	Phase 3	[105]

16	Fovista® (anti-PDGF-BB pegylated aptamer)	Therapeutic	NCT01940900	A phase 3 safety and efficacy study of Fovista® (E10030) intravitreous administration in combination with Lucentis® compared to Lucentis® monotherapy	Terminated	Age-related macular degeneration	Phase 3	[106]
17	Pegaptanib sodium (anti-VEGF pegylated aptamer)	Therapeutic	NCT00312351	A clinical trial to explore the safety and efficacy of three different doses of pegaptanib sodium in patients with wet age-related macular degeneration (AMD)	Terminated	Macular degeneration	Phase 4	[107]

(continued)

Table 3.1 (continued)

S. No.	Aptamer	Study type	NCT number	Study title	Study status	Disease conditions	Clinical trial phase	Study URL
18	Fovista® (anti-PDGF-BB pegylated aptamer) administered in combination with either Avastin® or Eylea® compared to Avastin® or Eylea®	Therapeutic	NCT01940887	A phase 3 safety and efficacy study of Fovista® (E10030) intravitreous administration in combination with either Avastin® or Eylea® compared to Avastin® or Eylea® monotherapy	Terminated	Age-related macular degeneration	Phase 3	[108]
19	EYE001 (anti-VEGF pegylated aptamer)	Therapeutic	NCT00321997	A clinical trial to explore safety and efficacy of different doses of pegaptanib sodium, compared to sham, in patients with wet AMD	Completed	Age-related macular degeneration	Phase 2, phase 3	[109]
20	DNA aptamer	Diagnostic	NCT04974203	Saliva-based COVID-19 DNA aptamer test	Unknown	COVID-19	NA	[110]

21	Protein tyrosine kinase-7 (PTK7)	Diagnostic	NCT03385148	The clinical application of 68Ga-labeled ssDNA aptamer Sgc8 in healthy volunteers and colorectal patients	Unknown	Colorectal cancer	Early-phase 1	[111]
22	Zimura™ (anti-C5 aptamer)	Therapeutic	NCT05571267	Safety study of Zimura®, in combination with anti-VEGF therapy in patients with neovascular AMD	Terminated	Macular degeneration	Phase 2	[112]
23	NOX-E36	Therapeutic	NCT00976729	NOX-E36 first-in-human (FIH) study	Completed	Chronic inflammatory diseases, type 2 diabetes mellitus, systemic lupus erythematosus	Phase 1	[113]

(continued)

Table 3.1 (continued)

S. No.	Aptamer	Study type	NCT number	Study title	Study status	Disease conditions	Clinical trial phase	Study URL
24	NOX-A12 stromal cell–derived factor-1 (SDF-1) L-oligonucleotide aptamerSpiegelmer	Therapeutic	NCT00976378	NOX-A12 first-in-human (FIH) study	Completed	Autologous stem cell transplantation	Phase 1	[114]
25	NOX-A12 stem cell transplantation SDF-1 L-oligonucleotide aptamerSpiegelmerhematopoietic stem cells	Therapeutic	NCT01194934	NOX-A12 multiple ascending dose study in healthy volunteers	Completed	Hematopoietic stem cell transplantation	Phase 1	[115]
26	Pegaptanib sodium (anti-VEGFpegylated aptamer)	Therapeutic	NCT00215670	Study of the safety, tolerability, and pharmacokinetics of 1 mg/eye and 3 mg/eye pegaptanib sodium in patients with exudative age-related macular degeneration (AMD)	Completed	Age-related macular degeneration	Phase 2, phase 3	[116]

27	AST-201	Therapeutic	NCT06687941	A study to evaluate the tolerability, safety, and pharmacokinetics (PK) of AST-201 in patients with GPC3-positive advanced solid tumors	Not yet recruiting	Neoplasms, hepatocellular carcinoma, non-small cell lung carcinoma, liver neoplasms	Phase 1	[117]
28	EYE001 (anti-VEGF pegylated aptamer)	Therapeutic	NCT00040313	Pegaptanib sodium compared to sham injection in patients Diabetic macular edema (DME) involving the center of the macula	Completed	Diabetic macular edema	Phase 2	[118]

3.7 Challenges and Future Perspectives

Despite their promising attributes, such as low immunogenicity and straightforward synthesis, aptamers face several significant hurdles on their path to widespread therapeutic adoption.

3.7.1 Current Limitations

3.7.1.1 Delivery Challenges

The efficient delivery of aptamers remains a formidable obstacle in therapeutic applications. Their inherent negative charge creates a barrier to cellular entry, significantly limiting their access to intracellular targets. When aptamers are taken up nonspecifically by unintended cells, therapeutic efficacies diminish and the risk of side effects increases [119]. Researchers are actively developing specialized aptamer delivery systems to enhance target specificity, particularly for RNA interference therapies where aptamers serve as delivery vehicles for small interfering RNAs to specific cell populations [120, 121].

3.7.1.2 Stability Issues

RNA aptamers exhibit high vulnerability to nuclease degradation in biological environments. These enzymes rapidly break down RNA molecules in blood serum and other bodily fluids, severely compromising the therapeutic window and in vivo efficacy of aptamer treatments [122]. This instability also affects diagnostic applications, particularly electrochemical aptamer-based (E-AB) sensors, where degradation can compromise detection accuracy and reliability [123].

3.7.1.3 Manufacturing Considerations

The clinical utility of aptamers hinges significantly on production protocols that influence their stability, specificity, and pharmacokinetic profile. While aptamers offer the advantage of minimal batch-to-batch variation—crucial for clinical consistency—manufacturing processes require careful optimization to preserve their structural integrity and functional properties [124, 125]. Developing efficient production and modification techniques remains essential for their successful integration into therapeutic and diagnostic platforms.

3.7.1.4 Regulatory Hurdles

The regulatory framework for aptamer-based therapeutics continues to evolve. A primary challenge lies in their classification into different regulatory systems. In the European Union, aptamers may be categorized as gene therapy products depending on their specific characteristics, affecting approval pathways and safety requirements [126]. The lack of global regulatory harmonization further complicates market entry, with different regions imposing varying standards for RNA-based therapeutics [126]. Additionally, the integration of artificial intelligence in aptamer development introduces new ethical and regulatory considerations, particularly regarding data privacy and algorithmic transparency [127].

3.7.2 Emerging Solutions

3.7.2.1 Novel Delivery Strategies

To address delivery limitations, researchers are exploring conjugation with various carrier systems, including nanoparticles, liposomes, and hydrogels. These carriers provide protection against enzymatic degradation while extending circulation time in the bloodstream [128]. Aptamer–nanoparticle conjugates can be engineered with exceptional targeting specificity, ensuring therapeutic agents reach only diseased tissues while sparing healthy cells [129].

3.7.2.2 Advanced Modification Techniques

Chemical modifications have significantly improved aptamer stability and binding characteristics. Locked nucleic acids incorporate a methylene bridge that stabilizes the ribose structure, enhancing thermal stability and nuclease resistance. The LNA-modified DNA aptamer RNV66 targeting VEGF demonstrates substantially higher stability and binding affinity compared to its unmodified counterpart [67].

Spiegelmers represent another innovative approach. These mirror-image aptamers possess unnatural chirality that renders them highly resistant to enzymatic degradation while maintaining their binding properties in biological environments for extended periods [130].

3.7.2.3 Improved Selection Methods

SELEX techniques have advanced considerably, enhancing aptamer specificity and affinity. Next-generation sequencing technologies like high-throughput sequencing-fluorescent ligand interaction profiling (HiTS-FLIP) enable simultaneous analysis of millions of aptamer candidates, dramatically improving selection efficiency [131]. The Single-Round Capillary Electrophoresis (SR-CE) selection method, which integrates capillary electrophoresis with sequencing, further enhances reproducibility and precision in aptamer identification [132].

3.7.2.4 Manufacturing Innovations

Recent advances in solid-phase synthesis and automation have streamlined aptamer production, improving both quality and yield. These innovations facilitate the incorporation of complex modifications, enabling the development of functionalized aptamers with enhanced therapeutic properties. Solid-phase synthesis allows integration of anticancer agents directly into aptamers, improving their targeting and cytotoxic effects against tumor cells [133].

Asymmetric PCR offers a cost-effective approach for aptamer evaluation, as it eliminates the need for costly modifications such as biotinylation or fluorescent labeling [134].

3.8 Integration with Diagnostic Applications

Aptamers are useful in diagnostic and therapeutic applications. They have exceptional specificity and versatile binding capabilities and can be modified easily by chemical methods. Their success in diagnostics has paved the way for theranostic molecules that have both diagnostic and therapeutic functionalities.

3.8.1 Theranostic Approaches

3.8.1.1 Dual Therapeutic–Diagnostic Applications

Aptamers can bind disease biomarkers with high specificity, allowing for simultaneous disease monitoring and targeted therapy delivery. The adaptability of aptamer design could be exploited for recognizing and interacting with cancer biomarkers [46]. The use of aptamers in biosensors has made early cancer detection and prognosis possible [46, 135]. Additionally, the use of aptamer–nanomaterial conjugates or aptamer–drug conjugates enables precise targeting of cancer cells while minimizing damage to healthy tissues [46, 136].

3.8.1.2 Real-Time Monitoring Capabilities

The use of aptamers in biosensor platforms has made continuous and real-time monitoring of biomarkers a reality. With the help of aptamer-based theranostic approaches, patient outcomes could be improved.

Electrochemical aptamer-based (E-AB) sensors utilize the binding affinity of aptamers to detect and quantify biomarkers in real time. For example, a pendulum-type E-AB sensor has been developed to detect proteins like VEGF. This sensor has shown high-frequency data acquisition and resistance to signal degradation [137]. The Chronoamperometric Interrogation technique enables reagent-free, continuous biomarker monitoring, such as thrombin detection, with a broad dynamic range and rapid response times, as demonstrated in tetrahedral DNA nanostructure (TDN) pendulum-empowered E-AB sensors [137].

3.8.1.3 Personalized Treatment Strategies

Aptamers' high specificity and affinity for biological targets sometimes surpass traditional antibodies, allowing the detection of subtle biomarker variations essential for personalized medicine [138, 139]. Their inherent modifiability enables the development of tailored diagnostic tools adaptable to individual patient needs, making them particularly valuable in precision medicine applications [140].

3.8.2 Future Directions

3.8.2.1 Emerging Technologies

The integration of microfluidic chips and nanoparticles with aptamer-based diagnostics has transformed point-of-care testing, enhancing sensitivity, specificity, and speed [141]. Microfluidic chips provide precise control of small fluid volumes, making them ideal for portable, affordable diagnostic platforms capable of performing complex analyses. These systems streamline sample processing and analysis, reducing diagnostic time and minimizing user intervention [142]. Aptamer-functionalized quantum dots have emerged as powerful imaging tools, combining unique optical properties with aptamers' target specificity. They have successfully detected SARS-CoV-2 viral particles using fluorescence-based detection, without complex amplification steps [143]. In cancer imaging, aptamer-functionalized graphene quantum dots enable two-photon imaging with deep tissue penetration and high resolution [144].

3.8.2.2 Integration with Other Therapeutic Modalities

The combination of aptamers with CRISPR-associated proteins offers unprecedented precision in gene editing. The Pin-point™ base editing platform utilizes RNA aptamers to recruit DNA base–modifying enzymes, enabling precise modifications without double-strand breaks or homology-directed repair, thereby improving editing efficiency while minimizing chromosomal translocations [145, 146]. The Casilio-DRP approach employs aptamers attached to guide RNA to recruit RNA-binding proteins that tether DNA repair enzymes, enhancing homology-directed repair efficiency while reducing errors from nonhomologous end joining [147]. Similarly, the S1mplex strategy uses RNA aptamers to assemble CRISPR-Cas9 ribonucleoproteins with nucleic acid donor templates, significantly improving genome editing precision [148].

3.8.2.3 Path to Clinical Implementation

Optimizing aptamer-based diagnostics for clinical use requires addressing several key challenges related to stability, regulatory approval, and economic viability. Aptamers typically suffer from reduced serum stability and rapid renal excretion, limiting their in vivo effectiveness. Enhancing their stability remains crucial for successful clinical application [149]. The regulatory approval pathway is complex, requiring extensive validation to meet stringent standards set by agencies like the FDA and EMA [150]. Efforts to harmonize global regulatory standards could facilitate the faster adoption of aptamer-based diagnostics [151]. Recent legislative initiatives, such as the twenty-first Century Cures Act, aim to streamline approval processes for personalized medicine tools, including aptamer-based diagnostics [152]. Implementation challenges include requirements for specialized equipment and trained personnel, potentially limiting adoption in resource-constrained settings [153]. Securing insurance coverage represents another critical factor for widespread clinical adoption. Demonstrating clinical utility and cost-effectiveness to health insurers, such as Medicare and Medicaid in the United States, is essential for successful market entry [154]. The favorable cost-effectiveness profile of aptamer-based diagnostics compared to traditional methods strengthens their appeal to healthcare providers and insurers alike [153, 155].

3.9 Conclusion

Aptamers represent a transformative class of therapeutic molecules with exceptional potential for targeted interventions across various disease states, particularly in oncology. Their unique advantages—including high specificity, low immunogenicity, chemical stability, and versatile modification capabilities—position them as valuable alternatives to traditional antibody-based therapeutics. While challenges persist in delivery, stability, and regulatory pathways, significant advances in chemical modifications, conjugation strategies, and selection methodologies continue to address these limitations. The integration of aptamers with diagnostic platforms has further expanded their utility, enabling theranostic approaches that combine disease monitoring with targeted treatment. As manufacturing processes become more refined and cost-effective, aptamers are poised to play an increasingly important role in precision medicine. The continued evolution of aptamer technology, coupled with emerging innovations in delivery systems and combination therapies, suggests a promising future for these versatile molecules in addressing unmet medical needs through highly specific molecular targeting.

References

1. Ellington AD, Szostak JW. In vitro selection of RNA molecules that bind specific ligands. Nature. 1990;346(6287):818–22.
2. Tuerk C, Gold L. Systematic evolution of ligands by exponential enrichment: RNA ligands to bacteriophage T4 DNA polymerase. Science. 1979;249(4968):505–10.
3. Brody EN, Gold L. Aptamers as therapeutic and diagnostic agents. Rev Mol Biotechnol. 2000;74(1):5–13.
4. Santarpia G, Carnes E. Therapeutic applications of Aptamers. Int J Mol Sci. 2024;25(12):6742.
5. Katz B, Goldbaum M. Macugen (Pegaptanib sodium), a novel ocular therapeutic that targets vascular endothelial growth factor (VEGF). Int Ophthalmol Clin. 2006;46(4):141–54.
6. Sett A. Aptamers: magic bullet for Theranostic applications. In: Theranostics – an old concept in new clothing. IntechOpen; 2020.
7. Zhang HL, Lv C, Li ZH, Jiang S, Cai D, Liu SS, et al. Analysis of aptamer-target binding and molecular mechanisms by thermofluorimetric analysis and molecular dynamics simulation. Front Chem. 2023;11:11.
8. Adachi T, Nakamura Y. Aptamers: a review of their chemical properties and modifications for therapeutic application. Molecules. 2019;24(23):4229.
9. Chen Z, Luo H, Gubu A, Yu S, Zhang H, Dai H, et al. Chemically modified aptamers for improving binding affinity to the target proteins via enhanced non-covalent bonding. Front Cell Dev Biol. 2023;11:11.
10. Gowland R, Gowers DM. A lambda-exonuclease SELEX method for generating Aptamers to bacterial targets. In: DNA manipulation and analysis. New York: Springer; 2023. p. 145–61.
11. Manea I, Casian M, Hosu-Stancioiu O, et al. A review on magnetic beads-based SELEX technologies: applications from small to large target molecules. Anal Chim Acta. 2024;1297:342325.
12. Kohlberger M, Gadermaier G. SELEX: critical factors and optimization strategies for successful aptamer selection. Biotechnol Appl Biochem. 2022;69(5):1771–92.
13. Preeti K, Jain N, Sharma SK. Advances in SELEX methods. In: Aptasensors for food safety. Boca Raton: CRC Press; 2024. p. 93–105.
14. Pantier R, Chhatbar K, Alston G, Lee HY, Bird A. High-throughput sequencing SELEX for the determination of DNA-binding protein specificities in vitro. STAR Protoc. 2022;3(3):101490.
15. Quang NN, Miodek A, Cibiel A, Ducongé F. Selection of Aptamers against whole living cells: from cell-SELEX to identification of biomarkers. In: Synthetic antibodies: methods and protocols; 2017. p. 253–72.
16. Chen M, Yu Y, Jiang F, Zhou J, Li Y, Liang C, et al. Development of cell-SELEX technology and its application in cancer diagnosis and therapy. Int J Mol Sci. 2016;17(12):2079.

17. Song MY, Nguyen D, Hong SW, Kim BC. Broadly reactive aptamers targeting bacteria belonging to different genera using a sequential toggle cell-SELEX. Sci Rep. 2017;7(1):43641.
18. Derbyshire N, White SJ, Bunka DHJ, Song L, Stead S, Tarbin J, et al. Toggled RNA Aptamers against aminoglycosides allowing facile detection of antibiotics using Gold nanoparticle assays. Anal Chem. 2012;84(15):6595–602.
19. Zhao L, Yang G, Zhu C, Li L, Zhao Y, Luan Y, et al. Three-step evolutionary enhanced capillary electrophoresis-SELEX for aptamer selection of exosome vesicles. Talanta. 2024;267:125203.
20. Wang H, Zhang Y, Chu C, Dai W, Liu R, Jiang Y. Abstract 2058: identification of a specific RNA aptamer targeting non-small cell lung cancer by in vivo SELEX. Cancer Res. 2016;76(14_Supplement):2058.
21. Uemachi H, Kasahara Y, Tanaka K, Okuda T, Yoneda Y, Obika S. Hybrid-type SELEX for the selection of artificial nucleic acid Aptamers exhibiting cell internalization activity. Pharmaceutics. 2021;13(6):888.
22. Olsen T, Zhu J, Kim J, Pei R, Stojanovic MN, Lin Q. An integrated microfluidic SELEX approach using combined Electrokinetic and hydrodynamic manipulation. SLAS Technol. 2017;22(1):63–72.
23. Lin Y, Chen CY, Lin ZQ, Chen BH, Sun YC, Hung KF. Abstract 3761: a modified SELEX enables the efficient identification of DNA aptamers with potential for specific cancer targeting. Cancer Res. 2024;84(6_Supplement):3761.
24. Oliveira R, Pinho E, Azevedo NF, Almeida C. Post-SELEX modifications with locked nucleic acids (LNA) of a SEA-specific DNA aptamer assisted by *in silico* modelling. Mol Syst Des Eng. 2024;9(8):847–55.
25. Eremeeva E, Fikatas A, Margamuljana L, Abramov M, Schols D, Groaz E, et al. Highly stable hexitol based XNA aptamers targeting the vascular endothelial growth factor. Nucleic Acids Res. 2019;47(10):4927–39.
26. Amero P, Lokesh GLR, Chaudhari RR, Cardenas-Zuniga R, Schubert T, Attia YM, et al. Conversion of RNA Aptamer into modified DNA Aptamers provides for prolonged stability and enhanced antitumor activity. J Am Chem Soc. 2021;143(20):7655–70.
27. Riccardi C, Pérez de Carvasal K, Platella C, Meyer A, Smietana M, Morvan F, et al. Probing naphthalene diimide and 3-hydroxypropylphosphate as end-conjugating moieties for improved thrombin binding aptamers: structural and biological effects. Bioorg Chem. 2023;141:106917.
28. Sargazi S, et al. Aptamer-conjugated carbon-based nanomaterials for cancer and bacteria theranostics: a review. Chem Biol Interact. 2022;361:109964.
29. Zhu S, Gao H, Li W, He X, Jiang P, Xu F, et al. Stimuli-responsive Aptamer-drug conjugates for targeted drug delivery and controlled drug release. Adv Healthc Mater. 2024;
30. Manna S, Mahata R, Dey SK, Das Chaudhuri A, Choudhury SM. Multifunctional aptamer grafted targeted nano-drugs execute molecular cross-talks with cancer cells. Appl Res. 2024;3(4)
31. He X, Guo L, He J, Xu H, Xie J. Stepping library-based post-SELEX strategy approaching to the minimized Aptamer in SPR. Anal Chem. 2017;89(12):6559–66.
32. Vorobyeva M, Vorobjev P, Venyaminova A. Multivalent Aptamers: versatile tools for diagnostic and therapeutic applications. Molecules. 2016;21(12):1613.
33. Dhanya CR, Mary AS, Madhavan M. <scp>Aptamer-siRNA</scp> chimeras: promising tools for targeting <scp>HER2</scp> signaling in cancer. Chem Biol Drug Des. 2023;101(5):1162–80.
34. Subramanian N, Kanwar JR, Kanwar RK, Sreemanthula J, Biswas J, Khetan V, et al. EpCAM Aptamer-siRNA chimera targets and regress epithelial cancer. PLoS One. 2015;10(7):e0132407.
35. Alhamhoom Y, As Sobeai H, Alsanea S, Alhoshani A. Aptamer-based therapy for targeting key mediators of cancer metastasis (review). Int J Oncol. 2022;60(6):65.
36. Gao F, Yin J, Chen Y, Guo C, Hu H, Su J. Recent advances in aptamer-based targeted drug delivery systems for cancer therapy. Front Bioeng Biotechnol. 2022;10

37. Sujith S, Naresh R, Srivisanth BU, Sajeevan A, Rajaramon S, David H, et al. Aptamers: precision tools for diagnosing and treating infectious diseases. Front Cell Infect Microbiol. 2024:14.
38. Huang Z, Wang D, Zhang Q, Zhang Y, Peng R, Tan W. Leveraging Aptamer-based DNA nanotechnology for bioanalysis and cancer therapeutics. Acc Mater Res. 2024;5(4):438–52.
39. Di Mauro V, Lauta FC, Modica J, Appleton SL, De Franciscis V, Catalucci D. Diagnostic and therapeutic Aptamers. JACC Basic Transl Sci. 2024;9(2):260–77.
40. Liu Z, Liu Y. Aptamer-based drug delivery systems. In: Aptamers for medical applications. Singapore: Springer Singapore; 2021. p. 77–113.
41. Parashar A. Aptamers in therapeutics. J Clin Diagn Res. 2016;10:BE01.
42. Venkatesan S, Chanda K, Balamurali MM. Aptamers as useful tool for therapeutic and theranostic applications. In: Futuristic trends in chemical material sciences & nano technology, vol. 3. Iterative International Publishers, Selfypage Developers Pvt Ltd; 2024. p. 200–15.
43. Murray MT, Wetmore SD. Unlocking precision in aptamer engineering: a case study of the thrombin binding aptamer illustrates why modification size, quantity, and position matter. Nucleic Acids Res. 2024;52(18):10823–35.
44. Lakshmipriya T, Gopinath SCB. Aptamer: a versatile probe in medical diagnosis. INNOSC Theranost Pharmacol Sci. 2018;1(1):14–9.
45. Duan Q, Jia H, Chen W, Qin C, Zhang K, Jia F, et al. Multivalent Aptamer-based lysosome-targeting chimeras (LYTACs) platform for mono- or dual-targeted proteins degradation on cell surface. Adv Sci. 2024;11(17)
46. Mahmoudian F, Ahmari A, Shabani S, Sadeghi B, Fahimirad S, Fattahi F. Aptamers as an approach to targeted cancer therapy. Cancer Cell Int. 2024;24(1):108.
47. Liustrovaite V, Ratautaite V, Ramanaviciene A, Plikusiene I, Malinovskis U, Erts D, et al. Electrochemical sensor for vascular endothelial growth factor based on self-assembling DNA aptamer structure. Sci Total Environ. 2024;955:177151.
48. Chen K, Cai J, Wang S, Li Y, Yang C, Fu T, et al. Aptamer inhibits tumor growth by leveraging cellular proteasomal degradation system to degrade c-met in mice. Angew Chem. 2023;135(2)
49. Pan Q, Nie C, Hu Y, Yi J, Liu C, Zhang J, et al. Aptamer-functionalized DNA origami for targeted codelivery of antisense oligonucleotides and doxorubicin to enhance therapy in drug-resistant cancer cells. ACS Appl Mater Interfaces. 2020;12(1):400–9.
50. Kolovskaya OS, Zamay TN, Zamay AS, Glazyrin YE, Spivak EA, Zubkova OA, et al. DNA-aptamer/protein interaction as a cause of apoptosis and arrest of proliferation in Ehrlich ascites adenocarcinoma cells. Biochem (Mosc) Suppl Ser A Membr Cell Biol. 2014;8(1):60–72.
51. Qiao Y, Shi Y, Ji M, Wang Z, Bai X, Zhang K, et al. Selection and identification of a prohibitin 2-binding DNA aptamer for tumor tissue imaging and targeted chemotherapy. Int J Biol Macromol. 2024;259:129002.
52. Chen W, Cai X, Sun Q, Guo X, Liang C, Tang H, et al. Design and synthesis of aptamer-cyclometalated iridium(III) complex conjugate targeting cancer cells. Eur J Med Chem. 2022;236:114335.
53. Chen K, Cai J, Wang S, Li Y, Yang C, Fu T, et al. Aptamer inhibits tumor growth by leveraging cellular proteasomal degradation system to degrade c-met in mice. Angew Chem Int Ed. 2023;62(2)
54. Fang Y, Wu Q, Wang F, Liu Y, Zhang H, Yang C, et al. Aptamer-RIBOTAC strategy enabling tumor-specific targeted degradation of MicroRNA for precise cancer therapy. Small Methods. 2024;
55. Wei J, Song R, Sabbagh A, Marisetty A, Shukla N, Fang D, et al. Cell-directed aptamer therapeutic targeting for cancers including those within the central nervous system. Onco Targets Ther. 2022;11(1)
56. Safarzadeh Kozani P, Safarzadeh Kozani P, Rahbarizadeh F. Aptamer-assisted delivery of nucleotides with tumor-suppressing properties for targeted cancer therapies. Trends Med Sci. 2021;1(4)

57. Ayass MA, Tripathi T, Griko N, Okyay T, Ramankutty Nair R, Zhang J, et al. Dual checkpoint Aptamer immunotherapy: unveiling tailored cancer treatment targeting CTLA-4 and NKG2A. Cancers (Basel). 2024;16(5):1041.
58. Sun Y, Mo L, Hu X, Yu D, Xie S, Li J, et al. Bispecific Aptamer-based recognition-then-conjugation strategy for PD1/PDL1 Axis blockade and enhanced immunotherapy. ACS Nano. 2022;16(12):21129–38.
59. Zhang Q, Wu L, Zhang Y, Wang D, Sima Y, Wang Z, et al. Aptamer-based nongenetic reprogramming of CARs enables flexible modulation of T cell-mediated tumor immunotherapy. ACS Cent Sci. 2024;10:813.
60. Yang Q, Hu S, Wang Y, Zhong L, Yu X, Zhang Y, et al. Engineering M1 macrophages with targeting aptamers for enhanced adoptive immunotherapy by modifying the cell surface. 2024.
61. Zhao R, Bai Y, Guo Y, Feng F, Shuang S. Aptamer-modified tetrahedral DNA nanostructures as drug delivery system for cancer targeted therapy. Macromol Biosci. 2024;24(4):e2300420.
62. Liu M, Zhao L, Chen Y, Chen X, Li J, Chen Z, et al. Aptamer-modified Nb_2C multifunctional nanomedicine for targeted photothermal/chemotherapy combined therapy of tumor. Mol Pharm. 2024;21(8):4047–59.
63. Rodríguez Serrano AF, Hsing IM. Prediction of Aptamer–small-molecule interactions using metastable states from multiple independent molecular dynamics simulations. J Chem Inf Model. 2022;62(19):4799–809.
64. Eisen SR, Dauphin-Ducharme P, Johnson PE. Solution-based biophysical characterization of conformation change in structure-switching aptamers. Q Rev Biophys. 2024;57:e9.
65. Autiero I, Vitagliano L. Enhanced molecular dynamic simulation studies unravel long-range effects caused by sequence variations and partner binding in RNA aptamers. Mol Ther Nucleic Acids. 2023;34:102039.
66. Gruenke PR, Alam KK, Singh K, Burke DH. 2′-fluoro-modified pyrimidines enhance affinity of RNA oligonucleotides to HIV-1 reverse transcriptase. RNA. 2020;26(11):1667–79.
67. Pal R, Deb I, Sarzynska J, Lahiri A. LNA-induced dynamic stability in a therapeutic aptamer: insights from molecular dynamics simulations. J Biomol Struct Dyn. 2023;41(6):2221–30.
68. Schmidt KS. Application of locked nucleic acids to improve aptamer in vivo stability and targeting function. Nucleic Acids Res. 2004;32(19):5757–65.
69. Wang Y, Wang D, Lin J, Lyu Z, Chen P, Sun T, et al. A long-circulating vector for Aptamers based upon Polyphosphodiester-backboned molecular brushes. Angew Chem. 2022;134(41):e202204576.
70. Vu CQ, Rotkrua P, Tantirungrotechai Y, Soontornworajit B. Oligonucleotide hybridization combined with competitive antibody binding for the truncation of a high-affinity Aptamer. ACS Comb Sci. 2017;19(10):609–17.
71. Liu CC, Hsiao YC, Lai WJ, Chiou CC, Chu LJ, Lin YT, et al. Development and optimization of a DNA aptamer to delay β-bungarotoxin-induced lethality in a rodent model. Int J Biol Macromol. 2024;270:132240.
72. Wong KW, Wang Z, He D, Li HW. Programmed aptamer target chain reaction (ATCR) for smart therapeutic inhibitor development. Chem Eng J. 2024;483:149228.
73. Zamay GS, Zamay TN, Lukyanenko KA, Kichkailo AS. Aptamers increase biocompatibility and reduce the toxicity of magnetic nanoparticles used in biomedicine. Biomedicines. 2020;8(3):59.
74. Shraim AS, Abdel Majeed BA, Al-Binni MA, Hunaiti A. Therapeutic potential of Aptamer–protein interactions. ACS Pharmacol Transl Sci. 2022;5(12):1211–27.
75. Zhang GQ, Zhong LP, Yang N, Zhao YX. Screening of aptamers and their potential application in targeted diagnosis and therapy of liver cancer. World J Gastroenterol. 2019;25(26):3359–69.
76. Kapcan E, Lake BPM, Rullo AF. Orchestrating binding interactions and the emergence of avidity driven therapeutics. ACS Cent Sci. 2023;9(4):586–9.
77. Driscoll J, Gondaliya P, Ziemer A, Yan IK, Gupta Y, Patel T. In Silico Design of Novel EpCAM-binding Aptamers for targeted delivery of RNA therapeutics. Nano. 2024;14(21):1727.
78. Peng X, Liu Y, Peng F, Wang T, Cheng Z, Chen Q, et al. Aptamer-controlled stimuli-responsive drug release. Int J Biol Macromol. 2024;279:135353.

79. Wang GA, Wu X, Chen F, Shen C, Yang Q, Li F. Toehold-exchange-based activation of Aptamer switches enables high thermal robustness and programmability. J Am Chem Soc. 2023;145(5):2750–3.
80. Wong KY, Wong MS, Liu J. Aptamer-functionalized liposomes for drug delivery. Biom J. 2024;47(4):100685.
81. Li Y, Zhao J, Xue Z, Tsang C, Qiao X, Dong L, et al. Aptamer nucleotide analog drug conjugates in the targeting therapy of cancers. Front Cell Dev Biol. 2022;10
82. Li J, Yan A, Wang M, Li D. Aptamer and phosphorothioated DNA engineered liposomes as a targeted intracellular protein delivery system. Chin J Anal Chem. 2024;52(6):100400.
83. Lim DY, Hwang BH. Aptamer-modified tetrahedral DNA nanostructure-immobilized liposome for specific gene delivery and potential cancer theragnostic. Biotechnol J. 2024;19(1):e2300156.
84. Madhusudhana KC, Newsom RSB. Bevacizumab: a new hope? Eye. 2009;23(9):1755–7.
85. Shakeel L, Khan A, Akilimali A. Izervay (avacincaptad pegol): paving the way for vision preservation in geographic atrophy. Ann Med Surg. 2024;86:2413.
86. Moreno TA, Kim SJ. Ranibizumab (Lucentis) versus bevacizumab (Avastin) for the treatment of age-related macular degeneration: an economic disparity of eye health. Semin Ophthalmol. 2016;31(4):378–84.
87. Van den Avont A, Sharma-Walia N. Anti-nucleolin aptamer AS1411: an advancing therapeutic. Front Mol Biosci. 2023;10
88. Zboralski D, Hoehlig K, Eulberg D, Frömming A, Vater A. Increasing tumor-infiltrating T cells through inhibition of CXCL12 with NOX-A12 synergizes with PD-1 blockade. Cancer Immunol Res. 2017;5(11):950–6.
89. Povsic TJ, Wargin WA, Alexander JH, Krasnow J, Krolick M, Cohen MG, et al. Pegnivacogin results in near complete FIX inhibition in acute coronary syndrome patients: RADAR pharmacokinetic and pharmacodynamic substudy. Eur Heart J. 2011;32(19):2412–9.
90. Ayass MA, Griko N, Pashkov V, Tripathi T, Zhang J, Ramankutty Nair R, et al. New high-affinity thrombin Aptamers for advancing coagulation therapy: balancing thrombin inhibition for clot prevention and effective bleeding management with antidote. Cells. 2023;12(18):2230.
91. https://clinicaltrials.gov/study/NCT00709527 [Internet]. [cited 2025 Feb 21]. Available from: https://clinicaltrials.gov/study/NCT00709527
92. https://clinicaltrials.gov/study/NCT00021736. [cited 2025 Feb 21]; Available from: https://clinicaltrials.gov/study/NCT00021736
93. https://clinicaltrials.gov/study/NCT04870671. [cited 2025 Feb 21]; Available from: https://clinicaltrials.gov/study/NCT04870671
94. https://clinicaltrials.gov/study/NCT02957370. [cited 2025 Feb 21]; Available from: https://clinicaltrials.gov/study/NCT02957370
95. https://clinicaltrials.gov/study/NCT00113997. [cited 2025 Feb 24]; Available from: https://clinicaltrials.gov/study/NCT00113997
96. https://clinicaltrials.gov/study/NCT00950638. [cited 2025 Feb 21]; Available from: https://clinicaltrials.gov/study/NCT00950638
97. https://clinicaltrials.gov/study/NCT01089517. [cited 2025 Feb 21]; Available from: https://clinicaltrials.gov/study/NCT01089517
98. https://clinicaltrials.gov/study/NCT00056199. [cited 2025 Feb 21]; Available from: https://clinicaltrials.gov/study/NCT00056199
99. https://clinicaltrials.gov/study/NCT02397954.
100. https://clinicaltrials.gov/study/NCT00569140. [cited 2025 Feb 21]; Available from: https://clinicaltrials.gov/study/NCT00569140
101. https://clinicaltrials.gov/study/NCT01034410. [cited 2025 Feb 21]; Available from: https://clinicaltrials.gov/study/NCT01034410
102. https://clinicaltrials.gov/study/NCT02686658. [cited 2025 Feb 21]; Available from: https://clinicaltrials.gov/study/NCT02686658
103. https://clinicaltrials.gov/study/NCT02214628. [cited 2025 Feb 21]; Available from: https://clinicaltrials.gov/study/NCT02214628

104. https://clinicaltrials.gov/study/NCT02387957. [cited 2025 Feb 21]; Available from: https://clinicaltrials.gov/study/NCT02387957
105. https://clinicaltrials.gov/study/NCT01944839. [cited 2025 Feb 24]; Available from: https://clinicaltrials.gov/study/NCT01944839
106. https://clinicaltrials.gov/study/NCT01940900. [cited 2025 Feb 24]; Available from: https://clinicaltrials.gov/study/NCT01940900
107. https://clinicaltrials.gov/study/NCT00312351. [cited 2025 Feb 24]; Available from: https://clinicaltrials.gov/study/NCT00312351
108. https://clinicaltrials.gov/study/NCT01940887. [cited 2025 Feb 24]; Available from: https://clinicaltrials.gov/study/NCT01940887
109. https://clinicaltrials.gov/study/NCT00321997. [cited 2025 Feb 24]; Available from: https://clinicaltrials.gov/study/NCT00321997
110. https://clinicaltrials.gov/study/NCT04974203. [cited 2025 Feb 24]; Available from: https://clinicaltrials.gov/study/NCT04974203
111. https://clinicaltrials.gov/study/NCT03385148. [cited 2025 Feb 24]; Available from: https://clinicaltrials.gov/study/NCT03385148
112. https://clinicaltrials.gov/study/NCT05571267. [cited 2025 Feb 24]; Available from: https://clinicaltrials.gov/study/NCT05571267
113. https://clinicaltrials.gov/study/NCT00976729. [cited 2025 Feb 24]; Available from: https://clinicaltrials.gov/study/NCT00976729
114. https://clinicaltrials.gov/study/NCT00976378. [cited 2025 Feb 24]; Available from: https://clinicaltrials.gov/study/NCT00976378
115. https://clinicaltrials.gov/study/NCT01194934. [cited 2025 Feb 24]; Available from: https://clinicaltrials.gov/study/NCT01194934
116. https://clinicaltrials.gov/study/NCT00215670. [cited 2025 Feb 24]; Available from: https://clinicaltrials.gov/study/NCT00215670
117. https://clinicaltrials.gov/study/NCT06687941. [cited 2025 Feb 24]; Available from: https://clinicaltrials.gov/study/NCT06687941
118. https://clinicaltrials.gov/study/NCT00040313. [cited 2025 Feb 24]; Available from: https://clinicaltrials.gov/study/NCT00040313
119. Xie S, Sun W, Fu T, Liu X, Chen P, Qiu L, et al. Aptamer-based targeted delivery of functional nucleic acids. J Am Chem Soc. 2023;145(14):7677–91.
120. Goyal M, Citu SN, Singla V, Singla A. Aptamer: apt system for target-specific drug delivery. In: Aptamers. Singapore: Springer Singapore; 2019. p. 59–71.
121. Zhou J, Rossi JJ. Aptamer-targeted cell-specific RNA interference. Silence. 2010;1(1):4.
122. Santos-Cancel M, White RJ. Collagen membranes with ribonuclease inhibitors for long-term stability of electrochemical Aptamer-based sensors employing RNA. Anal Chem. 2017;89(10):5598–604.
123. Schoukroun-Barnes LR, Wagan S, Liu J, Leach JB, White RJ. Biocompatible hydrogel membranes for the protection of RNA aptamer-based electrochemical sensors. In: Cullum BM, ES ML, editors. Smart biomedical and physiological sensor technology X; 2013. p. 87190I.
124. Zhou H, Li Y, Wu W. Aptamers: promising reagents in biomedicine application. Adv Biol. 2024;8(6):e2300584.
125. Mili M, Bachu V, Kuri PR, Singh NK, Goswami P. Improving synthesis and binding affinities of nucleic acid aptamers and their therapeutics and diagnostic applications. Biophys Chem. 2024;309:107218.
126. Guerriaud M, Kohli E. RNA-based drugs and regulation: toward a necessary evolution of the definitions issued from the European union legislation. Front Med (Lausanne). 2022;9
127. Kumar S, Mohan A, Sharma NR, Kumar A, Girdhar M, Malik T, et al. Computational frontiers in aptamer-based nanomedicine for precision therapeutics: a comprehensive review. ACS Omega. 2024;9(25):26838–62.
128. Bohrmann L, Burghardt T, Rodríguez-Rodríguez C, Herth MM, Saatchi K, Häfeli UO. Quantitative evaluation of a multimodal Aptamer-targeted long-circulating polymer for tumor targeting. ACS Omega. 2023;8(12):11003–20.

129. Urmi R, Banerjee P, Singh M, Singh R, Chhillar S, Sharma N, et al. Revolutionizing biomedicine: Aptamer-based nanomaterials and nanodevices for therapeutic applications. Biotechnol Rep. 2024;42:e00843.
130. Gao J, Nutan B, Gargouri D, Pisal ND, Do V, Zubair M, et al. Unlocking the potential of chemically modified nucleic acid therapeutics. Adv Ther (Weinh). 2024;7(11)
131. Drees A, Fischer M. High-throughput selection and characterisation of Aptamers on optical next-generation sequencers. Int J Mol Sci. 2021;22(17):9202.
132. Saito S, Sakamoto T, Tanaka N, Watanabe R, Kamimura T, Ota K, et al. Single-round DNA Aptamer selection by combined use of capillary electrophoresis and next generation sequencing: an Aptaomics approach for identifying unique functional protein-binding DNA Aptamers. Chem Eur J. 2021;27(39):10058–67.
133. Wang D, Peng Y, Deng Z, Tan Y, Su Y, Kuai H, et al. Modularly engineered solid-phase synthesis of Aptamer-functionalized small molecule drugs for targeted cancer therapy. Adv Ther (Weinh). 2020;3(9)
134. Wen K, Meng X, Lara K, Lin Q. Cost-effective evaluation of Aptamer candidates in SELEX-based Aptamer isolation. Talanta. 2024;275:126103.
135. Li Q, Maier SH, Li P, Peterhansl J, Belka C, Mayerle J, et al. Aptamers: a novel targeted theranostic platform for pancreatic ductal adenocarcinoma. Radiat Oncol. 2020;15(1):189.
136. Zhu G, Qiu L, Meng H, Mei L, Tan W. Aptamers-guided DNA Nanomedicine for cancer Theranostics. In: Aptamers selected by cell-SELEX for Theranostics. Berlin, Heidelberg: Springer; 2015. p. 111–37.
137. Wang Y, Duan H, Yalikun Y, Cheng S, Li M. A pendulum-type electrochemical aptamer-based sensor for continuous, real-time and stable detection of proteins. Talanta. 2024;266:125026.
138. Sousa AP, Rocha AC, Almeida C, Carneiro MCCG, Pais PP, Viana R, et al. Moving towards personalized medicine – the broad use of Aptamers for targeted Theranostic. Appl Sci. 2023;13(21):11933.
139. Liu Y, Wang Z, Zhuo Y, Wu H, Peng Y, Wang T, et al. Aptamer-based multiparameter analysis for molecular profiling of hematological malignancies. Anal Chem. 2024;96(8):3429–35.
140. Chen L, Yang G, Qu F. Aptamer-based sensors for fluid biopsies of protein disease markers. Talanta. 2024;276:126246.
141. Kaushal A, Seth A, Kala D, Gupta S, Krishnia L, Verma V. Miniaturized devices for point-of-care testing/miniaturization and integration with microfluidic systems. In: Biosensor based advanced cancer diagnostics. Elsevier; 2022. p. 375–83.
142. Liu D, Wang Y, Li X, Li M, Wu Q, Song Y, et al. Integrated microfluidic devices for in vitro diagnostics at point of care. Aggregate. 2022;3(5)
143. Radrizzani M, Flores CY, Stupka J, D'Alessio C, Garate O, Mendoza Herrera LJ, et al. Aptamer-quantum dots platform for SARS-CoV-2 viral particle detection by fluorescence microscopy. Int J Biol Macromol. 2024;278:134839.
144. Yan H, Yang S, Liu M, Bao K, Ren W, Lin F, et al. Aptamer-functionalized two-photon SiO $_2$ @GQDs hybrid-based signal amplification strategy for targeted cancer imaging. Analyst. 2023;148(20):5124–32.
145. Porreca I, Blassberg R, Harbottle J, Joubert B, Mielczarek O, Stombaugh J, et al. An aptamer-mediated base editing platform for simultaneous knock-in and multiple gene knockout for allogeneic CAR-T cells generation. Mol Ther. 2023;32(8):2692–710.
146. Collantes JC, Tan VM, Xu H, Ruiz-Urigüen M, Alasadi A, Guo J, et al. Development and characterization of a modular CRISPR and RNA Aptamer Mediated Base editing system. CRISPR J. 2021;4(1):58–68.
147. Jillette N, Zhu JJ, Cheng AW. Local recruitment of DNA repair proteins enhances CRISPR-ssODN-HDR editing. 2022.
148. Carlson-Stevermer J, Abdeen AA, Kohlenberg L, Goedland M, Molugu K, Lou M, et al. Assembly of CRISPR ribonucleoproteins with biotinylated oligonucleotides via an RNA aptamer for precise gene editing. Nat Commun. 2017;8(1):1711.

149. Otte DM, Choukeife M, Patwari T, Mayer G. Nucleic acid Aptamers: from basic research to clinical applications. In: Handbook of chemical biology of nucleic acids. Singapore: Springer Nature Singapore; 2023. p. 747–71.
150. Zhang Y, Li Y. Clinical translation of Aptamers for COVID-19. J Med Chem. 2023;66(24):16568–78.
151. Rodriguez-Manzano J, Subramaniam S, Uchea C, Szostak-Lipowicz KM, Freeman J, Rauch M, et al. Innovative diagnostic technologies: navigating regulatory frameworks through advances, challenges, and future prospects. Lancet Digit Health. 2024;6(12):e934–43.
152. Hays P. Legislation, reimbursement, and the regulatory landscape. In: Advancing healthcare through personalized medicine. Cham: Springer International Publishing; 2021. p. 583–607.
153. Sheraz M, Sun XF, Wang Y, Chen J, Sun L. Recent developments in Aptamer-based sensors for diagnostics. Sensors. 2024;24(23):7432.
154. Herscovitch P. Regulatory approval and insurance reimbursement: the final steps in clinical translation of amyloid brain imaging. Clin Translat Imaging. 2015;3(1):75–7.
155. Kumar V, Yadav GS, Banerjee BD. Aptamer based diagnosis: a cost-effective and suitable point of care testing method against SARS Coronavirus-2 (SARs-CoV-2) and other rapidly spreading diseases. Curr Biotechnol. 2021;10(1):3–6.

Role of Biosensors in Transforming Cancer Diagnostics

4

Pougang Golmei, Shriyansh Srivastava, Laxmi Yadav, and Sachin Kumar

4.1 Introduction

One of the biggest health problems in the world today is cancer, and improving patient outcomes depends heavily on early detection. Traditional diagnostic methods, such as tissue biopsies, imaging modalities (such as MRI and CT scans), and serological assays, frequently have drawbacks like being intrusive and expensive and having low sensitivity for identifying cancers in their early stages. Biosensors have become an effective and cutting-edge tool for cancer diagnostics in response to these difficulties, providing quick, accurate, and affordable alternatives [1].

4.1.1 Biosensors

A biosensor is an analytical instrument that uses a biological recognition element (BRE) and a transducer to detect and quantify certain biomarkers. These biomarkers may comprise proteins, nucleic acids, metabolites, and exosomal components linked to cancer [2]. The interaction between the BRE and the target biomolecule is the basic idea behind a biosensor; this interaction produces a detectable signal that is correlated with the analyte's concentration [3].

Key Components and Principles

Biosensors normally comprise three main parts: a signal processing system, a physicochemical detector or transducer, and a biological sensing element, or BRE (Fig. 4.1) [4].

P. Golmei · S. Srivastava · L. Yadav · S. Kumar (✉)
Department of Pharmacology, Delhi Pharmaceutical Sciences and Research University (DIPSAR), Delhi Pharmaceutical Sciences and Research University (DPSRU), New Delhi, India

S. Srivastava et al. (eds.), *Biosensors and Aptamers*,
https://doi.org/10.1007/978-981-96-8387-1_4

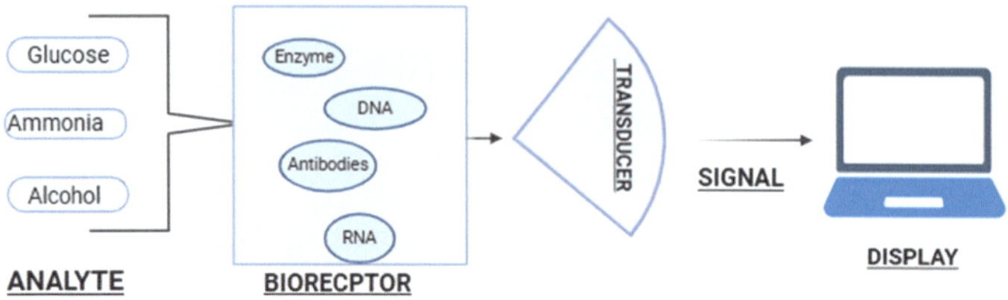

Fig. 4.1 Fundamental structure of a biosensor [5, 6]

Bioreceptor: Bioreceptors are biomolecules designed to recognize and bind to specific target substances (analytes). These biomolecules can include enzymes, aptamers, DNA, RNA, or antibodies [7, 8].

Transducer: A transducer converts a biorecognition event into a measurable signal, typically electrical, indicating the presence or amount of a target analyte. It generates signals proportional to analyte–bioreceptor interactions and can be classified into types like electrochemical, optical, thermal, electronic, and gravimetric based on its operation [9, 10].

Signal Processing System: The transduced signal is processed and formatted for display. The electrical signals from the transducer are amplified and converted into digital form, and the display unit then quantifies the processed signals [11].

Unique Advantages in Medical Diagnostics

Biosensors have transformed healthcare by providing cost-effective solutions for detecting contaminants, regulating biological processes, and diagnosing diseases. The high sensitivity and specificity of biosensors make it possible to identify biomarkers early on, allowing for prompt intervention and therapy. These tools facilitate individualized healthcare solutions, increase public health safety, and improve diagnostic accuracy [12–15].

Evolution of Biosensing Technologies

Over the past 40 years, the field of biosensors has seen substantial change, incorporating developments from electrical engineering, chemistry, physics, and microbiology [16]. Professor Leland C. Clark created the first biosensor in 1956 by introducing the idea of an electrochemical sensor based on enzymes [17]. Later developments resulted in the creation of different transducer technologies, DNA biosensors, and immunosensors [16]. To improve detection accuracy and usability, contemporary biosensors use artificial intelligence, microfluidics, and nanomaterials. Because of these developments, biosensors are now seen as a viable new area in cancer diagnosis.

4.1.2 Significance in Cancer Diagnostics

Limitations of Traditional Diagnostic Methods
Traditional cancer diagnoses are frequently expensive, time-consuming, and invasive [18]. Furthermore, blood-based assays might not have enough sensitivity for real-time monitoring, and imaging methods might not be able to identify cancers early enough [19, 20].

Potential for Early Detection
Biosensors can detect biomarkers in body fluids at the earliest stages of disease progression, potentially revolutionizing early cancer diagnosis [21]. This helps in increasing survival rates and permits prompt medical intervention [22].

Personalized Medicine Approach
Biosensors enable tailored treatment methods by assessing patient-specific biomarker profiles, which is becoming increasingly important in the field of personalized medicine. This enables the selection of the best therapeutic approaches and the tracking of treatment outcomes in real time [23].

Point-of-Care Testing Capabilities
Biosensor technology facilitates the development of portable diagnostic instruments, enabling on-site cancer screening in both clinical and nonclinical situations [24]. This is especially helpful in areas with low resources when access to cutting-edge diagnostic facilities is restricted [25].

4.2 Fundamental Principles of Biosensor Design

The design of biosensors for cancer diagnostics is rooted in fundamental principles that govern their sensitivity, specificity, and overall performance. To develop effective biosensors, it is crucial to understand their essential components, working mechanisms, and performance metrics [26].

4.2.1 Biosensor Components

Bioreceptors
The bioreceptor, also known as the detector element, is responsible for identifying the presence and concentration of the target analyte [27]. Biorecognition elements are categorized into natural and artificial substances. Natural elements include antibodies and enzymes, which rely on evolved physiological interactions to selectively identify analytes [28, 29]. Artificial biorecognition elements, such as DNA/RNA aptamers and molecularly imprinted polymers (MIPs), have been developed to enhance biosensor capabilities. Aptamers are short nucleic acid sequences that bind to specific targets through non-covalent interactions, serving as a versatile

alternative to antibodies. MIPs are synthetic polymers designed with specific binding sites that mimic natural receptors, offering high selectivity and stability [30].

Transduction Mechanisms
The transducer is a crucial component that converts the biochemical signal generated by the bioreceptor into a measurable output. Depending on the biosensor type, the transducer may operate through piezoelectric, optical, or electrochemical mechanisms [31].

Signal Processing Systems
The signal processing system amplifies and interprets this data, transforming it into a readable output that provides quantitative or qualitative information about the target analyte [32].

Performance Metrics
Clear performance metrics are crucial for assessing a sensor's efficiency in real-world scenarios and for making objective comparisons across different sensor types [33].

Selectivity: The biosensor must be able to distinguish the target analyte from other substances in a sample. This requires precise selection and immobilization of the bioreceptor [34, 35].

Sensitivity: The ability to detect low analyte concentrations is critical. Sensitivity can be enhanced through nanomaterials, which increase surface area and reactivity [34].

Specificity: Closely related to sensitivity, specificity ensures that the biosensor responds exclusively to the target biomolecule, minimizing false positives and improving reliability [36].

Stability and Reproducibility: A biosensor should maintain consistent performance over time and across multiple tests. Using robust materials and careful engineering can prevent degradation and ensure long-term reliability [37].

4.2.2 Types of Biosensors

Optical Biosensors
Optical biosensors measure output signals in the form of light. These sensors can be designed using optical diffraction or electrochemiluminescence (ECL) techniques. Optical transducers are particularly useful for label-free detection of bacterial pathogens, as they detect minute changes in refractive index or thickness when cells bind to the transducer's surface. Common optical detection methods include surface plasmon resonance (SPR), ellipsometry, resonant mirrors, and interferometers [38–40].

Electrochemical Biosensors

Electrochemical biosensors convert biochemical interactions into electrical signals, allowing for the sensitive detection of specific analytes in complex samples [41]. These biosensors are widely used for detecting hybridized DNA, DNA-binding drugs, and glucose concentrations. They can be classified based on the type of electrical parameter measured: conductimetric, amperometric, and potentiometric biosensors. Compared to optical biosensors, electrochemical biosensors offer lower capital costs and the ability to work with turbid samples, although they may exhibit slightly lower selectivity and sensitivity [42, 43].

Piezoelectric Biosensors

Piezoelectric biosensors utilize the piezoelectric effect, a phenomenon discovered by Jacques and Pierre Curie, to detect biological interactions. These sensors operate by measuring frequency changes resulting from mass variations or viscoelastic alterations on the sensor's surface. Quartz crystal microbalances (QCMs) are the most commonly used piezoelectric biosensor platforms. They enable label-free detection of biomolecular interactions such as antigen–antibody binding and DNA hybridization, making them valuable for disease diagnostics, environmental monitoring, and drug discovery. Advancements in nanostructures, hybrid films, nanoparticles, and enzymatic amplification cascades have significantly enhanced their sensitivity and broadened their applications [44, 45].

Thermal Biosensors

Thermal biosensors function by detecting temperature changes resulting from biological reactions. These sensors are constructed by integrating immobilized enzyme molecules with temperature sensors. When the target analyte interacts with the enzyme, the heat generated by the reaction is measured and correlated with the analyte concentration. Thermal biosensors are widely used for detecting pesticides and pathogenic bacteria in various environmental and clinical applications [40, 46].

Magnetic Biosensors

Magnetic biosensors detect changes in the magnetic properties of materials when exposed to external magnetic fields [47]. These sensors have gained significant attention in point-of-care (POC) applications due to their low cost, high detection efficiency, and minimal sample preparation requirements. By eliminating the need for expensive optical components, magnetic biosensors provide an efficient and cost-effective alternative for rapid diagnostics [48, 49].

4.3 Biomarker Detection Strategies

Detecting biomarkers presents a complex challenge due to the diverse chemical properties of biomolecules, requiring specialized strategies for accurate identification. Biomarkers, which include proteins, nucleic acids, and small metabolites, vary in chemical structure, size, and solubility. For instance, proteins often necessitate specific antibodies for detection, while nucleic acids can be identified through hybridization techniques. This diversity underscores the need for tailored detection methods suited to each biomarker's unique characteristics [50].

4.3.1 Molecular Biomarkers

Genetic Biomarkers

Genetic mutations and alterations serve as essential cancer biomarkers, offering insights into disease progression and treatment options. Notable examples include the BRAF V600E mutation in melanoma [51], epidermal growth factor receptor (EGFR) mutations in non-small cell lung cancer (NSCLC) [52], *KRAS* mutations in colorectal cancer [53], and BRCA1/BRCA2 mutations in breast and ovarian cancers [54], all of which influence therapeutic decisions. *HER2* gene amplification indicates aggressive breast and gastric cancers [55], while *IDH* mutations serve as diagnostic and prognostic markers in gliomas [56].

Gene Expression Profiles

Gene expression profiling is a powerful approach to understanding tumor behavior, prognosis, and treatment response. For instance, the Oncotype DX test evaluates 16 genes to predict disease recurrence risk and guide treatment for early-stage hormone receptor–positive breast cancer [57].

Protein Biomarkers

Proteins play a critical role in cell function and cancer progression, making them valuable biomarkers [58, 59]. Certain pancreatic cancer–associated proteins present in body fluids hold potential for early detection, staging, prognosis, and treatment monitoring. Many FDA-approved cancer biomarkers, such as human chorionic gonadotropin (HCG), alpha-fetoprotein (AFP), and lactate dehydrogenase (LDH), are single proteins used for staging cancers, while others, like HER2/NEU, provide additional diagnostic value [60].

Circulating Tumor DNA

Circulating tumor DNA is an emerging biomarker found at higher levels in cancer patients than in healthy individuals [61]. Elevated ctDNA levels correlate with tumor burden and poorer survival outcomes in colorectal, breast, ovarian, lung, and liver cancers. As a minimally invasive tool, ctDNA enables early detection, real-time monitoring of treatment response, and post-therapy tumor burden assessment [62]. Studies suggest that TP53 mutations in ctDNA provide more reliable treatment monitoring than traditional biomarkers like cancer antigen 125 (CA-125), enhancing personalized cancer therapy [63, 64].

Exosomal Markers

Exosomes, extracellular vesicles ranging from 40–150 nm in size, are lipid bilayer-encapsulated structures containing proteins, nucleic acids, glycoconjugates, and lipids [65, 66]. Due to their stability, exosomes protect their cargo from degradation, allowing them to serve as biomarkers for cancer detection, prognosis, and treatment monitoring [67]. Notably, the glioblastoma-specific variant of the epidermal growth factor receptor (EGFRvIII) has been identified in serum exosomes from glioblastoma patients, highlighting its potential as a diagnostic marker [68–70].

4.3.2 Detection Technologies

Nanomaterial-Enhanced Detection

Nanomaterials such as gold nanoparticles (AuNPs), carbon nanotubes (CNTs), quantum dots (QDs), and graphene have unique properties that enhance biosensor performance. These materials improve sensitivity, specificity, and reliability, making them ideal for portable point-of-care (POC) diagnostics. AuNPs facilitate signal transduction by enabling biomolecule immobilization [71], while CNTs enhance electron transfer, expediting sensor response times [72]. QDs, conjugated with biomolecules, target cancer markers with high specificity [73]. Graphene derivatives improve sensor performance through superior electrical properties and high surface area, optimizing biomolecule immobilization [74, 75].

Multiplexed Detection Systems

Multiplexed detection enables the simultaneous identification of multiple biomarkers, improving diagnostic accuracy, efficiency, and cost-effectiveness while reducing patient discomfort. Technologies such as Clustered Regularly Interspaced Short Palindromic Repeats (CRISPR)-based biosensors exhibit exceptional sensitivity and specificity in detecting pathogen-related nucleic acids, making them invaluable for rapid clinical diagnostics. The programmability of CRISPR/Cas systems allows simultaneous targeting of multiple biomarkers, enhancing disease monitoring and management [76, 77].

Ultrasensitive Detection Techniques

Ultrasensitive detection technologies identify analytes at concentrations significantly lower than conventional methods, often reaching femtomolar or attomolar levels. These methods employ advanced signal amplification techniques, including nanoparticle labeling, enzymatic amplification, and CRISPR-based strategies, to enhance detection capabilities. Additionally, integrating nanomaterials, such as gold nanoparticles and carbon nanotubes, boosts sensor performance by increasing signal strength and reliability [78].

Signal Amplification Strategies

Signal amplification techniques enhance biosensor sensitivity, enabling highly precise biomarker detection. Two primary approaches include target-based and signal-based amplification. Target-based amplification increases the number of detectable analytes, improving the limit of detection (LOD). Techniques such as nucleic acid amplification (polymerase chain reaction (PCR) and loop-mediated isothermal amplification (LAMP)) facilitate the detection of low-abundance biomarkers, crucial for early disease diagnosis [79, 80]. Signal-based amplification, on the other hand, strengthens detectable signals without increasing target molecule numbers. Strategies such as integrating gold or silver nanoparticles improve electroactive surface areas and signal-to-noise ratios, enhancing biosensor sensitivity [81]. For instance, a SARS-CoV-2 RNA sensor incorporating gold nanoparticles achieved an LOD of 200 copies/mL [82]. Furthermore, nanostructured impedance-based biosensors improve sensitivity by increasing the active surface area for analyte interactions, ensuring precise and reliable biomarker detection [82].

4.4 Advanced Biosensing Platforms

Biosensor development has seen significant advancements in healthcare, biomedicine, and food processing. The integration of nanotechnology and nanomaterials has greatly enhanced biosensor sensitivity, specificity, and versatility across various applications [83].

4.4.1 Nanotechnology-Enabled Biosensors

Nanomaterial Integration

Nanoparticle-based biosensors have gained considerable attention due to their broad applications across various scientific and technological fields. Metallic nanoparticles, owing to their unique optical and electronic properties, have found applications in multiple domains, including molecular positioning within electrode gaps [84]. Carbon nanotubes (CNTs) modified with biorecognition elements are particularly effective in designing nanostructured surfaces for sensor devices [85]. Additionally, nanophotonic devices, which manipulate light at sub-wavelength scales to enhance light–matter interactions, have led to the development of highly sensitive biosensors that address the limitations of traditional bioanalytical methods [86]. Micro-light-emitting diode (μLED) technology, incorporating nanomaterials and III-nitride nanostructures, has contributed to the creation of high-efficiency micro-LED displays [87].

Quantum Dot–Based Sensors

Quantum dot–based photoelectrochemical (PEC) sensors have emerged as powerful tools for detecting chemicals and biomolecules. These sensors operate by attaching quantum dots (QDs) to an electrode using a linker molecule. Upon illumination, QDs generate a photocurrent that corresponds to the type and concentration of the analyte present [88]. Fluorescent quantum dots, typically less than 10 nm in diameter, have played a foundational role in nanoscience and nanotechnology [89].

Incorporating QDs into three-dimensional (3D) hydrogel networks has proven highly effective, producing QD/hydrogel composites applicable in healthcare, energy, and environmental fields. These composites combine polymer and QD properties, facilitating applications in catalysis, energy storage, nanomedicine, electronic skin, and separation technologies [90]. Colloidal quantum dot (CQD)-based image sensors also provide unique advantages, such as solution processability, simple bandgap tunability across the short-wave infrared (SWIR) spectrum, and large-scale manufacturing feasibility, making them ideal for light-emission applications, including displays [91].

Nanoparticle Signal Enhancement

Nanoparticle signal enhancement strategies have substantially improved detection limits in biosensing platforms. The incorporation of metallic nanoparticles, particularly in surface plasmon resonance (SPR)-based sensors, has enabled single-molecule detection capabilities [92]. Beyond nanomaterial benefits, leveraging phase information from reflected light further enhances SPR sensitivity. Phase-sensitive SPR sensors detect subtle changes in external target properties that conventional SPR methods cannot [92]. Additionally, advances in nanomaterial-based electrochemiluminescence (ECL) systems focus on signal enhancement strategies, discussing their mechanisms and biosensing applications. These developments suggest future improvements in ECL signal performance, further strengthening biosensing capabilities [93].

Biosensor Miniaturization

The demand for point-of-care (POC) testing and wearable applications has driven the miniaturization of biosensors. Miniaturization enhances the signal-to-noise ratio by increasing signal density and reducing background noise, improving biosensor sensitivity and accuracy [94, 95]. Miniaturized biosensors enable lightweight, portable, and cost-effective diagnostic systems. Reduced material and manufacturing costs facilitate multiplexed and automated analyses. Innovations such as active fluidics, surface-based signal transduction, and distributed systems enhance biosensor efficiency, making them highly effective for real-time, high-precision applications [95]. Microfluidic biosensors, in particular, offer portability, controllability, and operational transparency, providing faster and more cost-effective sensing solutions compared to traditional bulky devices [96].

4.4.2 Emerging Sensing Platforms

Lab-on-a-Chip Technologies

Lab-on-a-chip (LOC) technology miniaturizes laboratory functions onto small chips, integrating processes such as polymerase chain reaction (PCR) and DNA sequencing. This miniaturization enhances cost-effectiveness, reduces reagent volumes, and enables high-parallelization, fast diagnostics, and high sensitivity [97]. LOC devices can be integrated with smartphones, creating portable and efficient systems for personalized medicine. This integration allows real-time diagnostics and monitoring, making healthcare more accessible and tailored to individual needs [98].

Microfluidic Biosensors

Microfluidics, a multidisciplinary technology, facilitates the manipulation of small fluid volumes in microscale channels, enhancing applications in diagnostics and medical devices. These structures provide a stable environment for biosensing reactions, improving sensitivity and reliability [99]. Recent advancements focus on electrochemical immunosensors and aptamer sensors, particularly for detecting diseases like melanoma. These microfluidic devices incorporate immunosensors to detect circulating tumor cells (CTCs) with high sensitivity. Utilizing pore-sized channel filters, these devices allow CTCs to pass while blocking larger cells. The detection of melanoma cells is achieved through antibody–antigen complexes, leading to electrochemical signal changes that enable precise disease monitoring [22, 100].

Wearable Diagnostic Devices

Wearable biosensors (WBSs) integrate sensors into body-worn devices such as tattoos, gloves, clothing, or implants. These devices facilitate real-time, noninvasive physiological monitoring [101]. Recent research has led to miniaturized wearable biosensors capable of detecting various physiological and biochemical markers, including glucose, dopamine, and ions, in biofluids like sweat, saliva, and tears. First-generation wearable biosensors primarily tracked biophysical parameters, such as heart rate and body temperature, while second-generation biosensors incorporate more invasive methods like microneedles and injectable devices for enhanced physiological data collection [102].

Wearable devices are increasingly used for remote clinical trial monitoring, particularly in cancer research. A study evaluating wearable interventions for lung cancer patients post-surgery found that patients using wearable devices exhibited improved physical function, reduced dyspnea, and less pain, highlighting their potential in patient recovery and rehabilitation [103].

Digital Health Integration

Digital health leverages technology to improve diagnosis, treatment, and health management through wearable devices, mobile apps, and telemedicine. Biosensors play a critical role in analyzing biomarkers in body fluids, enabling rapid and accurate diagnostics [104].

Machine learning (ML) and deep learning (DL) techniques are increasingly utilized for biomarker discovery. The integration of digital biomarkers, combining biological, neurological, socioeconomic, and environmental data, offers comprehensive disease analysis. Advances in next-generation sequencing and genomic research further enhance biomarker discovery, particularly in oncology, paving the way for improved early detection and personalized treatment [105].

4.5 Specific Cancer Diagnostic Applications

Early detection and continuous monitoring represent critical factors in improving cancer patient outcomes. Biosensor technologies have emerged as powerful tools addressing these fundamental clinical needs, offering innovative solutions for both initial diagnosis and disease progression tracking [106].

4.5.1 Early Cancer Detection

Screening Strategies

Early cancer detection through biosensor technologies has transformed screening approaches, particularly in high-risk populations.

Advanced screening strategies now incorporate ultrasensitive biosensors capable of detecting cancer biomarkers at previously undetectable levels [107, 108]. These platforms enable the identification of disease markers before conventional imaging techniques can reveal structural changes, significantly improving early intervention possibilities [109].

Ultra-Early Biomarker Identification

Ultra-early biomarker identification has become increasingly precise through the integration of multiplexed biosensor systems [110]. These platforms can simultaneously monitor multiple cancer-specific markers, including circulating tumor DNA, protein signatures, and metabolic indicators. This comprehensive approach significantly reduces false-positive rates while maintaining high sensitivity, addressing a long-standing challenge in cancer diagnostics [111].

High-Risk Population Monitoring

High-risk population monitoring has benefited substantially from the development of rapid, cost-effective biosensor platforms [112, 113]. These systems enable regular screening programs that were previously impractical due to cost or complexity constraints. The implementation of point-of-care biosensors has made routine screening more accessible, particularly in resource-limited settings [113, 114].

Minimally Invasive Detection Approaches

Minimally invasive detection approaches have expanded through the development of liquid biopsy–compatible biosensors [115]. These platforms can detect cancer markers in blood, urine, or saliva samples, reducing the need for traditional tissue biopsies and enabling more frequent monitoring without patient discomfort [116, 117].

4.5.2 Cancer Progression Monitoring

Treatment Response Tracking
Treatment response tracking has been revolutionized by real-time biosensor monitoring capabilities. These systems enable clinicians to assess therapeutic efficacy promptly, allowing for rapid adjustment of treatment strategies when necessary. Continuous monitoring of cancer markers provides immediate feedback on treatment effectiveness, potentially improving patient outcomes through more responsive care protocols [118].

Recurrence Detection
Recurrence detection has become more reliable through the implementation of highly sensitive biosensor platforms. These systems can detect minimal residual disease markers, enabling earlier identification of cancer recurrence and more timely intervention. Regular monitoring using biosensors has proven particularly valuable during the critical posttreatment period [119, 120].

Metastasis Monitoring
Metastasis monitoring through biosensor technology has enhanced the ability to track disease spread. Advanced biosensing platforms can detect circulating tumor cells and other metastasis-associated markers, providing crucial information about disease progression and potential secondary site development [121].

Personalized Treatment Guidance
Personalized treatment guidance has been significantly enhanced by biosensor data integration with patient-specific factors. These platforms enable real-time monitoring of individual patient responses to therapy, facilitating more precise treatment adjustment [122]. The combination of biosensor data with other clinical parameters has improved the ability to predict treatment outcomes and optimize therapeutic strategies [123].

4.6 Technological Challenges and Innovations

The development of biosensor technologies for cancer diagnostics faces several significant technological challenges while simultaneously benefiting from innovative solutions that continue to emerge. Understanding these challenges and their potential solutions is crucial for advancing the field and improving clinical outcomes [124, 125].

4.6.1 Current Limitations

Sensitivity Constraints

Sensitivity constraints remain a primary challenge in biosensor development. Despite significant advances, detecting extremely low concentrations of cancer biomarkers in complex biological samples continues to be difficult. This challenge becomes particularly acute in early-stage cancer detection, where biomarker concentrations may be below current detection thresholds [126, 127].

Specificity Challenges

Specificity challenges persist due to the complex nature of biological samples and the presence of potentially interfering substances. Achieving highly specific detection while maintaining sensitivity has proven challenging, especially in multiplex detection systems where cross-reactivity between different biomarkers can occur [128, 129].

Sample Preparation Complexities

Sample preparation complexities present significant obstacles to widespread biosensor implementation. The need for complex sample processing steps can limit the practical utility of biosensors, particularly in point-of-care settings. Additionally, variations in sample quality and composition can affect sensor performance and reliability [14, 130, 131].

Standardization Issues

Standardization issues continue to impact biosensor development and clinical implementation. The lack of standardized protocols for biosensor validation and calibration has led to difficulties in comparing results across different platforms and laboratories. This challenge particularly affects the clinical translation of promising biosensor technologies [132].

4.6.2 Emerging Solutions

Advanced Signal Processing

Advanced signal processing techniques have emerged as powerful tools for addressing sensitivity and specificity limitations. Digital signal processing algorithms can now effectively filter out background noise and enhance genuine signals, improving overall detection capabilities [133]. These approaches have particularly benefited from the integration of artificial intelligence and machine learning technologies.

Machine Learning Integration

Machine learning integration has revolutionized data analysis in biosensor applications. Advanced algorithms can now identify subtle patterns in biosensor signals that might be imperceptible through conventional analysis methods. This capability has significantly improved both the sensitivity and specificity of biosensor platforms [134].

Artificial Intelligence in Biomarker Analysis
Artificial intelligence in biomarker analysis has enabled more sophisticated interpretation of complex biosensor data. AI systems can now correlate multiple biomarker signals with clinical outcomes, improving diagnostic accuracy and reliability. These systems have proven particularly valuable in identifying early disease indicators and predicting disease progression [135].

Computational Prediction Models
Computational prediction models have enhanced biosensor design and optimization. These models can simulate biosensor performance under various conditions, enabling more efficient development cycles and improved sensor designs [136]. Additionally, predictive modeling has facilitated the identification of optimal operating parameters and potential performance limitations [137]. These technological innovations continue to drive improvements in biosensor performance and reliability. The integration of advanced computational approaches with traditional biosensing principles has created new opportunities for overcoming long-standing challenges in cancer diagnostics. As these technologies mature, they are expected to enable increasingly sophisticated and reliable cancer detection and monitoring capabilities.

4.7 Clinical Translation and Validation

The successful translation of biosensor technologies from laboratory development to clinical implementation requires careful consideration of regulatory requirements, validation protocols, and implementation strategies [138].

4.7.1 Regulatory Considerations

FDA Approval Processes
FDA approval processes for biosensor-based diagnostic devices follow stringent pathways that evaluate safety, efficacy, and reliability. These processes typically require extensive documentation of analytical validation, clinical performance data, and quality control measures. Medical device classifications determine the specific regulatory requirements, with most cancer diagnostic biosensors falling under class II or III categories, necessitating thorough premarket approval [139, 140].

Clinical Validation Protocols
Clinical validation protocols must demonstrate both analytical and clinical validity. These protocols evaluate sensitivity, specificity, reproducibility, and reliability under actual clinical conditions. The validation process includes rigorous testing

across diverse patient populations and comparison with existing gold standard diagnostic methods to establish clinical equivalence or superiority [141–143].

Ethical Considerations

Ethical considerations in biosensor implementation encompass patient privacy, data security, and informed consent requirements. The collection and storage of genetic and molecular diagnostic information require robust protection measures and clear protocols for data handling and patient confidentiality [144].

Standardization Frameworks

Standardization frameworks ensure consistency in biosensor performance across different clinical settings. These frameworks establish quality control measures, calibration protocols, and performance metrics that enable a reliable comparison of results between different facilities and laboratories [35, 145].

4.7.2 Translational Research

From Bench to Bedside

The path from bench to bedside requires coordinated efforts across multiple disciplines. Successful translation depends on close collaboration between bioengineers, clinicians, and healthcare administrators to address practical implementation challenges and optimize device performance in clinical settings [146, 147].

Interdisciplinary Collaboration

Interdisciplinary collaboration brings together expertise from various fields, including biomedical engineering, oncology, pathology, and healthcare informatics. This collaborative approach ensures that biosensor development addresses real clinical needs while maintaining technical feasibility and practical utility [148].

Economic Considerations

Economic considerations significantly influence the adoption of new biosensor technologies. Cost-effectiveness analyses must demonstrate clear value propositions, considering factors such as device costs, operational expenses, and potential healthcare savings through improved early detection and monitoring capabilities [130].

Implementation Strategies

Implementation strategies focus on integrating biosensor technologies into existing clinical workflows. These strategies address practical aspects such as staff training, quality control procedures, and integration with current laboratory information systems. Successful implementation requires careful planning to minimize disruption while maximizing the benefits of new diagnostic capabilities [149]. The continued advancement of biosensor technologies in clinical settings relies on maintaining a balance between innovation and practical implementation considerations. As these technologies mature, established validation frameworks and implementation strategies will facilitate their broader adoption in cancer diagnostics and monitoring [150].

4.8 Future Perspectives

The future of biosensor-based cancer diagnostics presents unprecedented opportunities for transforming healthcare delivery and patient outcomes [151].

4.8.1 Emerging Technologies

Artificial intelligence integration continues to advance rapidly, with machine learning algorithms becoming increasingly sophisticated in interpreting complex biosensor data patterns. These developments promise to enhance diagnostic accuracy and enable predictive analytics for disease progression. The integration of quantum computing may further revolutionize data processing capabilities, allowing for real-time analysis of complex biomarker patterns [152–154]. Quantum sensing technologies represent a frontier in biosensor development, potentially offering unprecedented sensitivity levels through quantum effects. These advanced sensing mechanisms could enable single-molecule detection with perfect specificity, revolutionizing early cancer detection capabilities [155–157]. Personalized diagnostic platforms are evolving toward fully integrated systems that can account for individual genetic profiles and environmental factors. These platforms will likely incorporate multiple sensing modalities and real-time data analysis, providing comprehensive health monitoring solutions [158].

4.8.2 Transformative Potential

Precision oncology will benefit significantly from these technological advances, enabling truly personalized treatment approaches based on continuous, real-time monitoring of cancer biomarkers. This capability will allow for immediate treatment adjustments and improved patient outcomes. Early intervention strategies will be transformed by the ability to detect cancer at increasingly earlier stages. Ultrasensitive biosensors, combined with advanced data analytics, will enable intervention before traditional symptoms appear, potentially revolutionizing cancer survival rates [159]. Cost-effective diagnostics will become increasingly accessible as manufacturing technologies advance and economies of scale take effect. This development will particularly impact global healthcare delivery, making advanced cancer diagnostics available in resource-limited settings. The global healthcare impact of these advances promises to be substantial, potentially reducing cancer mortality rates through earlier detection and more effective treatment monitoring. As these technologies mature, they will likely reshape the landscape of cancer diagnostics and treatment strategies worldwide [162].

4.9 Conclusion

Biosensors have become revolutionary instruments in the field of cancer diagnosis, filling important gaps left by conventional diagnostic techniques. They present previously unheard-of possibilities for early detection, real-time monitoring, and individualized treatment strategies due to their great sensitivity and specificity in identifying cancer biomarkers. The efficiency, portability, and accessibility of biosensor technologies have been further improved by developments like the incorporation of nanomaterials, artificial intelligence, and microfluidics. These developments have unlocked access to cutting-edge cancer care by making noninvasive detection and point-of-care diagnostics more practical, especially in environments with limited resources. Although issues like sensitivity, specificity, and standardization still exist, new developments in downsizing, machine learning, and signal amplification hold hope for overcoming these constraints. With further development, biosensor technologies have the potential to transform cancer diagnosis and eventually improve patient outcomes by enabling earlier interventions, more accurate treatments, and improved disease management techniques. Their incorporation into standard clinical practice around the world has enormous potential for the future.

References

1. Bhardwaj H, Archana, Noumani A, Himanshu JK, Chakravorty S, Solanki PR. Recent advancement in the detection of potential cancer biomarkers using the nanomaterial integrated electrochemical sensing technique: a detailed review. Mater Adv. 2024;5:475–503.
2. Varnakavi N, Lee N. A review on biosensors and recent development of nanostructured materials-enabled biosensors. Sensors. 2021;21:1109.
3. Karunakaran C, Rajkumar R, Bhargava K. Introduction to biosensors. In: Biosensors and bioelectronics. Elsevier; 2015. p. 1–68.
4. Thomas S, Saji KJ, Jayaraj MK. An introduction to biosensors. In: Nanomaterials for sensing and optoelectronic applications. Elsevier; 2022. p. 91–107.
5. Tetyana P, Shumbula M, Njengele-Tetyana Z. Biosensors: design, development and applications.
6. Korotkaya E. Biosensors: design, classification, and applications in the food industry. Foods Raw Mater. 2014;2:161–71.
7. Tripathi MK, Nickhil C, Kate A, Srivastva RM, Mohapatra D, Jadam RS, Yadav A, Modhera B. Biosensor: fundamentals, biomolecular component, and applications. In: Advances in biomedical polymers and composites. Elsevier; 2023. p. 617–33.
8. Chadha U, Bhardwaj P, Agarwal R, et al. Recent progress and growth in biosensors technology: a critical review. J Ind Eng Chem. 2022;109:21–51.
9. Atta NF, Galal A, Ali S. Nanobiosensors for health care. In: Biosensors for Health, Environment and Biosecurity; 2011. https://doi.org/10.5772/17996.
10. Yadav S, Saini A, Devi R, Lata S. Transducers in biosensors. In: Biomaterials-based sensors. Singapore: Springer; 2023. p. 101–25.
11. Kumar Kundu B. Introduction to sensors and types of biosensors. In: Multifaceted biosensing technology. Elsevier; 2023. p. 1–12.
12. Lino C, Barrias S, Chaves R, Adega F, Martins-Lopes P, Fernandes JR. Biosensors as diagnostic tools in clinical applications. Biochimica Biophysica Acta Rev Cancer. 2022;1877:188726.
13. Haleem A, Javaid M, Singh RP, Suman R, Rab S. Biosensors applications in medical field: a brief review. Sensors International. 2021;2:100100.

14. Bhatia D, Paul S, Acharjee T, Ramachairy SS. Biosensors and their widespread impact on human health. Sensors International. 2024;5:100257.
15. Shafiee A, Ghadiri E, Kassis J, Pourhabibi Zarandi N, Atala A. Biosensing technologies for medical applications, manufacturing, and regenerative medicine. Curr Stem Cell Rep. 2018;4:105–15.
16. Mascini M. A brief story of biosensor technology. In: Biotechnological applications of photosynthetic proteins: biochips, biosensors and biodevices. Springer; 2007. p. 4–10.
17. Clark LC, Kaplan S, Matthews EC, Edwards PK, Helmsworth JA. Monitor and control of blood oxygen tension and pH during total body perfusion. Journal of Thoracic Surgery. 1958;36:488–96.
18. Liu X, Jiang H, Wang X. Advances in cancer research: current and future diagnostic and therapeutic strategies. Biosensors (Basel). 2024;14:100.
19. Bi WL, Hosny A, Schabath MB, et al. Artificial intelligence in cancer imaging: clinical challenges and applications. CA Cancer J Clin. 2019;69:127–57.
20. Haber DA, Velculescu VE. Blood-based analyses of cancer: circulating tumor cells and circulating tumor DNA. Cancer Discov. 2014;4:650–61.
21. Elbasiony AM, Alharthi S, Mohamady Ghobashy M, Boraie WE, Attia MS, Madani M, Ali Al-Gahtany S, Darwesh R, Shaban M, Sharshir AI. Development and application of novel biosensors for enhanced detection in medical diagnostics. Microchem J. 2024;207:111938.
22. Liu Z, Zhou Y, Lu J, Gong T, Ibáñez E, Cifuentes A, Lu W. Microfluidic biosensors for biomarker detection in body fluids: a key approach for early cancer diagnosis. Biomark Res. 2024;12:153.
23. Pandey A, Gupta SP. Personalized medicine: a comprehensive review. Orient J Chem. 2024;40:933–44.
24. Purohit B, Kumar A, Mahato K, Chandra P. Smartphone-assisted personalized diagnostic devices and wearable sensors. Curr Opin Biomed Eng. 2020;13:42–50.
25. Kim J, Jeong J, Ko SH. Electrochemical biosensors for point-of-care testing. Biodes Manuf. 2024;7:548–65.
26. Huang C-W, Lin C, Nguyen MK, Hussain A, Bui X-T, Ngo HH. A review of biosensor for environmental monitoring: principle, application, and corresponding achievement of sustainable development goals. Bioengineered. 2023;14:58–80.
27. Chaubey A, Malhotra BD. Mediated biosensors. Biosens Bioelectron. 2002;17:441–56.
28. Wu Q, Zhang Y, Yang Q, Yuan N, Zhang W. Review of electrochemical DNA biosensors for detecting food borne pathogens. Sensors. 2019;19:4916.
29. Wahid Anwar A, Anwar Z, Dildar I, Ali N, Uzba, Ahsan K. Biosensing basics; 2024. https://doi.org/10.5772/intechopen.113771.
30. Sande MG, Rodrigues JL, Ferreira D, Silva CJ, Rodrigues LR. Novel biorecognition elements against pathogens in the design of state-of-the-art diagnostics. Biosensors (Basel). 2021;11:418.
31. Thévenot DR, Toth K, Durst RA, Wilson GS. Electrochemical biosensors: recommended definitions and classification1International Union of Pure and Applied Chemistry: Physical Chemistry Division, Commission I.7 (Biophysical Chemistry); Analytical Chemistry Division, Commission V.5 (Electroanalytical Chemistry).1. Biosens Bioelectron. 2001;16:121–31.
32. Chandrasekar S. Core components of a biosensor biosensors consist of three primary components: the bioreceptor, transducer, and signal.
33. Schackart KE, Yoon J-Y. Machine learning enhances the performance of bioreceptor-free biosensors. Sensors. 2021;21:5519.
34. Haniff Bin Ghazali M, Vajravelu A, Binti Othman N, Muhammad Hazli Bin Mazlan T, Ahmed Gilani Mohamed M, Onn Malaysia H, Pahat B. Fundamentals of biosensor-an introduction with its applications in the engineering perspective. International Journal of Advances in Engineering and Management (IJAEM). 2021;3:249.
35. Bhalla N, Jolly P, Formisano N, Estrela P. Introduction to biosensors. Essays Biochem. 2016;60:1–8.

36. Senveli SU, Tigli O. Biosensors in the small scale: methods and technology trends. IET Nanobiotechnol. 2013;7:7–21.
37. Malhotra S, Verma A, Tyagi N, Kumar V. Bionsensors: principle, types and applications. 2017.
38. Lazcka O, Del Campo FJ, Muñoz FX. Pathogen detection: a perspective of traditional methods and biosensors. Biosens Bioelectron. 2007;22:1205–17.
39. Watts HJ, Lowe CR, Pollard-Knight DV. Optical biosensor for monitoring microbial cells. Anal Chem. 1994;66:2465–70.
40. Davis J, Bunglavan SJ. Biosensors: a novel approach for pathogen detection.
41. Grieshaber D, Mackenzie R, Vörös J, Reimhult E. Electrochemical biosensors-sensor principles and architectures. Sensors. 2008;8:1400–58.
42. Kazemi-Darsanaki R, Azizzadeh A, Nourbakhsh M, Raeisi G, AzizollahiAliabadi M. Biosensors: functions and applications. Journal of Biology and Today's World. 2013; https://doi.org/10.15412/j.jbtw.01020105.
43. Huet A-C, Delahaut P, Fodey T, Haughey SA, Elliott C, Weigel S. Advances in biosensor-based analysis for antimicrobial residues in foods. TrAC Trends Anal Chem. 2010;29:1281–94.
44. Skládal P. Piezoelectric biosensors. TrAC Trends Anal Chem. 2016;79:127–33.
45. Pohanka M. The piezoelectric biosensors: principles and applications, a review. Int J Electrochem Sci. 2017;12:496–506.
46. Sivarajasekar N, Dharshni RA, Dharshini R. Thermal biosensors and their applications. American International Journal of Research in Science. 2019;50
47. Rivero G, Multigner M, Spottorno J. Magnetic sensors for biomedical applications. In: Magnetic sensors – principles and applications; 2012. https://doi.org/10.5772/37285.
48. Llandro J, Palfreyman JJ, Ionescu A, Barnes CHW. Magnetic biosensor technologies for medical applications: a review. Med Biol Eng Comput. 2010;48:977–98.
49. Wang C, Liu M, Wang Z, Li S, Deng Y, He N. Point-of-care diagnostics for infectious diseases: from methods to devices. Nano Today. 2021; https://doi.org/10.1016/j.nantod.2021.101092.
50. Nimse SB, Sonawane MD, Song K-S, Kim T. Biomarker detection technologies and future directions. Analyst. 2016;141:740–55.
51. Tangella LP, Clark ME, Gray ES. Resistance mechanisms to targeted therapy in BRAF-mutant melanoma – a mini review. Biochim Biophys Acta (BBA) General Subjects. 2021;1865:129736.
52. Passaro A, Mok T, Peters S, Popat S, Ahn M-J, de Marinis F. Recent advances on the role of EGFR tyrosine kinase inhibitors in the management of NSCLC with uncommon, non exon 20 insertions, EGFR mutations. J Thorac Oncol. 2021;16:764–73.
53. Zenonos K. RAS signaling pathways, mutations and their role in colorectal cancer. World J Gastrointest Oncol. 2013;5:97.
54. Pujol P, Barberis M, Beer P, et al. Clinical practice guidelines for BRCA1 and BRCA2 genetic testing. Eur J Cancer. 2021;146:30–47.
55. Amisha F, Malik P, Saluja P, Gautam N, Patel TH, Roy AM, Singh SRK, Malapati SJ. A comprehensive review on the role of human epidermal growth factor receptor 2 (HER2) as a biomarker in extra-mammary and extra-gastric cancers. Onco. 2023;3:96–124.
56. Ma R, de Pennington N, Hofer M, Blesing C, Stacey R. Diagnostic and prognostic markers in gliomas – an update. Br J Neurosurg. 2013;27:311–5.
57. Das S, Dey MK, Devireddy R, Gartia MR. Biomarkers in cancer detection, diagnosis, and prognosis. Sensors. 2023;24:37.
58. Anderson NL, Anderson NG. The human plasma proteome. Mol Cell Proteomics. 2002;1:845–67.
59. Colantonio DA, Chan DW. The clinical application of proteomics. Clin Chim Acta. 2005;357:151–8.
60. Pérez-Ibave DC, Burciaga-Flores CH, Elizondo-Riojas MÁ. Prostate-specific antigen (PSA) as a possible biomarker in non-prostatic cancer: a review. Cancer Epidemiol. 2018;54:48–55.

61. Rashid S, Sun Y, Ali Khan Saddozai U, Hayyat S, Munir MU, Akbar MU, Khawar MB, Ren Z, Ji X, Ihsan Ullah Khan M. Circulating tumor DNA and its role in detection, prognosis and therapeutics of hepatocellular carcinoma. Chin J Cancer Res. 2024;36:195–214.
62. Markus H, Chandrananda D, Moore E, Mouliere F, Morris J, Brenton JD, Smith CG, Rosenfeld N. Refined characterization of circulating tumor DNA through biological feature integration. Sci Rep. 2022;12:1928.
63. Xu J, Gao H, Guan X, Meng J, Ding S, Long Q, Yi W. Circulating tumor DNA: from discovery to clinical application in breast cancer. Front Immunol. 2024; https://doi.org/10.3389/fimmu.2024.1355887.
64. Parkinson CA, Gale D, Piskorz AM, et al. Exploratory Analysis of TP53 Mutations in Circulating Tumour DNA as Biomarkers of Treatment Response for Patients with Relapsed High-Grade Serous Ovarian Carcinoma: A Retrospective Study. PLoS Med. 2016;13:e1002198.
65. Kim J-H, Kim E, Lee MY. Exosomes as diagnostic biomarkers in cancer. Mol Cell Toxicol. 2018;14:113–22.
66. Nedaeinia R, Manian M, Jazayeri MH, et al. Circulating exosomes and exosomal microRNAs as biomarkers in gastrointestinal cancer. Cancer Gene Ther. 2017;24:48–56.
67. Jiang L, Gu Y, Du Y, Liu J. Exosomes: diagnostic biomarkers and therapeutic delivery vehicles for cancer. Mol Pharm. 2019;16:3333–49.
68. Makler A, Narayanan R. Mining exosomal genes for pancreatic cancer targets. Cancer Genomics Proteomics. 2017;14:161–72.
69. Boukouris S, Mathivanan S. Exosomes in bodily fluids are a highly stable resource of disease biomarkers. Proteomics Clin Appl. 2015;9:358–67.
70. Falcon-Perez J. Exosome profiling: potential in cancer diagnosis and stratification. Endocr Abstr. 2017; https://doi.org/10.1530/endoabs.49.NSA2.
71. Arora T, Kaur M, Nand P. Nanomaterial-enhanced sensors for biomarker detection: improving accuracy and feasibility for point-of-care early detection devices. 2025.
72. Rathinavel S, Priyadharshini K, Panda D. A review on carbon nanotube: An overview of synthesis, properties, functionalization, characterization, and the application. Mater Sci Eng B. 2021;268:115095.
73. Wagner MK, Li F, Li J, Li X-F, Le XC. Use of quantum dots in the development of assays for cancer biomarkers. Anal Bioanal Chem. 2010;397:3213–24.
74. Saharan R, Paliwal SK, Tiwari A, Tiwari V, Singh R, Beniwal SK, Dahiya P, Sagadevan S. Exploring graphene and its potential in delivery of drugs and biomolecules. J Drug Deliv Sci Technol. 2023;84:104446.
75. Magne TM, de Oliveira Vieira T, Alencar LMR, et al. Graphene and its derivatives: understanding the main chemical and medicinal chemistry roles for biomedical applications. J Nanostructure Chem. 2022;12:693–727.
76. Wu Y, Zhou Y, Leng Y, Lai W, Huang X, Xiong Y. Emerging design strategies for constructing multiplex lateral flow test strip sensors. Biosens Bioelectron. 2020;157:112168.
77. Dincer C, Bruch R, Kling A, Dittrich PS, Urban GA. Multiplexed point-of-care testing – xPOCT. Trends Biotechnol. 2017;35:728–42.
78. Kelley SO. What are clinically relevant levels of cellular and biomolecular analytes? ACS Sens. 2017;2:193–7.
79. Bao C, Deng L, Huang F, Yang M, Li X. Signal amplification strategies in photoelectrochemical sensing of carcinoembryonic antigen. Biosens Bioelectron. 2024;262:116543.
80. Cajigas S, Soto D, Orozco J. Biosensors: biosensors with signal amplification. In: Encyclopedia of sensors and biosensors. Elsevier; 2023. p. 429–57.
81. Yang L, Zhang S, Liu X, Tang Y, Zhou Y, Wong DKY. Detection signal amplification strategies at nanomaterial-based photoelectrochemical biosensors. J Mater Chem B. 2020;8:7880–93.
82. Zhou X, Schuh DA, Castle LM, Furst AL. Recent advances in signal amplification to improve electrochemical biosensing for infectious diseases. Front Chem. 2022; https://doi.org/10.3389/fchem.2022.911678.

83. Mohankumar P, Ajayan J, Mohanraj T, Yasodharan R. Recent developments in biosensors for healthcare and biomedical applications: a review. Measurement. 2021;167:108293.
84. Dahman Y. Nanoparticles**By Yaser Dahman, Hoda Javaheri, Jiafu Chen, and Basel Al-Chikh Sulaiman. In: Nanotechnology and functional materials for engineers. Elsevier; 2017. p. 93–119.
85. Boujtita M. Chemical and biological sensing with carbon nanotubes (CNTs). In: Nanosensors for chemical and biological applications. Elsevier; 2014. p. 3–27.
86. Altug H, Oh S-H, Maier SA, Homola J. Advances and applications of nanophotonic biosensors. Nat Nanotechnol. 2022;17:5–16.
87. Mishra RK, Verma K, Chianella I, Goel S, Nezhad HY. Nanomaterial integration in micro LED technology: enhancing efficiency and applications. Next Nanotechnology. 2024;5:100056.
88. Yue Z, Lisdat F, Parak WJ, Hickey SG, Tu L, Sabir N, Dorfs D, Bigall NC. Quantum-dot-based photoelectrochemical sensors for chemical and biological detection. ACS Appl Mater Interfaces. 2013;5:2800–14.
89. Farzin MA, Abdoos H. A critical review on quantum dots: From synthesis toward applications in electrochemical biosensors for determination of disease-related biomolecules. Talanta. 2021;224:121828.
90. Zhang J, Jin J, Wan J, Jiang S, Wu Y, Wang W, Gong X, Wang H. Quantum dots-based hydrogels for sensing applications. Chem Eng J. 2021;408:127351.
91. Goossens S, Konstantatos G, Oikonomou A. Colloidal quantum dot image sensors: technology and marketplace opportunities. Inf Disp (1975). 2021;37:18–23.
92. Mohammadzadeh-Asl S, Keshtkar A, Ezzati Nazhad Dolatabadi J, de la Guardia M. Nanomaterials and phase sensitive based signal enhancement in surface Plasmon resonance. Biosens Bioelectron. 2018;110:118–31.
93. Yin F, Sun Q, Huang X, Wu G, Zhang Y, Shen Y. Recent progress in signal enhancement of nanomaterials-based electrochemiluminescence systems. TrAC Trends Anal Chem. 2023;169:117376.
94. Liu D, Wang J, Wu L, Huang Y, Zhang Y, Zhu M, Wang Y, Zhu Z, Yang C. Trends in miniaturized biosensors for point-of-care testing. TrAC Trends Anal Chem. 2020;122:115701.
95. Soleymani L, Li F. Mechanistic challenges and advantages of biosensor miniaturization into the nanoscale. ACS Sens. 2017;2:458–67.
96. Kulkarni MB, Ayachit NH, Aminabhavi TM. Biosensors and microfluidic biosensors: from fabrication to application. Biosensors (Basel). 2022;12:543.
97. Yılmaz B, Yılmaz F. Lab-on-a-chip technology and its applications. In: Omics technologies and bio-engineering. Elsevier; 2018. p. 145–53.
98. Kuru Cİ, Ulucan-Karnak F, Akgöl S. Lab-on-a-chip sensors. In: Fundamentals of sensor technology. Elsevier; 2023. p. 65–98.
99. Wang J, Ren L, Li L, Liu W, Zhou J, Yu W, Tong D, Chen S. Microfluidics: a new cosset for neurobiology. Lab Chip. 2009;9:644–52.
100. Anu Prathap MU, Castro-Pérez E, Jiménez-Torres JA, Setaluri V, Gunasekaran S. A flow-through microfluidic system for the detection of circulating melanoma cells. Biosens Bioelectron. 2019;142:111522.
101. Sharma A, Badea M, Tiwari S, Marty JL. Wearable Biosensors: An Alternative and Practical Approach in Healthcare and Disease Monitoring. Molecules. 2021;26:748.
102. Erdem A, Eksin E, Senturk H, Yildiz E, Maral M. Recent developments in wearable biosensors for healthcare and biomedical applications. TrAC Trends Anal Chem. 2024;171:117510.
103. Lee J, Kong S, Shin S, Lee G, Kim HK, Shim YM, Cho J, Kang D, Park HY. Wearable device-based intervention for promoting patient physical activity after lung cancer surgery: a nonrandomized clinical trial. JAMA Netw Open. 2024;7:e2434180.
104. Fatehi F, Samadbeik M, Kazemi A. What is digital health? Review of definitions. 2020. https://doi.org/10.3233/SHTI200696.
105. Wasilewski T, Kamysz W, Gębicki J. AI-assisted detection of biomarkers by sensors and biosensors for early diagnosis and monitoring. Biosensors (Basel). 2024;14:356.

106. Milner DA, Lennerz JK. Technology and future of multi-cancer early detection. Life. 2024;14:833.
107. Chaudhry G-S, Akim AM, Safdar N, Yasmin A, Begum S, Sung YY, Muhammad TST. Cancer and disease diagnosis – biosensor as potential diagnostic tool for biomarker detection. J Adv Pharm Technol Res. 2022;13:243–7.
108. Mikaeeli Kangarshahi B, Naghib SM, Rabiee N. DNA/RNA-based electrochemical nanobiosensors for early detection of cancers. Crit Rev Clin Lab Sci. 2024;61:473–95.
109. Azab MY, Hameed MFO, Obayya SSA. Overview of optical biosensors for early cancer detection: fundamentals, applications and future perspectives. Biology (Basel). 2023;12:232.
110. Silva P, Homer JJ, Slevin NJ, Musgrove BT, Sloan P, Price P, West CML. Clinical and biological factors affecting response to radiotherapy in patients with head and neck cancer: a review. Clin Otolaryngol. 2007;32:337–45.
111. Budnik B, Amirkhani H, Forouzanfar MH, Afshin A. Novel proteomics-based plasma test for early detection of multiple cancers in the general population. BMJ Oncology. 2024;3:e000073.
112. Lowry KP, Lee JM, Kong CY, et al. Annual screening strategies in *BRCA1* and *BRCA2* gene mutation carriers. Cancer. 2012;118:2021–30.
113. Bevers TB, Niell BL, Baker JL, et al. NCCN Guidelines® insights: breast cancer screening and diagnosis, version 1.2023. J Natl Compr Cancer Netw. 2023;21:900–9.
114. Antoniou A, Pharoah PDP, Narod S, et al. Average risks of breast and ovarian cancer associated with BRCA1 or BRCA2 mutations detected in case series unselected for family history: a combined analysis of 22 studies. Am J Hum Genet. 2003;72:1117–30.
115. Gonzalez MA, Coleman N, Laskey RA. New minimally invasive approaches to early cancer detection. Eur Oncol Haematol. 2007:122.
116. Shen Y, Yang W, Liu J, Zhang Y. Minimally invasive approaches for the early detection of endometrial cancer. Mol Cancer. 2023; https://doi.org/10.1186/s12943-023-01757-3.
117. Porcaro F, Paolucci A, Porcaro P, Cardinale G, Romitelli A, Cozzolino D, Voccola S. Minimally invasive and emerging diagnostic approaches in endometrial cancer: epigenetic insights and the promise of DNA methylation. Diagnostics. 2024;14:2575.
118. Iqbal MJ, Javed Z, Herrera-Bravo J, et al. Biosensing chips for cancer diagnosis and treatment: a new wave towards clinical innovation. Cancer Cell Int. 2022; https://doi.org/10.1186/s12935-022-02777-7.
119. Hou JY, Chapman JS, Kalashnikova E, et al. Circulating tumor DNA monitoring for early recurrence detection in epithelial ovarian cancer. Gynecol Oncol. 2022;167:334–41.
120. Balasan N, Kharrat F, Di Lorenzo G, et al. Sensitive detection of gynecological cancer recurrence using circulating tumor DNA and digital PCR: a comparative study with serum biochemical markers. Int J Mol Sci. 2024;25:11997.
121. Prasad R, Peng B, Mendes BB, Kilian HI, Gorain M, Zhang H, Kundu GC, Xia J, Lovell JF, Conde J. Biomimetic bright optotheranostics for metastasis monitoring and multimodal image-guided breast cancer therapeutics. J Control Release. 2024;367:300–15.
122. Puccetti M, Pariano M, Schoubben A, Giovagnoli S, Ricci M. Biologics, theranostics, and personalized medicine in drug delivery systems. Pharmacol Res. 2024;201:107086.
123. Koulis C, Yap R, Engel R, Jardé T, Wilkins S, Solon G, Shapiro JD, Abud H, McMurrick P. Personalized medicine – current and emerging predictive and prognostic biomarkers in colorectal cancer. Cancers (Basel). 2020;12:812.
124. Sen M, Seth S. Current challenges and future prospects of biosensors. In: Fundamentals of biosensors in healthcare. Elsevier; 2025. p. 721–41.
125. Deshmukh A V, Hasbe SS, Hajare SS, Jadhav AS, Yadav AR. Current research trends, future challenges and limitations of biosensor technology. 2022.
126. Thusu R. Biosensors are poised for accelerated growth through 2025. 2021.
127. Shah SS, Senapati S, Klacsmann F, Miller DL, Johnson JJ, Chang HC, Stack MS. Current technologies and recent developments for screening of HPV-associated cervical and oropharyngeal cancers. Cancers (Basel). 2016; https://doi.org/10.3390/cancers8090085.
128. Wilkins E, Atanasov P. Glucose monitoring: state of the art and future possibilities. Med Eng Phys. 1996;18:273–88.

129. Polatoğlu İ, Aydın L, Nevruz BÇ, Özer S. A novel approach for the optimal design of a biosensor. Anal Lett. 2020;53:1428–45.
130. Sin ML, Mach KE, Wong PK, Liao JC. Advances and challenges in biosensor-based diagnosis of infectious diseases. Expert Rev Mol Diagn. 2014;14:225–44.
131. Kabay G, DeCastro J, Altay A, Smith K, Lu H, Capossela AM, Moarefian M, Aran K, Dincer C. Emerging biosensing technologies for the diagnostics of viral infectious diseases. Adv Mater. 2022; https://doi.org/10.1002/adma.202201085.
132. Wang S, Zheng Y, Wang Q. Technical standardization and total factor productivity in innovation-driven development: evidence from China. PLoS One. 2023;18:e0287109.
133. Beadle A. New breakthrough could lead to all-purpose biosensors moving away from single-analyte testing.
134. Cui F, Yue Y, Zhang Y, Zhang Z, Zhou HS. Advancing biosensors with machine learning. ACS Sens. 2020;5:3346–64.
135. Sarvesh Raikar G, Raikar AS, Somnache SN. Advancements in artificial intelligence and machine learning in revolutionising biomarker discovery. Braz J Pharm Sci. 2023; https://doi.org/10.1590/s2175-97902023e23146.
136. Khoshbin Z, Housaindokht MR, Izadyar M, Bozorgmehr MR, Verdian A. Recent advances in computational methods for biosensor design. Biotechnol Bioeng. 2021;118:555–78.
137. Aghajani J, Farnia P, Farnia P, Ghanavi J, Velayati AA. Molecular dynamic simulations and molecular docking as a potential way for designed new inhibitor drug without resistance. Tanaffos. 2022;21:1–14.
138. Fenster A. Clinical translation. In: Handbook of medical image computing and computer assisted intervention. Elsevier; 2020. p. 893–907.
139. Joshi G, Jain A, Araveeti SR, Adhikari S, Garg H, Bhandari M. FDA-approved artificial intelligence and machine learning (AI/ML)-enabled medical devices: an updated landscape. Electronics (Basel). 2024;13:498.
140. Van Norman GA. Drugs, devices, and the FDA: part 2. JACC Basic Transl Sci. 2016;1:277–87.
141. Goldsack JC, Coravos A, Bakker JP, et al. Verification, analytical validation, and clinical validation (V3): the foundation of determining fit-for-purpose for Biometric Monitoring Technologies (BioMeTs). NPJ Digit Med. 2020;3:55.
142. Gruson D, Cobbaert C, Dabla PK, Stankovic S, Homsak E, Kotani K, Samir Assaad R, Nichols JH, Gouget B. Validation and verification framework and data integration of biosensors and in vitro diagnostic devices: a position statement of the IFCC Committee on Mobile Health and Bioengineering in Laboratory Medicine (C-MBHLM) and the IFCC Scientific Division. Clinical Chemistry and Laboratory Medicine (CCLM). 2024;62:1904–17.
143. Ulrich CM, Demiris G, Kennedy R, Rothwell E. The ethics of sensor technology use in clinical research. Nurs Outlook. 2020;68:720–6.
144. Giorgi G, Tonello S. Wearable biosensor standardization: how to make them smarter. Standards. 2022;2:366–84.
145. Chandra P. Personalized biosensors for point-of-care diagnostics: from bench to bedside applications. Nano. 2023;7:210–5.
146. Fan C, Tamiya E. Editorial: translating the advances of biosensors from bench to bedside. Biotechnol J. 2016;11:727–8.
147. Patel S, Nanda R, Sahoo S, Mohapatra E. Biosensors in health care: the milestones achieved in their development towards lab-on-chip-analysis. Biochem Res Int. 2016;2016:1–12.
148. Devine JK, Schwartz LP, Hursh SR. Technical, regulatory, economic, and trust issues preventing successful integration of sensors into the mainstream consumer wearables market. Sensors. 2022;22:2731.
149. Prabowo BA, Cabral PD, Freitas P, Fernandes E. The Challenges of Developing Biosensors for Clinical Assessment: A Review. Chemosensors. 2021;9:299.
150. Fatima A, Younas I, Ali MW. An overview on recent advances in biosensor technology and its future application. Arch Pharm Pract. 2022;13:5–10.
151. Jin X, Liu C, Xu T, Su L, Zhang X. Artificial intelligence biosensors: challenges and prospects. Biosens Bioelectron. 2020;165:112412.

152. Flynn CD, Chang D. Artificial intelligence in point-of-care biosensing: challenges and opportunities. Diagnostics. 2024;14:1100.
153. Vo D-K, Trinh KTL. Advances in wearable biosensors for healthcare: current trends, applications, and future perspectives. Biosensors (Basel). 2024;14:560.
154. Aslam N, Zhou H, Urbach EK, Turner MJ, Walsworth RL, Lukin MD, Park H. Quantum sensors for biomedical applications. Nature Reviews Physics. 2023;5:157–69.
155. Bakhshandeh S. Quantum sensing goes bio. Nat Rev Mater. 2022;7:254.
156. Chicago Quantum Exchange. Quantum biosensing: medicine at the smallest scales. 2021.
157. Calabretta MM, Zangheri M, Lopreside A, Marchegiani E, Montali L, Simoni P, Roda A. Precision medicine, bioanalytics and nanomaterials: toward a new generation of personalized portable diagnostics. Analyst. 2020;145:2841–53.
158. Lawler M, Keeling P, Kholmanskikh O, et al. Empowering effective biomarker-driven precision oncology: a call to action. Eur J Cancer. 2024;209:114225.
159. AlDoughaim M, AlSuhebany N, AlZahrani M, AlQahtani T, AlGhamdi S, Badreldin H, Al Alshaykh H. Cancer biomarkers and precision oncology: a review of recent trends and innovations. Clin Med Insights Oncol. 2024; https://doi.org/10.1177/11795549241298541.

Aptamer-Based Biosensors for Cancer Diagnosis

5

Mayank Mishra, Sarasa Meenakshi, Santosh Kumar, and Nitesh Kumar

Abbreviations

LMICs	Low- and middle-income countries
NF-κB	Nuclear factor kappa B
SPR	Surface plasmon resonance
HER2	Human epidermal growth factor receptor 2
CTC	Circulating tumor cell
TISS	Target-induced structure switching
TID	Target-induced dissociation
CRC	Colorectal cancer
ELISA	Enzyme-linked immunosorbent assay
HRP	Horseradish peroxidase
AuNP	Gold nanoparticle

The original version of the chapter has been revised. A correction to this chapter can be found at https://doi.org/10.1007/978-981-96-8387-1_15

Authors Mayank Mishra and Sarasa Meenakshi have equally contributed to this chapter.

M. Mishra · N. Kumar (✉)
Department of Pharmacology and Toxicology, National Institute of Pharmaceutical Education and Research (NIPER), Hajipur, Bihar, India

S. Meenakshi
Department of Pharmacy Practice, National Institute of Pharmaceutical Education and Research (NIPER), Hajipur, Bihar, India

S. Kumar
Division of Cardiovascular Medicine, Carver College of Medicine, University of Iowa, Iowa City, IA, USA
e-mail: santosh-kumar@uiowa.edu

S. Srivastava et al. (eds.), *Biosensors and Aptamers*,
https://doi.org/10.1007/978-981-96-8387-1_5

HCC	Hepatocellular carcinoma
NAB	Nanoparticle albumin-bound
siRNA	Small interfering RNA
SARS-CoV	Severe acute respiratory syndrome coronavirus 2
MERS-CoV	Middle East respiratory syndrome coronavirus
AI	Artificial intelligence
ssDNA	Single-stranded DNA
PCR	Polymerase chain reaction
AFP	Alpha-fetoprotein
CEA	Carcinoembryonic antigen

Overview
This chapter examines the critical role of "aptamer-driven biosensors" in enhancing cancer diagnosis. Aptamers are known for their exceptional specificity, stability, and versatility and are revolutionizing the detection of cancer biomarkers, such as human epidermal growth factor receptor 2 (HER2), alpha-fetoprotein (AFP), and carcinoembryonic antigen (CEA). The chapter describes the methods by which these biosensors enable precise, timely, and economical cancer detection. Their applications in point-of-care (POC) portable diagnostic devices, noninvasive liquid biopsies, and the early detection of diseases are reviewed. Aptamer-based biosensors offer innovative possibilities for treating cancer with personalized strategies through the advantages of biosensing over conventional detection methods. It is underlined how essential these are for patient outcomes and accurate diagnosis worldwide.

5.1 Introduction

Despite its growing influence on public health, cancer has been generally ignored by international funders and policymakers for many years. Cancer is responsible for the death of about 8.8 million people every year, which means one in six. Low- and middle-income countries (LMICs) have the most significant burden in terms of cancer-related deaths, reaching 75%. These developing regions also have the highest number of cases of cancer diagnosed globally [1]. In 2020, approximately 19.3 million new cases of cancer were reported, and the disease accounted for almost ten million deaths, GLOBOCAN reports. It is estimated that by 2040, there will be 28.4 million cases of cancer [2]. The most frequently diagnosed cancer is female breast cancer, which accounts for 11.7% of cases, surpassing lung cancer by 11.4%, This is followed by colorectal cancer (CRC) at 10.0%, prostate cancer at 7.3%, and stomach cancer at 5.6%. Lung cancer continues to dominate as the leading cause of death among cancer cases, with 1.8 million deaths, at 18%. The second leading cancer is colorectal cancer at 9.4%, followed by liver and stomach cancers, both ranking at 7.7%, and the fifth cancer is female breast cancer at 6.9%. Lung, prostate, and colorectal cancers are the most common in men, while breast, colorectal, and lung cancers are the most common in women. Worldwide, the top ten malignancies account for 70% of cancer-related deaths and more than 60% of cancer diagnoses [3]. The first thing is to establish and implement effective cancer preventive technologies, especially for the most common cancers, including colorectal, lung, prostate, and breast cancers. When the local prevalence of cancers is high, appropriate targeted screening programs should be implemented in a region, such as oral cancer screening in India [4].

In most cases, traditional diagnostic methods, such as inspection and biopsy, often fail to detect oral malignancies at early and manageable stages. This flaw delays the diagnosis, negatively affecting patient outcomes [5]. Biosensors are highly accurate in converting specific biological activity into quantitative signals and provide clear advantages over more traditional analytical techniques, such as chromatography and enzyme-linked immunosorbent assay (ELISA), especially in terms of specificity for targets, high sensitivity, and the capability to detect changes in real time during biological processes [6, 7]. Aptamers have been used mainly in developing test techniques, especially in molecular analysis, disease diagnosis, and targeted drug delivery. When identifying protein biomarkers, aptamers are conjugated with proteins to create an aptamer–protein complex [8, 9].

5.2 Aptamers: A Revolutionary Biorecognition Element

5.2.1 Definition, Structure, Discovery, and Features of Aptamers

Aptamers are single-stranded oligonucleotides capable of folding into stable three-dimensional structures, and they are highly versatile in binding to a broad range of molecular targets with impressive affinity and specificity. In many aspects, aptamers are similar to antibodies as their capability to bind to their protein target and affect its function is identical. A closer look shows that high affinity and particular interactions between oligonucleotides and proteins are crucial to many biological processes, including transcription, translation, and RNA interference, even though the concept of oligonucleotides acting in this manner might seem surprising at first [10, 11]. Aptamers tend to recognize the positively charged surfaces of the target proteins due to contacts in their architecture. Because of the negatively charged backbones, electrostatic contacts have been observed between protein and aptamer complexes in crystal structures, including structures of thrombin, MS2 bacteriophage capsid, and nuclear factor kappa B (NF-κB) [12]. In these instances, thrombin has a positively charged surface where it binds to an aptamer, but that same surface must be available for binding heparin. At the same time, the nucleic acid–binding domains of NF-κB and the MS2 protein are available as sites for aptamer binding [13]. Altogether, these structures suggest that electrostatic forces are key to the strong affinity of aptamers toward their target. Several of their advantages, like physicochemical characteristics, ease of synthesis and manufacturing, cost-effectiveness, flexibility in structure, lower degree of immunogenicity, and increased stability, make aptamers an attractive substitute for biological ligands such as peptides and antibodies [14].

5.2.2 SELEX: Key Technique in Aptamer Selection

Szostak and Gold published the first studies describing aptamers generated by the in vitro selection method, otherwise known as the Systematic Evolution of Ligands by Exponential Enrichment (SELEX), in 1990 [15, 16]. Aptamers take on the most complex higher-order structure (three-dimensional form) through intramolecular interactions, such as a zipper of base-phosphate hairpin loops, bulges, G-quadruplexes (G4), double helices, and triplexes [17]. These complex structures allow them to contact target molecules due to electrostatic interactions, possibly involving phosphate groups, hydrogen bonding, and hydrophobic interactions mediated by their sugar and nucleobase groups [18]. A brief process of the SELEX technique can be visually understood in Fig. 5.1. Aptamer sequences are selected in the SELEX process either from an RNA library or an initial random single-stranded DNA (ssDNA) library by transcription. Such libraries usually consist of sequences of two primer

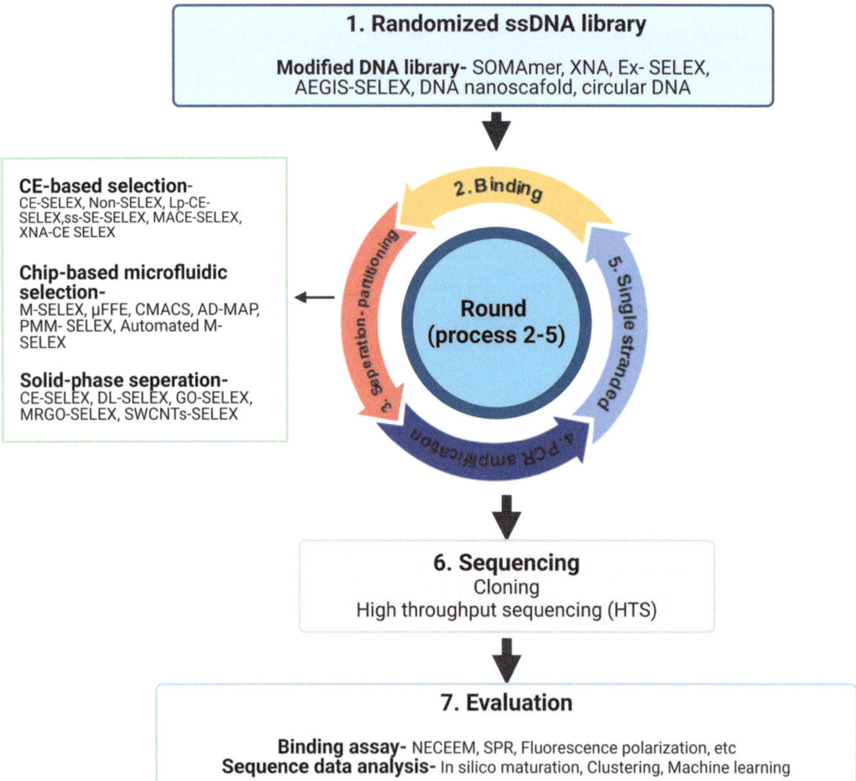

Fig. 5.1 SELEX process and aptamer development for biosensors. The Systematic Evolution of Ligands by Exponential Enrichment (SELEX) process for aptamer development involves iterative rounds of selection and amplification to identify high-affinity aptamers. These aptamers are engineered to target-specific cancer biomarkers with precision. The figure illustrates the key steps of SELEX and its application in biosensor design for cancer diagnostics

arms of about 20 bases each at the 3′ and 5′ ends, separated by a randomly variable N-base region of 20 to 60 bases, and are usually supplied by reagent providers. The sequences are amplified by polymerase chain reaction (PCR) amplification. A theoretical N-base randomized library area should accommodate 4^N distinct sequences. However, in practice the number of sequences that can be handled is limited to around 10^{11}–10^{15} which is significantly lower than the theoretical 4^n possibilities. Target molecules are incubated with the library in order to allow for the formation of target–DNA or target–RNA complexes. Target-bound sequences, known as the selection pool, are amplified by PCR once these complexes have been removed from unattached molecules. Before additional rounds of selection, RNA aptamers undergo reverse transcription. A cycle includes binding, separation, amplification, and processing. Adverse selection eliminates sequences that bind too avidly to non-targets; however, trace amounts of sequences specific to the target accumulate over multiple selection rounds. The particular sequences are identified using the process of cloning, electrophoretic sequencing, or next-generation sequencing. Binding affinity is measured by dissociation rate constant (k_{off}) and dissociation equilibrium constant (Kd) with the help of surface plasmon resonance (SPR), capillary electrophoresis, or bio-layer interferometry [18].

5.2.3 Comparative Advantages of Aptamers over Antibodies for Biosensor Applications

Aptamers offer several distinct advantages over antibodies, making them highly suitable for biosensor applications:

(a) **Stability and Resistance to Denaturation**: Even under severe conditions, which include pH and temperature fluctuations, aptamers are highly stable. Though antibodies denature and also tend to lose their functionality after a short period due to harsh conditions, which include pH and temperature variations, aptamers carry on for long periods despite such conditions [19, 20].

(b) **Ease of Synthesis and Modification**: Aptamers are very repetitive and flexible because they are chemically synthesized. The manufacturing process of aptamers is much faster and easier than that involved in the complicated biological processes applied in the preparation of antibodies. Furthermore, aptamers are easy to modify by incorporating functional groups to enhance their affinity properties for easy incorporation into biosensor systems [19, 20].

(c) **Lower Immunogenicity**: Aptamers are safer for in vivo applications since they have a lower immunogenicity than antibodies. This characteristic reduces the risk of adverse immunological responses, which is desirable for therapeutic and diagnostic purposes [19, 20].

(d) **Cost-Effectiveness**: Aptamer synthesis is cheap because it does not necessitate animals or complicated cell culture methods. This capability to scale significantly reduces the cost of developing biosensors, and it is especially applicable to large-volume applications [19].

(e) **High Specificity and Versatility**: One good reason is that aptamers may be designed to selectively target almost any type of molecule—anything from proteins or even ions to small molecules and intact cells. They also achieve relatively high binding selectivities and make excellent candidates for wide-scale biosensing analyses [20].
(f) **Adaptability to Novel Platforms**: Due to their small size and structure, aptamers are compatible with contemporary biosensor technologies, such as optical, electrochemical, and mass-sensitive sensors. Their versatility allows them to be used in creating portable, real-time detection systems [19, 20].
(g) **Reusability and Regeneration**: Aptamers in biosensor applications can be reused often and used several times. Due to their reversible denaturation, they can be reused after regaining functionality, thereby increasing usability and reducing the costs of operation [19, 20].

5.3 Biosensors: A Framework for Precision Diagnostics

Cammann coined the term "biosensors," which refer to analytical instruments that convert a biological reaction into an electrical signal. The device is expected to have high specificity, reusability, and continued functioning under environmental conditions such as pH and temperature [21]. Practical biosensor production involves making and immobilizing biomolecules and integrating them with a transducer system. The interdisciplinary approach of the above project allows for creative engineering solutions at the chemistry–biology interface boundary [22].

5.3.1 Basic Components of Biosensors

Based on their functional mechanisms, the materials used in biosensors can be categorized into four groups:

(a) Enzymes: Used in biocatalytic biosensors to catalyze particular biological reactions.
(b) Bio-affinity-Based Biosensors: Biomolecules, such as nucleic acids, antigens, or antibodies, detect specific targets.
(c) Microbial Biosensors: In this type of biosensor, microbes monitor environmental factors or analytes.
(d) Nanosensors: Biosensors embedded with nanoparticles (NPs) can increase sensitivity and specificity, thereby diagnosing illnesses at an early stage [23–25].

These biosensors can accurately detect hormones, drugs, poisons, pollutants, heavy metals, pesticides, etc. This work instead incorporates several types of biosensors, ranging from enzyme-based biosensors, immunosensors, DNA biosensors, and nano-specific biosensors, among which the latter is especially imperative in the medical field. They have helpful applications in treatments and diagnostic procedures [26].

The components of a generic biosensor are as follows:

I. **Analyte:** It is the material to be detected for diabetes monitoring, such as glucose. This is the target material, and it is the one that must be found.
II. **Bioreceptor:** A biomolecule, such as glucose-detecting enzymes, selectively identifies and attaches to the analyte. This step is known as biorecognition.
III. **Transducer:** Signalization is the process of transforming the biorecognition event into a measurable signal.
IV. **Electronics:** The electronics process the signal from the transducer and give a readable output.
V. **Display:** An LCD is often used along with hardware and software to present biosensor results in a user-friendly manner for analysis.

This configuration easily allows for the detection and precise quantification of specific analytes by biosensors [27].

5.3.2 Categories of Biosensors Tailored for Cancer Diagnosis

Translational medicine is always trying to innovate new methods of accurate staging, early cancer detection, and the assessment of how well a tumor responds to chemotherapy. For clinical applications, these instruments are a must. Biosensors are a crucial part of the study of cancer biology as they help determine the effectiveness of cytotoxic and antiproliferative drugs and the novel features of metastatic diseases [28].

Biosensors translate the signals they detect into electrical signals (electrochemical) that transducers could evaluate to identify specific biological analytes, such as proteins, nucleotides, metabolites, or whole cells [29]. There are two categories of electrochemical biosensors: potentiometric and amperometric. Potentiometric biosensors utilize ion-selective electrodes to determine changes in electrical potential caused by molecular recognition events. Amperometric biosensors measure the current that flows when two electrodes are held at an applied voltage. These concepts have been applied to create a range of biosensors, including genosensors, immunosensors, electrochemiluminescence (ECL) sensors, impedance-based sensors, and microfluidic platforms. Some of the merits of electrochemical sensing systems include low sample needs, excellent repeatability, remarkable sensitivity, cost-effectiveness, quick detection, ease of downsizing, and user-friendly operation [30, 31].

Optical biosensors convert metabolic reactions into measurable output signals based on optical principles. The transducer's optical properties, such as intensity, phase, and polarization, are modified by these interactions at the sensor surface. Any alteration in any of the optical properties, such as absorption, fluorescence, luminescence, or refractive index, can be used for detection. Optical biosensors have significantly influenced the analytical technologies designed to detect chemical and biological contaminants. They have become a focus for many researchers as they substitute or complement traditional analysis techniques by eliminating expensive, complex, and time-consuming detection processes [32–34]. The optical waveguide is the essential element of any optical biosensor. Initially developed for use in telecommunications to provide mechanical stability, variable geometry, noise immunity, and the ability to transmit light over large distances, these properties make them highly suitable for sensor applications [35]. Because optical fibers are small, low in cost, and flexible in shape, they have been the dominant form of optical waveguide sensors for a long time. However, the lack of customization ability of optical fibers means that the users have to adapt to what is already made. Planar and channel optical waveguides have become more popular for sensor development as their use outnumbers that of optical fiber sensors [33].

The physical phenomenon that is sometimes called piezoelectricity or the piezoelectric effect occurs in some materials, producing a voltage when subjected to mechanical stress. If a voltage is applied across a piezoelectric material's surface, there will be mechanical stress or oscillation with changes in voltage. Thus, it also acts the other way around. Examples of anisotropic crystals that are not centrosymmetric and show piezoelectric behavior include all ferroelectric minerals. Some of the most common piezoelectric materials include crystallized topaz ($Al_2SiO_4(F, OH)_2$), zinc oxide, aluminum phosphate (berlinite), aluminum nitride, barium and lead titanate, gallium orthophosphate, quartz (SiO_2), tartrate tetrahydrate (Rochelle salt), polyvinylidene fluoride, and polylactic acids [36–38]. The biorecognition element used in such biosensors is an antibody, and the overall specificity of the immunosensor largely depends on the specificity of the antibody. Suppose the selected antibody is specifically selective and the piezoelectric material's electrode and other sensitive parts are resistant to nonspecific interactions of interfering chemicals. In that case, a piezoelectric immunosensor generally shows specificity. In the other configuration, a physically immobilized antibody detects antigens in immunosensors. On the other hand, the immobilized antigen can be used as the target molecule, where the immunosensor used to detect antibodies contains the immobilized antigen. Immobilized antigen–based piezoelectric immunosensors are highly applicable in diagnosing infectious diseases [39].

5.3.3 The Integration of Aptamers into Biosensors: Enhancing Accuracy and Efficiency

Aptamer-based biosensors offer several key advantages over traditional biosensors that use natural receptors like antibodies and enzymes [40]:

- **Broad Applicability:** The key advantage of developing aptamers in the lab is that thousands of different biosensors can be created, sensing virtually anything from large proteins to tiny compounds and even whole cells [41].
- **Reproducibility and Stability:** Aptamers are produced with high purity and reproducibility compared to enzymes and antibodies. Moreover, their chemical stability is higher than protein-based receptors [20].

- **Conformational Change and Sensitivity:** Like other molecular recognition elements, aptamers exhibit dramatic conformational changes when they bind to their targets. Utilizing this property of aptamers, very sensitive and selective biosensors have recently been developed [20]. It can be understood clearly from Table 5.1.

Many new bioassay techniques appeared, along with the latest research into the structure and characteristics of the aptamers and their binding properties [42].

Table 5.1 Comparison of traditional methods vs. aptamer-driven biosensors for cancer diagnostics (accuracy, efficiency, cost, etc.)

Aspect	Traditional methods	Aptamer-driven biosensors
Accuracy	Traditional approaches, such as ELISA, often suffer from cross-reactivity, leading to inaccurate outcomes and compromising diagnostic reliability.	Aptamer-based biosensors have higher specificity and selectivity, resulting in fewer false positives and negatives.
Efficiency	Traditional methods, such as biopsy analysis and immunohistochemistry, can be highly time-consuming.	Aptamer-based biosensors enable real-time detection and rapid analysis due to aptamers' binding kinetics.
Cost	Traditional methods are often expensive due to the need for antibodies, reagents, and sophisticated equipment.	Aptamer-based biosensors are cost-effective as aptamers are cheaper and do not require animals for production.
Sensitivity	Traditional methods have moderate sensitivity, sometimes requiring higher sample volumes.	Aptamer-based biosensors have high sensitivity; they can detect low concentrations of biomarkers in small sample volumes.
Stability	Antibodies and enzymes used in traditional methods are prone to denaturation under extreme pH or temperature.	Aptamers are highly stable and resistant to harsh conditions like high temperatures.
Reusability	Traditional methods have limited reusability due to the degradation of biological components after use.	Aptamer-based biosensors are reusable due to aptamer stability and reversible binding.
Ease of modification	Modifying antibodies using traditional methods without affecting their binding properties is difficult.	Aptamers are readily modifiable with functional groups to enhance detection or conjugation.
Multiplexing capability	Traditional immunoassays have limited multiplexing capability.	Aptamer-based biosensors allow the simultaneous detection of multiple biomarkers using aptamer arrays.
Invasiveness	Traditional methods often require invasive procedures like biopsies.	Aptamer-based biosensors enable noninvasive detection through blood or liquid biopsy samples.
Portability	Traditional methods require bulky laboratory equipment, restricting use to clinical settings.	Aptamer-based biosensors are compact, portable devices ideal for point-of-care (POC) testing.

5.4 Aptamer-Driven Biosensors in Cancer Detection

5.4.1 Mechanisms: How Aptamers Improve Biomarker Detection

Aptamers have emerged as significant tools for biomarker discovery due to the extraordinary affinities and selectivities that these single-stranded DNA or RNA molecules exhibit towards specifically binding to particular target molecules. Their unique properties provide notable benefits over the conventional recognition components, such as antibodies, enhancing the sensitivity of the diagnostic assays and their selectivities, together with better flexibility. A general mechanism of aptamers in detecting biomarkers is shown in Fig. 5.2.

More discussion on how the aptamers contribute to improving the biomarker detection is provided below:

(a) **High Affinity and Specificity**
SELEX is an iterative in vitro method of generating aptamers. Using this method, several cycles of binding, separation, and amplification can result in highly effective aptamers possessing extraordinary affinity and specificity toward their target molecules. These molecules may be any protein, peptide, nucleic acid, tiny molecule, or a complete cell. It is versatile for identifying many biomarkers, and aptamers are easily engineered to target several different types of molecules [15].

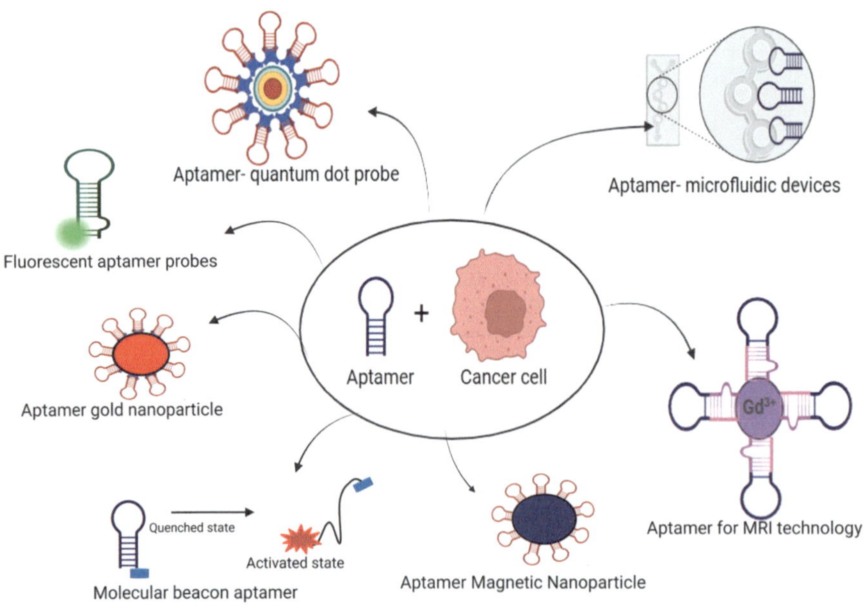

Fig. 5.2 The aptamer selectively binds to the target biomarker, triggering a measurable signal. The figure demonstrates the integration of aptamers into biosensor platforms, showcasing their specificity and sensitivity in cancer diagnostics

(b) **Conformational Change upon Binding**

Aptamers undergo conformational changes as well when they bind to target molecules. This is also a necessity in the transduction of the signal in biosensors. There are a few methods by which this conformational change may be utilized:

- **Direct Signaling:** The binding event can directly result in a detectable signal, either a fluorescence change or an electrochemical current alteration. For example, when the target binds to the aptamer, it can change the environment around it so that the attached fluorophore alters its fluorescence intensity [43].
- **Indirect Signaling:** It can be coupled with other signal transduction pathways through the conformational change. For instance, it may trigger an enzyme reaction that generates a measurable product or results in the release of a quencher molecule, which places a fluorophore and quencher closer together.

(c) **Chemical Stability and Ease of Synthesis**

Aptamers are chemically stable molecules. They can tolerate extreme temperatures and can be kept for a very long time. This stability is of immense utility in making portable and durable biosensors. In addition, aptamers can be produced in bulk by chemical synthesis at an affordable price, with great purity and reproducibility, thereby ensuring test reliability [44].

(d) **Versatile Modifications and Functionalization**

Aptamers are easily exchanged with various functional groups, which include fluorophores, enzymes, nanoparticles, or solid supports, without affecting the binding properties of aptamers. This characteristic can lead to different types of signal transduction methods and tests. For example, aptamers can be anchored onto surfaces for surface plasmon resonance measurement or gold nanoparticles (AuNPs) for colorimetric assays [45].

(e) **Multiplexed Detection**

Multiplexed assays can be efficiently designed by combining aptamers and detecting several biomarkers simultaneously. Such an approach is highly useful for identifying complex disorders where several biomarkers are typically involved. Aptamers are perfect for developing such assays because they can produce aptamers for a wide range of targets and are easy to modify [46].

(f) **In Vivo Applications**

Other applications for aptamers include targeted drug delivery and in vivo biomarker detection. These are suitable for systemic administration because of their small size and ability to target-specific biomarkers. They can also be engineered to carry therapeutic payloads or imaging agents for theranostic use.

5.4.2 Examples of Cancer Biomarkers Detected by Aptamer-Based Biosensors

A brief idea can be drawn from Table 5.2, which highlights aptamer-based biosensors and their applications in detecting cancer types.

Table 5.2 List of aptamer-based biosensors and their applications in detecting cancer types

Cancer type	Biomarker	Aptamer-driven biosensor detection method	Application	References
Breast cancer	Human epidermal growth factor receptor 2 (HER2)	Electrochemical aptasensor with gold nanoparticles	Enhanced sensitivity for HER2 detection in serum	[47]
Breast cancer	Mucin 1 (MUC1)	Fluorescent aptasensor using quantum dots	Sensitive detection of MUC1, a breast cancer marker	[48, 49]
Colorectal cancer	Carcinoem-bryonic antigen (CEA)	SPR-based aptasensor	Label-free detection of CEA in serum	[50]
Colorectal cancer	Kirsten Rat Sarcoma viral oncogene homolog (KRAS) mutation	Aptamer-based PCR assay	Detection of KRAS mutations in circulating tumor DNA	[51]
Liver cancer	Alpha-fetoprotein (AFP)	Aptamer-based ELISA-like assay	Improved sensitivity for AFP detection	[52]
Liver cancer	Glypican-3 (GPC3)	Electrochemical aptasensor with graphene oxide	Enhanced detection of GPC3 in hepatocellular carcinoma (HCC)	[53]
Lung cancer	Cytokeratin 19 fragment (CYFRA 21-1)	Chemiluminescence aptasensor	Sensitive detection of CYFRA 21-1 in serum	[54]
Lung cancer	Epidermal growth factor receptor (EGFR)	Aptamer-based flow cytometry	Detection of EGFR in lung cancer cells	[55]
Prostate cancer	Prostate-specific antigen (PSA)	Electrochemical aptasensor with carbon nanotubes	Improved sensitivity for PSA detection	[56]
Prostate cancer	Prostate-specific membrane antigen (PSMA)	Fluorescent aptasensor with molecular beacons	Detection of PSMA in prostate cancer cells	[57]
Leukemia	Nucleolin	Aptamer-based magnetic bead separation and detection	Isolation and detection of leukemia cells	[58]

(continued)

Table 5.2 (continued)

Cancer type	Biomarker	Aptamer-driven biosensor detection method	Application	References
Leukemia	Breakpoint Cluster Region–Abelson murine leukemia (BCR-ABL) fusion gene	Aptamer-based biosensor with rolling circle amplification	Highly sensitive detection of BCR-ABL mRNA (messenger Ribonucleic Acid)	[59]
Melanoma	S100B	Aptamer-based lateral flow assay	Rapid and point-of-care detection of S100B	[60]
Ovarian cancer	Cancer antigen 125 (CA125)	Electrochemical aptasensor with DNA nanostructures	Enhanced signal amplification for CA125 detection	[61]
Gastric cancer	Carcinoem-bryonic antigen–related cell adhesion molecule 5 (CEACAM5)	Aptamer-based biosensor with surface-enhanced Raman spectroscopy (SERS)	Highly sensitive detection of CEACAM5	[62]
Bladder cancer	Survivin	Aptamer-based biosensor with quantum dots and magnetic beads	Sensitive detection of survivin in urine	[63]
Cervical cancer	Human papillomavirus (HPV) DNA	Aptamer-based biosensor with electrochemical impedance spectroscopy	Detection of HPV DNA associated with cervical cancer	[64]
Brain cancer	Glioblastoma multiforme–associated antigen (GMAA)	Aptamer-based biosensor with bioluminescence resonance energy transfer (BRET)	Detection of GMAA in brain tumor cells	[65]
Multiple cancers	Circulating tumor cells (CTCs)	Aptamer-based capture and release of CTCs	Enrichment and detection of CTCs from blood	[66]

5.4.2.1 HER2 for Breast Cancer

Approximately 20–30% of patients reporting breast cancer have overexpressed HER2 (15–75 ng/mL), which is significantly higher than in the case of healthy people, for whom it is around 4–15 ng/mL [67]. Serum HER2 testing has turned out to be an important prognostic marker for the treatment of breast cancer and plays a considerable role in the monitoring of breast cancer metastasis [68]. Techniques directed at the application of antibodies, including immunohistochemistry [69], ELISA [70], and electrochemical immunosensors, are used today in the majority of

HER2 diagnostic processes [71]. However, since antibodies are expensive and their modification is challenging, such approaches fail frequently. This challenge was overcome when the field of aptasensors for protein detection was extended into three-dimensional tetrahedral DNA nanostructures (TDNs), with excellent rigidity and stability [72]. This approach targets HER2 effectively by combining TDNs with aptamers, providing a well-structured sensing interface.

Recently, nanomaterials such as graphene, metal oxides, noble metals, and metal-organic frameworks have received significant interest owing to their excellent thermal stability, multifunctionality, and facility of fabrication as novel types of nanocarriers for the enhancement of biosensor sensitivity [73, 74]. From the above materials, MnO_4 and Pd@Pt flower-like nanozymes were identified by the biomedical community owing to their large surface area, superior stability, special biocompatibility, and catalase-like activity [75, 76].

5.4.2.2 CEA for Colorectal Cancer

A human glycoprotein, called carcinoembryonic antigen (CEA), is a protein expressed during embryonic development and associated with cell adhesion functions. It is produced by normal fetal intestinal tissue and epithelial tumors, but nonmalignant diseases, like inflammatory bowel disease, are associated with elevated serum levels [77]. In healthy subjects, the levels of CEA expression are severely reduced after birth, leading to very low plasma levels [78]. Abnormal CEA expression has been found to occur in many cancers, including colorectal, gastric, breast, ovarian, lung, and pancreatic cancers [79]. The correlation of serum level of serum Carcinoembryonic Antigen (sCEA) with CRC is reported to be significant in 95% of all cases with pronounced CEA expression [80]. Thus, CEA measurement is essential for assessment and use in monitoring and differential diagnosis.

Some fields in which optical biosensors are applied include medical diagnostics, environmental monitoring, life sciences, and food safety due to significant developments [81]. Long-used platforms for optical biosensors include colorimetric, surface plasmon resonance, fluorescence, and chemiluminescence. Aptamer-based optical technologies have gained much attention in colorimetry due to low readout costs and the possibility of visual inspection [82]. The analyte is detected quickly by label-free colorimetric biosensors, as the colorimetric changes of the sensor are readily observable. These include horseradish peroxidase (HRP)–mimicking DNAzyme and gold nanoparticle (AuNP) sensors [83]. These are good candidates for commercialized detection because they are portable and easy to use and do not require additional measurement devices.

The sensitivity of SPR biosensors to changes in the local refractive index because of the evanescent field makes them highly appealing for biosensing applications. SPR is characterized by intense electron–electron oscillations at the metal/dielectric interface, and its first successful utilization was in 1983 to develop biosensors for detecting biomolecular interactions [84]. This technology has gained much attention because it is label-free, highly selective, and direct and has real-time detection capabilities [85]. It is exceptional in its ability to sense the refractive index of materials near the thin metal film, which permits the observation of the interactions between biological molecules on the surface in real time with great accuracy [86].

5.4.2.3 AFP for Liver Cancer

The five members of the albuminoid gene family are alpha-albumin, albumin, vitamin D–binding (Gc) protein, AFP, and Afamin, and it is also known as an adaptable glycoprotein, which develops in the liver and yolk sac throughout fetal development to become the most common plasma protein of the fetal stage. Infants typically exhibit high blood concentrations of AFP at birth, which decline to very low concentrations by one year of life. With the three domains of intramolecular loops stabilized through disulfide bridges, it is a single-chain glycoprotein with a tertiary V-shaped conformational structure [87].

AFP, an important tumor marker for HCC, the most common type of liver cancer, can be detected using aptamer-based biosensors [88]. These biosensors employ the unique features of aptamers, single-stranded DNA or RNA molecules that bind to specific targets with strong affinity and specificity [89]. A general review of their application in AFP detection is as follows:

(a) Aptamer Selection: Systematic Evolution of Ligands by Exponential Enrichment (SELEX) is an in vitro selection procedure to identify aptamers specific to AFP.
(b) Biosensor Design: Various biosensor formats employ the selected aptamers. Common approaches include:
   i. Electrochemical sensors immobilize aptamers on an electrode surface [90]. Electrical current or impedance varies upon AFP binding [88].
   ii. Optical Sensors: These utilize changes in the properties of light. These include:
      - Fluorescence-Based: Fluorescence is altered by binding to an aptamer of the dye or nanoparticle [91].
      - Colorimetric: Aptamer binding changes color with gold nanoparticles [92].
      - Surface Plasmon Resonance (SPR): This measures AFP binding–induced changes in refractive index at the sensor surface [93].
(c) Detection: A biosensor needs to generate electrical or optical signals proportional to the concentration of AFP to be used for quantitation [88].

5.5 Unlocking New Possibilities in Cancer Diagnostics

5.5.1 Real-Time, Point-of-Care Testing Enabled by Aptamer-Driven Biosensors

Aptasensors are frequently used in point-of-care test systems for faster diagnostics at a point-of-care test center. They give reliable, cost-effective, and accurate detection. An aptamer-based biosensor offers unique advantages over those using natural receptors, such as enzymes and antibodies. The development of point-of-care (POC) technologies will allow for quick, self-supported testing in remote or outpatient settings, enhancing clinical diagnostics. Low-cost tests integrated with digital devices transmitting data remotely promise real-time public health interventions.

Aptasensors may be a promising route to transition traditional diagnostics into faster POC tests in personalized medicine [94]. The World Health Organization predicts 15 million cancer cases by 2020, a 50% increase. Early detection remains a significant challenge in clinical practice. To address this, rapid, sensitive, and affordable cancer detection methods using nanoparticle albumin-bound (NAB) technology and DNA/RNA probes show potential for cost-effective monitoring of various cancers. The technology of using RNA-based biosensors is developing, and there is a specific interest in oncology diagnostics: cancer diagnosis specificity. Nanoparticle-based miRNA biosensors also promise to detect various cancer types, even lung and ovarian cancers [95].

5.5.2 Role in Noninvasive Diagnostics, e.g., Liquid Biopsies

The attention given to "liquid biopsy" is based on the fact that cancer cells shed fragments of their DNA, or circulating free DNA (cfDNA), into the bloodstream. These fragments may contain genetic mutations, rearrangements, amplifications, and gene copy variations, all reflecting the genomic changes present in tumors [96]. RNA analysis from external vesicles such as exosomes and platelets can provide valuable biological insights. Exosomes are nanoscale vesicles containing proteins and nucleic acids found in bodily fluids, which offer the potential for noninvasive molecular diagnostics and novel therapeutic delivery methods. Recent clinical studies have emphasized the use of circulating tumor cell (CTC) counts as prognostic and predictive markers, especially in breast and prostate cancers. Although isolating CTCs from whole blood is difficult, they offer valuable information at the DNA, RNA, and protein levels. Functional assessments of CTCs in vitro and in vivo have been attempted in some patients. cfDNA and CTCs as major constituents of liquid biopsies [97].

5.5.3 Advances in Miniaturization for Portable and Wearable Diagnostics

Microfluidics and lab-on-a-chip technologies have permitted the identification of circulating cancer biomarkers, such as exosomes, CTCs, and cfDNA, using minimally invasive, miniaturized platforms. These point-of-care cancer diagnostic strategies require fewer sample volumes using cost-effective and less invasive standards [98]. Miniature liquid biopsy instruments use blood, urine, plasma, or serum samples to analyze genomic and proteomic changes related to cancer spread. Microfluidic devices require minimal sample preparation, offer reduced sample volumes, and enable rapid, specific, and sensitive results, attracting significant research interest. Targeted protein–based diagnostics will likely elevate biomolecular information for diagnosis, especially in cancer therapeutics. Biomarker panels make treatments even more tailored [99]. Classical immunoassays, like ELISA, test one biomarker at a time, whereas multiplex technologies, such as the bead-based Luminex platform, can detect several protein targets simultaneously and offer tremendous diagnostic potential [100]. A fully automated sandwich test with silicon photonic sensors could simultaneously detect eight cancer biomarkers in serum. The test takes about an hour to complete and offers a speedy, efficient mechanism for early disease identification. Using integrated arrays increases sensitivity, allowing reliable detection of biomarkers to monitor their dynamics for prognostic assessment [101].

5.6 Advantages of Aptamer-Driven Biosensors for Accuracy and Efficiency

5.6.1 High Specificity and Sensitivity for Cancer Biomarkers

Aptamers are synthetic DNA or RNA receptors with high affinity and selectivity to bind to macromolecules like proteins or small chemical substrates. They were first discovered in 1990 and hold great promise and are being produced for a wide range of targets using in vitro, animal-independent techniques for applications in both medicine and the environmental monitoring [102]. Aptamers are used in diagnostics for cancer, heart diseases, and many other diseases through aptamer-based biosensors. Aptamers are stable in harsh chemical environments due to their chemical nature, which renders them resistant to alkaline hydrolysis, nuclease activity, and thermal instability, thus having a longer shelf life [103]. Because of their small size and high binding affinity, these can detect tiny compounds in a particular manner. The sensors function through different modes, including sandwich, target-induced structure switching (TISS), target-induced dissociation (TID), and competitive, to quickly create flexible biosensors that detect tiny compounds [104].

5.6.2 Enhanced Signal Amplification Using Nanotechnology

Aptamers are chemically stable in buffer conditions like $MgCl_2$, with maintained bioactivity and reversibility of thermal denaturation. They target biomolecules, such as amino acids, proteins, metal ions, and cells. In point-of-care (POC) testing, aptamers show high sensitivity, selectivity, stability, and accuracy, binding to a wide range of targets with strong affinity and aiding in precise diagnostics [105]. Highly programmable, synthetic aptamers can selectively recognize a wide variety of targets. Their sensitivity is considerably enhanced through cooperative binding to target molecules, and even in complex mixtures, target detection is feasible through binding-induced structure switching. These artificial ligand materials can be easily integrated into various devices because of the availability of chemical synthesis and functional changes, and the modularity of the aptamer-based biosensors enables them to diversify detectable targets and signaling pathways [106].

5.7 Challenges and Limitations

5.7.1 Stability of Aptamers in Complex Biological Samples

The application of aptamers in in vivo imaging and sensing may be severely hampered by nucleic acids' susceptibility to in vivo conditions, such as aggregation with plasma proteins and destruction by ubiquitous nucleases. Aptamers' small size can occasionally be a drawback; their employment in vivo may also be hampered by renal filtration and quick bloodstream clearance. Aptamer generation is complex; the present SELEX technologies, which are typically labor-intensive and time-consuming, have an inadequate success rate in discovery. Aptamers, particularly RNA strands, are readily degraded under biological conditions. Many aptamers have been shown to degrade in blood in less than a few minutes, which is far too short for most medical applications [107]. Aptamers have been chemically modified to extend their half-life in circulation in vivo. They can resist exonucleases by changing the 3′- and 5′-termini or adding Polyethylene Glycol (PEG) ligands [108]. Considering recent advances in aptameric biosensing technologies, there is an urgent need to develop a fast and efficient technique for generating the necessary aptamers.

Aptamers can be used as novel biological receptors to speed up the creation of valuable biosensors. Other than a few well-known exceptions, such as glucose and lactate biosensors, aptasensors can overcome most biosensors' functional and storage stability deficiencies due to their remarkably high stability, selectivity, and sensitivity. Aptamers can be combined with many different biosensor principles, for example, mass-sensitive, optical, and electrochemical principles, to be utilized as biological receptors [109].

5.7.2 Regulatory Challenges and Market Adoption Hurdles

Low market acceptance compared to antibodies will probably limit the market expansion of aptamers. Ethical concerns around aptamers will limit the market's range of applications because they are derived from animals. Another issue impeding market expansion will be strict laws governing the usage and application of aptamers. The lack of qualified specialists will further slow the market growth rate. An unstructured regulatory framework and a limited technology capacity in low- and middle-class economies will further hamper the market expansion. One of the primary disadvantages of aptamers is their poor affinity. Aptamers are limited by their oligonucleotide structure, limiting their ability to interact with the target. The presence of liver uptake, spleen uptake, nuclease degradation, and renal filtration further limits their utility. Although aptamers have advantages over antibodies, these limitations limit commercial acceptance and market expansion potential.

5.8 Emerging Trends and Future Innovations

5.8.1 Integration with Nanomaterials to Enhance Sensor Performance

Nanomaterials are nanometric and exhibit enhanced properties and chemical reactivity compared to their larger counterparts. Biomedical applications in disease diagnosis, prevention, and treatment are enormous, with benefits like increased sensitivity, specificity, faster action, and lower cost and invasiveness [110]. Cancer nanotechnology offers promising, less invasive treatments to address the high death rates from conventional chemotherapy and radiation. It enables early detection of molecular alterations and targeted therapy, which preserves healthy cells. Multifunctional systems can simultaneously detect and treat, with nanoscale devices providing in vivo reports on drug effectiveness [111].

Nanotechnology, including drug delivery and imaging techniques, has dramatically changed cancer treatment. Passively targeted nanoparticles (50–100 nm) take advantage of enhanced penetration and retention in the tumor. Nanocomposites can provide direct therapeutic or signaling agents to cancer cells for improved diagnosis and treatment effectiveness [112]. Active targeting enhances nanoparticle (NP) therapy by functionalizing NPs with ligands, such as antibodies, lectins, or peptides, targeting tumor cells. These NPs are internalized via endocytosis, releasing drugs intracellularly for a potent antitumor effect. This approach reduces drug delivery frequency and minimizes cytotoxicity to healthy tissue, with triggers like temperature, specific analytes, or an acidic tumor microenvironment activating drug release [113]. Using polymeric coatings, stealth particle technology makes nanocarriers invisible to the immune system, enhancing circulation, stability, and bioavailability. This approach allows for tumor-selective applications in detection, phototherapy, and theranostics. Several FDA-approved nanocarriers are under development, promising hope for improving the quality and longevity of cancer patients' lives [114].

5.8.2 AI and Machine Learning in Improving Diagnostic Accuracy

Artificial intelligence (AI) is helping advance cancer research and care through drug discovery, surveillance, mechanisms, screening, diagnosis, and healthcare delivery. Large language models are helping improve knowledge extraction from scientific literature, advance understanding of how cancer develops, spreads, and metastasizes; and support the development of advanced computational tools for researchers in the field. AI is helping in the cancer screening and detection process by making techniques faster and more accurate. The FDA-approved AI software helps pathologists identify cancerous areas in prostate biopsies. Moreover, AI imaging algorithms improve mammography detection and predict long-term risks of invasive breast cancer, thus saving time for radiologists to perform other tasks. AI advances cancer treatment through drug discovery, repurposing, and patient response prediction. National Cancer Institute (NCI) researchers use machine learning to anticipate T cell responses to tumors, improving immunotherapies. Additionally, AI techniques are employed to better understand the molecular processes behind medication responses.

5.8.3 Prospects of Aptamer-Based Biosensors in Personalized Cancer Diagnosis and Treatment

Precision oncology tailors cancer treatment based on tumor information, such as biomarkers, using advanced AI techniques to analyze large datasets. AI can accelerate genetic subtyping of brain tumor tissue during surgery, accelerating treatment decisions. NCI-funded researchers developed an AI model that predicts survival outcomes in nonmetastatic breast cancer, improving clinical decision-making by integrating diverse patient data sources. Cancer surveillance encompasses the collection of patient data and cancer statistics. AI techniques identify trends and accelerate information extraction. AI algorithms automatically extract tumor traits from unstructured clinical data, saving time and improving the understanding of treatment impacts on patient outcomes. AI can mitigate cancer health disparities by providing high-quality care to patients in low-resource areas or remote locations. Researchers have been studying chatbots for cancer treatment, and various studies indicate that they may provide information tailored to specific needs and assist in generating doctors' responses to patients' questions.

5.8.4 Development of Hybrid Biosensors Combining Aptamers with Other Biorecognition Elements

Aptamers are novel probes for cancer targeting in diagnostics and treatment. Their short half-lives limit them because of renal and nuclease-mediated clearance. Thus, advanced biochemistry techniques were used to design modified aptamers to improve stability, pharmacokinetics, and pharmacodynamics. A wide range of modifications, including functional optimization, multimerization, and truncation, enhances the stability and makes aptamers more binding and effective [115]. The various conjugation techniques, linking schemes, and chemical modifications enhance their functionality and stability. Chimeric aptamers combining aptamers with other molecules, such as small interfering RNA (siRNA), proteins, or drugs, show increased stability and resist nucleases. This technology permits the construction of diverse chemical or biological multifunctional structures, thus advancing aptamer technology toward its application in cancer treatment [116].

5.9 Real-World Applications and Success Stories

5.9.1 Examples of Aptamer-Based Biosensors Used in Clinical Diagnostics

As bio-components, aptamers present many diagnostic test opportunities in infectious microorganism identification, cancer clinical testing, and biomarker detection. Aptasensors detect substances such as immunoglobulin (Ig) E and thrombin by studying biomarkers in bodily fluids, such as blood and urine. One technique amplifies the detection of thrombin using conjugates of aptamer–gold nanoparticle–horseradish peroxidase (aptamer–AuNP–HRP) in a sandwich electrochemical aptasensor assay for early disease diagnosis and biomarkers detection. The aptamers were coupled to the appropriate probes [117]. Initially, aptamer1 (Apt1), after immobilization on core/shell Fe_3O_4/Au magnetic nanoparticles (AuMNPs), is used as the capture probe; then, with dual labeling of HRP and AuNPs, aptamer2 (Apt2) is used as the detection probe [118].

Cancer is the second leading cause of death across the globe and, therefore, needs early detection for survival and a better prognosis. Detection of tumor cells depends on identifying markers only present on cancer cells, as in cases of leukemia and lymphoma. Aptamers have successfully targeted free DNA and plasma proteins in blom,-++++od cells, key markers for cancer diagnosis. There has also been the use of N-(aminobutyl)-N-ethylisoluminol functionalized gold nanoparticles (ABEI-AuNPs) and aptamers to construct a highly sensitive, cost-effective ECL aptasensor for the cancer biomarker PDGF-BB. This approach immobilized biotinylated aptamer probes on a streptavidin-coated gold nanoparticle electrode to make a sandwich conjugate with the target for detection [119].

Microbial pathogen detection and viral diagnosis are important for public health protection. The identification of infected cells is based on the detection of viral proteins using infection detection probes. Although probes for specific viral targets on host cell surfaces are limited, several aptasensors have been developed to detect viral proteins and bacteria effectively. Tombelli et al. designed a piezoelectric quartz crystal microgravimetry (QCM)-based aptasensor platform to detect HIV-1 Tat protein. They used the shift in oscillation frequency induced by receptor–target interactions for label-free detection by immobilizing an RNA aptamer on the crystal [120]. Aptamers that bind to various pathogens are very valuable in the fight against infectious diseases, including respiratory viruses. Previous outbreaks, such as Middle East respiratory syndrome coronavirus (MERS-CoV), H5N1, severe acute respiratory syndrome coronavirus 2 (SARS-CoV), and H1N1, have inspired the development of aptamers targeting MERS-CoV and SARS-CoV.

5.9.2 Success Stories: From Research to Commercialization

Recent developments have discovered aptamers targeting SARS-CoV-2, especially the S protein, which is the key to treating COVID-19. Most therapeutic aptamers prevent viral infection by binding to the Receptor Binding Domain (RBD) domain, thereby blocking the interaction of the Angiotensin-Converting Enzyme 2 (ACE2) receptor. Examples include aptamer-1, nCoV-S1-Apt1, and CoV2-6C3, which disrupt the RBD–ACE2 interaction [121]. NOX-E36 is a 40-nucleotide PEGylated L-RNA aptamer, or Spiegelmer, with a high affinity for human chemokines. It is thus linked to the inflammatory chemokine CCL2/MCP-1, critical for monocyte invasion, and is implicated in several inflammatory diseases, offering an attractive therapy target. NOXXON Pharma developed NOX-E36 for diabetic nephropathy and completed a phase 2a study of 76 patients who have type 2 diabetes. The drug, tested at a dose of 0.5 mg/kg, was safe and well-tolerated and had the potential for renoprotection [122]. Aptamers have been clinically tested to treat a range of diseases such as Age-related Macular Degeneration (AMD), acute myeloid leukemia (AML), hemophilia, cardiac disease, von Willebrand disease (VWD), type 2 diabetes mellitus, thrombosis, acute coronary syndrome, and metastatic renal cell carcinoma. Only a handful of aptamer companies have translated their research into commercially viable diagnostic products or chemicals. Neo Ventures Biotechnology Inc. (Ontario, Canada); SomaLogic, Inc. (Boulder, CO, USA); Aptamer Sciences Inc. (AptSci, South Korea); and Base Pair (Houston, TX, USA) are a few examples of these successful aptamer companies that have gone commercial [123].

5.10 Conclusion

5.10.1 Summary of the Transformative Role of Aptamer-Driven Biosensors in Cancer Diagnostics

Cancer remains a significant global health issue, necessitating the development of new diagnostic tools that can bypass the limitations of traditional methods, such as low sensitivity, high cost, and time-consuming procedures. A groundbreaking solution to these problems is aptamer-driven biosensors, which provide a new approach to cancer diagnosis. These biosensors are based on aptamers, single-stranded oligonucleotides with excellent specificity and affinity for cancer biomarkers. They offer several advantages over traditional antibodies, such as improved stability, lower cost, and ease of alteration.

A transducer, signal processor, and bioreceptor (the aptamer), when combined, allow aptamer-based biosensors to detect the biomarkers very sensitively and with high specificity. These biosensors allow for proper, noninvasive, real-time detection tailored toward different cancer biomarkers, like AFP for liver cancer, CEA for colorectal cancer, and HER2 for breast cancer. Aptamers significantly raise the detection accuracy when employed in biosensors, thus contributing to early detection and better patient care.

5.10.2 Long-Term Potential for Improving Early Detection and Treatment Outcomes

Aptamer-driven biosensors have a gigantic long-term potential in the diagnostics of cancer. They provide promising techniques for early cancer detection, maybe even prior to clinical signs, which could prompt intervention and higher survival rates. One significant advantage lies in their ability to perform point-of-care testing in real time, particularly in low-resource settings. In addition, multiplex detection and downsizing advances will allow for simultaneous analysis of several biomarkers, making these biosensors invaluable tools for tracking cancer treatment and individualized diagnosis. Their noninvasive nature makes them an even more attractive prospect for routine clinical applications, predominantly liquid biopsy applications.

5.11 Future Research and Development

Aptamer-based biosensors have a bright future. Further developments in nanotechnology, such as applying graphene and gold nanoparticles, will improve sensor performance and yield even greater sensitivity and quicker results. Combining machine learning and artificial intelligence (AI) will improve diagnostic accuracy, allowing more effective data processing and interpretation. Hybrid biosensors based on aptamers and other biorecognition components may also lead to more comprehensive diagnostic platforms. Removing barriers like aptamer instability and regulatory barriers will be of utmost importance in the technology, enabling broad clinical acceptance as it grows, thus improving cancer diagnosis and treatment results.

Acknowledgments The authors are thankful to the Department of Pharmaceuticals, Ministry of Chemicals and Fertilizers, Government of India. All the figures are from https://www.biorender.com.

Credit Authorship Contribution Statement
Sarasa Meenakshi and Mayank Mishra: Conceptualization.
Mayank Mishra and Sarasa Meenakshi: Writing: original draft preparation.
Nitesh Kumar: Visualization and supervision.
Santosh Kumar and Nitesh Kumar: Editing the final draft.

Declaration of Competing Interests The authors declare no competing or financial interests relevant to this article.

Consent for Publication None to declare.

References

1. Prager GW, Braga S, Bystricky B, Qvortrup C, Criscitiello C, Esin E, et al. Global cancer control: responding to the growing burden, rising costs and inequalities in access. ESMO open. 2018;3(2):e000285.
2. Sung H, Ferlay J, Siegel RL, Laversanne M, Soerjomataram I, Jemal A, Bray F. Global cancer statistics. 2020:209–49.
3. Deo S, Sharma J, Kumar S. GLOBOCAN 2020 report on global cancer burden: challenges and opportunities for surgical oncologists. Ann Surg Oncol. 2022;29(11):6497–500.
4. D'Cruz AK, Vaish R. Risk-based oral cancer screening—lessons to be learnt. Nat Rev Clin Oncol. 2021;18(8):471–2.
5. Siegel RL, Miller KD, Jemal A. Cancer statistics, 2018. CA Cancer J Clin. 2018;68(1):7–30.
6. Salek-Maghsoudi A, Vakhshiteh F, Torabi R, Hassani S, Ganjali MR, Norouzi P, et al. Recent advances in biosensor technology in assessment of early diabetes biomarkers. Biosens Bioelectron. 2018;99:122–35.
7. Hernandez-Vargas G, Sosa-Hernández JE, Saldarriaga-Hernandez S, Villalba-Rodríguez AM, Parra-Saldivar R, Iqbal HM. Electrochemical biosensors: a solution to pollution detection with reference to environmental contaminants. Biosensors. 2018;8(2):29.
8. Li W, Zhang Q, Zhou H, Chen J, Li Y, Zhang C, et al. Chemiluminescence detection of a protein through the aptamer-controlled catalysis of a porphyrin probe. Anal Chem. 2015;87(16):8336–41.
9. Qureshi A, Gurbuz Y, Niazi JH. Capacitive aptamer–antibody based sandwich assay for the detection of VEGF cancer biomarker in serum. Sensors Actuators B Chem. 2015;209:645–51.
10. Proske D, Blank M, Buhmann R, Resch A. Aptamers – basic research, drug development, and clinical applications. Appl Microbiol Biotechnol. 2005;69:367–74.
11. Kaur G, Roy I. Therapeutic applications of aptamers. Expert Opin Investig Drugs. 2008;17(1):43–60.
12. Huang D-B, Vu D, Cassiday LA, Zimmerman JM, Maher LJ III, Ghosh G. Crystal structure of NF-**κ**B (p50) 2 complexed to a high-affinity RNA aptamer. Proc Natl Acad Sci. 2003;100(16):9268–73.
13. Long SB, Long MB, White RR, Sullenger BA. Crystal structure of an RNA aptamer bound to thrombin. RNA. 2008;14(12):2504–12.
14. Zhou J, Rossi J. Aptamers as targeted therapeutics: current potential and challenges. Nat Rev Drug Discov. 2017;16(3):181–202.
15. Ellington AD, Szostak JW. In vitro selection of RNA molecules that bind specific ligands. Nature. 1990;346(6287):818–22.
16. Tuerk C, Gold L. Systematic evolution of ligands by exponential enrichment: RNA ligands to bacteriophage T4 DNA polymerase. Science. 1990;249(4968):505–10.
17. Troisi R, Napolitano V, Spiridonova V, Russo Krauss I, Sica F. Several structural motifs cooperate in determining the highly effective anti-thrombin activity of NU172 aptamer. Nucleic Acids Res. 2018;46(22):12177–85.
18. Saito S. SELEX-based DNA aptamer selection: a perspective from the advancement of separation techniques. Anal Sci. 2021;37(1):17–26.
19. Arshavsky-Graham S, Urmann K, Salama R, Massad-Ivanir N, Walter J-G, Scheper T, et al. Aptamers vs. antibodies as capture probes in optical porous silicon biosensors. Analyst. 2020;145(14):4991–5003.
20. Song K-M, Lee S, Ban C. Aptamers and their biological applications. Sensors. 2012;12(1):612–31.
21. Mehrotra P. Biosensors and their applications–a review. J Oral Biol Craniofac Res. 2016;6(2):153–9.
22. Bhalla N, Jolly P, Formisano N, Estrela P. Introduction to biosensors. Essays Biochem. 2016;60(1):1–8.

23. Byrne B, Stack E, Gilmartin N, O'Kennedy R. Antibody-based sensors: principles, problems and potential for detection of pathogens and associated toxins. Sensors. 2009;9(6):4407–45.
24. Holford TR, Davis F, Higson SP. Recent trends in antibody based sensors. Biosens Bioelectron. 2012;34(1):12–24.
25. Rocchitta G, Spanu A, Babudieri S, Latte G, Madeddu G, Galleri G, et al. Enzyme biosensors for biomedical applications: Strategies for safeguarding analytical performances in biological fluids. Sensors. 2016;16(6):780.
26. Metkar SK, Girigoswami K. Diagnostic biosensors in medicine–a review. Biocatal Agric Biotechnol. 2019;17:271–83.
27. Kazemi-Darsanaki R, Azizzadeh A, Nourbakhsh M, Raeisi G, AzizollahiAliabadi M. Biosensors: functions and applications. J Biol Today's World. 2013;2(1):53–61.
28. Zhang Z, Li Q, Du X, Liu M. Application of electrochemical biosensors in tumor cell detection. Thoracic Cancer. 2020;11(4):840–50.
29. Hassan RY, Wollenberger U. Direct determination of bacterial cell viability using carbon nanotubes modified screen-printed electrodes. Electroanalysis. 2019;31(6):1112–7.
30. Mahato K, Wang J. Electrochemical sensors: from the bench to the skin. Sensors Actuators B Chem. 2021;344:130178.
31. Anusha T, Bhavani KS, Kumar JS, Brahman PK, Hassan RY. Fabrication of electrochemical immunosensor based on GCN-β-CD/Au nanocomposite for the monitoring of vitamin D deficiency. Bioelectrochemistry. 2022;143:107935.
32. Ramsay G, Wolpert SM. Utility of wiring nitrate reductase by alkylpyrroleviologen-based redox polymers for electrochemical biosensor and bioreactor applications. Anal Chem. 1999;71(2):504–6.
33. Kooyman R, Lechuga L. Immunosensors based on total internal reflectance, chapter 8. In: Kress-Rogers E, editor. Handbook of biosensors: medicine, food and the environment. Florida: CRC Press; 1997.
34. Scheller F. Present state and frontiers in biosensors. In: Scheller FW, Schubert F, Fedrowitz J, editors. Frontiers in biosensorics I. Berlin: Birkhäuser; 1997.
35. Ligler FS, Taitt CR. Fluorescence lifetime biosensing: entering the mainstream. In: Optical biosensors: today and tomorrow; 2008. p. 287.
36. Hagood NW, Von Flotow A. Damping of structural vibrations with piezoelectric materials and passive electrical networks. J Sound Vib. 1991;146(2):243–68.
37. Meyers FN, Loh KJ, Dodds JS, Baltazar A. Active sensing and damage detection using piezoelectric zinc oxide-based nanocomposites. Nanotechnology. 2013;24(18):185501.
38. Fukada E. History and recent progress in piezoelectric polymers. IEEE Trans Ultrason Ferroelectr Freq Control. 2000;47(6):1277–90.
39. Pohanka M. Overview of piezoelectric biosensors, immunosensors and DNA sensors and their applications. Materials. 2018;11(3):448.
40. İnce B, Kavacık M, Sezgintürk MK. Electrochemical aptamer-based biosensors for disease biomarkers. Essential Chem. 2024;1(1):1–23.
41. White RR, Sullenger BA, Rusconi CP. Developing aptamers into therapeutics. J Clin Invest. 2000;106(8):929–34.
42. Domsicova M, Korcekova J, Poturnayova A, Breier A. New insights into aptamers: an alternative to antibodies in the detection of molecular biomarkers. Int J Mol Sci. 2024;25(13):6833.
43. Nutiu R, Li Y. Aptamers with fluorescence-signaling properties. Methods. 2005;37(1):16–25.
44. Jayasena SD. Aptamers: an emerging class of molecules that rival antibodies in diagnostics. Clin Chem. 1999;45(9):1628–50.
45. Song S-H, Gao Z-F, Guo X, Chen G-H. Aptamer-based detection methodology studies in food safety. Food Anal Methods. 2019;12:966–90.
46. McCauley TG, Hamaguchi N, Stanton M. Aptamer-based biosensor arrays for detection and quantification of biological macromolecules. Anal Biochem. 2003;319(2):244–50.
47. Aiello F, Carullo G, Giordano F, Spina E, Nigro A, Garofalo A, et al. Identification of breast cancer inhibitors specific for G protein-coupled estrogen receptor (GPER)-expressing cells. ChemMedChem. 2017;12(16):1279–85.

48. Liu M, Yu X, Chen Z, Yang T, Yang D, Liu Q, et al. Aptamer selection and applications for breast cancer diagnostics and therapy. J Nanobiotechnol. 2017;15:1–16.
49. Wei W, Pan X, Li D, Qian J, Yin L, Pu Y, et al. Detection of MUC-1 protein and MCF-7 cells based on fluorescence resonance energy transfer from quantum dots to graphene oxide. J Nanosci Nanotechnol. 2012;12(10):7685–91.
50. Tombelli S, Minunni M, Mascini M. Analytical applications of aptamers. Biosens Bioelectron. 2005;20(12):2424–34.
51. Diehl F, Schmidt K, Durkee KH, Moore KJ, Goodman SN, Shuber AP, et al. Analysis of mutations in DNA isolated from plasma and stool of colorectal cancer patients. Gastroenterology. 2008;135(2):489–98. e7
52. Li G. Nano-inspired biosensors for protein assay with clinical applications. Elsevier; 2018.
53. Dong L, Zhou H, Zhao M, Gao X, Liu Y, Liu D, et al. Phosphorothioate-modified AP613-1 specifically targets GPC3 when used for hepatocellular carcinoma cell imaging. Mol Ther-Nucleic Acids. 2018;13:376–86.
54. Roointan A, Mir TA, Wani SI, Hussain KK, Ahmed B, Abrahim S, et al. Early detection of lung cancer biomarkers through biosensor technology: A review. J Pharm Biomed Anal. 2019;164:93–103.
55. Ruiz Ciancio D, Vargas MR, Thiel WH, Bruno MA, Giangrande PH, Mestre MB. Aptamers as diagnostic tools in cancer. Pharmaceuticals. 2018;11(3):86.
56. Lin DW. Beyond PSA: utility of novel tumor markers in the setting of elevated PSA. In: Urologic oncology: seminars and original investigations. Elsevier; 2009.
57. Lupold SE, Hicke BJ, Lin Y, Coffey DS. Identification and characterization of nuclease-stabilized RNA molecules that bind human prostate cancer cells via the prostate-specific membrane antigen. Cancer Res. 2002;62(14):4029–33.
58. Bates PJ, Kahlon JB, Thomas SD, Trent JO, Miller DM. Antiproliferative activity of G-rich oligonucleotides correlates with protein binding. J Biol Chem. 1999;274(37):26369–77.
59. Duan M-H, Li H, Cai H. A rare e13a3 (b2a3) BCR-ABL1 fusion transcript with normal karyotype in chronic myeloid leukemia: the challenges in diagnosis and monitoring minimal residual disease (MRD). Leuk Res. 2017;59:8–11.
60. Pultar J. Protein microarray for detection of sepsis-and melanoma relevant biomarkers: na. 2008.
61. Zhao J, Tan W, Zheng J, Su Y, Cui M. Aptamer nanomaterials for ovarian cancer target theranostics. Front Bioeng Biotechnol. 2022;10:884405.
62. Beauchemin N, Arabzadeh A. Carcinoembryonic antigen-related cell adhesion molecules (CEACAMs) in cancer progression and metastasis. Cancer Metastasis Rev. 2013;32:643–71.
63. Wu M-L, Li H, Yu L-J, Chen X-Y, Kong Q-Y, Song X, et al. Short-term resveratrol exposure causes in vitro and in vivo growth inhibition and apoptosis of bladder cancer cells. PLoS One. 2014;9(2):e89806.
64. Mahmoodi P, Rezayi M, Rasouli E, Avan A, Gholami M, Ghayour Mobarhan M, et al. Early-stage cervical cancer diagnosis based on an ultra-sensitive electrochemical DNA nanobiosensor for HPV-18 detection in real samples. J Nanobiotechnol. 2020;18:1–12.
65. Gao M, Yu F, Lv C, Choo J, Chen L. Fluorescent chemical probes for accurate tumor diagnosis and targeting therapy. Chem Soc Rev. 2017;46(8):2237–71.
66. Tang Z, Parekh P, Turner P, Moyer RW, Tan W. Generating aptamers for recognition of virus-infected cells. Clin Chem. 2009;55(4):813–22.
67. Shen C, Zeng K, Luo J, Li X, Yang M, Rasooly A. Self-assembled DNA generated electric current biosensor for HER2 analysis. Anal Chem. 2017;89(19):10264–9.
68. Li X, Shen C, Yang M, Rasooly A. Polycytosine DNA electric-current-generated immunosensor for electrochemical detection of human epidermal growth factor receptor 2 (HER2). Anal Chem. 2018;90(7):4764–9.
69. Takehana T, Kunitomo K, Kono K, Kitahara F, Iizuka H, Matsumoto Y, et al. Status of c-erbB-2 in gastric adenocarcinoma: a comparative study of immunohistochemistry, fluorescence in situ hybridization and enzyme-linked immuno-sorbent assay. Int J Cancer. 2002;98(6):833–7.

70. Konecny G, Pauletti G, Pegram M, Untch M, Dandekar S, Aguilar Z, et al. Quantitative association between HER-2/neu and steroid hormone receptors in hormone receptor-positive primary breast cancer. J Natl Cancer Inst. 2003;95(2):142–53.
71. Sharma S, Zapatero-Rodríguez J, Saxena R, O'Kennedy R, Srivastava S. Ultrasensitive direct impedimetric immunosensor for detection of serum HER2. Biosens Bioelectron. 2018;106:78–85.
72. Rinker S, Ke Y, Liu Y, Chhabra R, Yan H. Self-assembled DNA nanostructures for distance-dependent multivalent ligand–protein binding. Nat Nanotechnol. 2008;3(7):418–22.
73. Zheng T, Zhang Q, Feng S, Zhu J-J, Wang Q, Wang H. Robust nonenzymatic hybrid nano-electrocatalysts for signal amplification toward ultrasensitive electrochemical cytosensing. J Am Chem Soc. 2014;136(6):2288–91.
74. Chen B, Chen D, Li F, Lin X, Huang Q. Graphitic porous carbon: efficient synthesis by a combustion method and application as a highly selective biosensor. J Mater Chem B. 2018;6(46):7684–91.
75. Singh N, Savanur MA, Srivastava S, D'Silva P, Mugesh G. A redox modulatory Mn3O4 nanozyme with multi-enzyme activity provides efficient cytoprotection to human cells in a Parkinson's disease model. Angew Chem. 2017;129(45):14455–9.
76. Fang Y, Li C, Bo J, Henzie J, Yamauchi Y, Asahi T. Chiral sensing with mesoporous Pd@ Pt nanoparticles. ChemElectroChem. 2017;4(8):1832–5.
77. Chen C-H, Hsieh M-C, Lai C-C, Yeh C-Y, Chen J-S, Hsieh P-S, et al. Lead time of carcino-embryonic antigen elevation in the postoperative follow-up of colorectal cancer did not affect the survival rate after recurrence. Int J Color Dis. 2010;25:567–71.
78. Hensel JA, Khattar V, Ponnazhagan S. Recombinant AAV-CEA tumor vaccine in combination with an immune adjuvant breaks tolerance and provides protective immunity. Mol Ther-Oncolytics. 2019;12:41–8.
79. Blumenthal RD, Leon E, Hansen HJ, Goldenberg DM. Expression patterns of CEACAM5 and CEACAM6 in primary and metastatic cancers. BMC Cancer. 2007;7:1–15.
80. Yang KM, Park IJ, Kim CW, Roh SA, Cho D-H, Kim JC. The prognostic significance and treatment modality for elevated pre-and postoperative serum CEA in colorectal cancer patients. Ann Surg Treat Res. 2016;91(4):165–71.
81. Nguyen V-T, Kwon YS, Gu MB. Aptamer-based environmental biosensors for small molecule contaminants. Curr Opin Biotechnol. 2017;45:15–23.
82. Qu F, Li T, Yang M. Colorimetric platform for visual detection of cancer biomarker based on intrinsic peroxidase activity of graphene oxide. Biosens Bioelectron. 2011;26(9):3927–31.
83. Feng C, Dai S, Wang L. Optical aptasensors for quantitative detection of small biomolecules: a review. Biosens Bioelectron. 2014;59:64–74.
84. Liedberg B, Nylander C, Lunström I. Surface plasmon resonance for gas detection and biosensing. Sensors Actuators. 1983;4:299–304.
85. Wijaya E, Lenaerts C, Maricot S, Hastanin J, Habraken S, Vilcot J-P, et al. Surface plasmon resonance-based biosensors: From the development of different SPR structures to novel surface functionalization strategies. Curr Opinion Solid State Mater Sci. 2011;15(5):208–24.
86. Wang H, Wang X, Wang J, Fu W, Yao C. A SPR biosensor based on signal amplification using antibody-QD conjugates for quantitative determination of multiple tumor markers. Sci Rep. 2016;6(1):33140.
87. Lakhi NA, Mizejewski GJ. Alpha-fetoprotein and Fanconi anemia: relevance to DNA repair and breast cancer susceptibility. Fetal Pediatr Pathol. 2017;36(1):49–61.
88. Liu L, Wang H, Xie B, Zhang B, Lin Y, Gao L. Detection of alpha-fetoprotein using aptamer-based sensors. Biosensors. 2022;12(10):780.
89. Canoura J, Alkhamis O, Liu Y, Willis C, Xiao Y. High-throughput quantitative binding analysis of DNA aptamers using exonucleases. Nucleic Acids Res. 2023;51(4):e19-e.
90. Oberhaus FV, Frense D, Beckmann D. Immobilization techniques for aptamers on gold electrodes for the electrochemical detection of proteins: a review. Biosensors. 2020;10(5):45.
91. Trachman RJ III, Ferre-D'Amare AR. Tracking RNA with light: selection, structure, and design of fluorescence turn-on RNA aptamers. Q Rev Biophys. 2019;52:e8.

92. Davydova A, Vorobyeva M. Aptamer-based biosensors for the colorimetric detection of blood biomarkers: paving the way to clinical laboratory testing. Biomedicines. 2022;10(7):1606.
93. Sequeira-Antunes B, Ferreira HA. Nucleic acid aptamer-based biosensors: a review. Biomedicines. 2023;11(12):3201.
94. Prante M, Segal E, Scheper T, Bahnemann J, Walter J. Aptasensors for point-of-care detection of small molecules. Biosensors. 2020;10(9):108.
95. Catuogno S, Esposito CL, Quintavalle C, Cerchia L, Condorelli G, De Franciscis V. Recent advance in biosensors for microRNAs detection in cancer. Cancers. 2011;3(2):1877–98.
96. Alix-Panabières C, Pantel K. Clinical applications of circulating tumor cells and circulating tumor DNA as liquid biopsy. Cancer Discov. 2016;6(5):479–91.
97. Schwarzenbach H, Nishida N, Calin GA, Pantel K. Clinical relevance of circulating cell-free microRNAs in cancer. Nat Rev Clin Oncol. 2014;11(3):145–56.
98. Rana A, Zhang Y, Esfandiari L. Advancements in microfluidic technologies for isolation and early detection of circulating cancer-related biomarkers. Analyst. 2018;143(13):2971–91.
99. Washburn AL, Shia WW, Lenkeit KA, Lee S-H, Bailey RC. Multiplexed cancer biomarker detection using chip-integrated silicon photonic sensor arrays. Analyst. 2016;141(18):5358–65.
100. Etzioni R, Urban N, Ramsey S, McIntosh M, Schwartz S, Reid B, et al. The case for early detection. Nat Rev Cancer. 2003;3(4):243–52.
101. Sawyers CL. The cancer biomarker problem. Nature. 2008;452(7187):548–52.
102. Gewirtz AM, Sokol DL, Ratajczak MZ. Nucleic acid therapeutics: state of the art and future prospects. Blood. 1998;92(3):712–36.
103. Dalirirad S, Steckl AJ. Aptamer-based lateral flow assay for point of care cortisol detection in sweat. Sens Actuators B Chem. 2019;283:79–86.
104. Daprà J, Lauridsen LH, Nielsen AT, Rozlosnik N. Comparative study on aptamers as recognition elements for antibiotics in a label-free all-polymer biosensor. Biosens Bioelectron. 2013;43:315–20.
105. Shan W, Pan Y, Fang H, Guo M, Nie Z, Huang Y, et al. An aptamer-based quartz crystal microbalance biosensor for sensitive and selective detection of leukemia cells using silver-enhanced gold nanoparticle label. Talanta. 2014;126:130–5.
106. Nutiu R, Li Y. Structure-switching signaling aptamers. J Am Chem Soc. 2003;125(16):4771–8.
107. Sun H, Zu Y. A highlight of recent advances in aptamer technology and its application. Molecules. 2015;20(7):11959–80.
108. Padilla R, Sousa R. Efficient synthesis of nucleic acids heavily modified with non-canonical ribose 2′-groups using a mutant T7 RNA polymerase (RNAP). Nucleic Acids Res. 1999;27(6):1561–3.
109. Strehlitz B, Nikolaus N, Stoltenburg R. Protein detection with aptamer biosensors. Sensors. 2008;8(7):4296–307.
110. Woolley AT. Biomedical microdevices and nanotechnology. Trends Biotechnol. 2001;19(2):38–9.
111. Brigger I, Dubernet C, Couvreur P. Nanoparticles in cancer therapy and diagnosis. Adv Drug Deliv Rev. 2012;64:24–36.
112. Heath JR, Davis ME. Nanotechnology and cancer. Annu Rev Med. 2008;59(1):251–65.
113. Misra R, Acharya S, Sahoo SK. Cancer nanotechnology: application of nanotechnology in cancer therapy. Drug Discov Today. 2010;15(19–20):842–50.
114. Brannon-Peppas L, Blanchette JO. Nanoparticle and targeted systems for cancer therapy. Adv Drug Deliv Rev. 2004;56(11):1649–59.
115. Kanwar JR, Roy K, Kanwar RK. Chimeric aptamers in cancer cell-targeted drug delivery. Crit Rev Biochem Mol Biol. 2011;46(6):459–77.
116. Cho Y, Lee YB, Lee J-H, Lee DH, Cho EJ, Yu SJ, et al. Modified AS1411 aptamer suppresses hepatocellular carcinoma by up-regulating galectin-14. PLoS One. 2016;11(8):e0160822.
117. Wang Y, Yuan R, Chai Y, Yuan Y, Bai L, Liao Y. A multi-amplification aptasensor for highly sensitive detection of thrombin based on high-quality hollow CoPt nanoparticles decorated graphene. Biosens Bioelectron. 2011;30(1):61–6.

118. Zhao J, Zhang Y, Li H, Wen Y, Fan X, Lin F, et al. Ultrasensitive electrochemical aptasensor for thrombin based on the amplification of aptamer–AuNPs–HRP conjugates. Biosens Bioelectron. 2011;26(5):2297–303.
119. Chai Y, Tian D, Gu J, Cui H. A novel electrochemiluminescence aptasensor for protein based on a sensitive N-(aminobutyl)-N-ethylisoluminol-functionalized gold nanoprobe. Analyst. 2011;136(16):3244–51.
120. Tombelli S, Minunni M, Luzi E, Mascini M. Aptamer-based biosensors for the detection of HIV-1 Tat protein. Bioelectrochemistry. 2005;67(2):135–41.
121. Zhang Y, Juhas M, Kwok CK. Aptamers targeting SARS-COV-2: a promising tool to fight against COVID-19. Trends Biotechnol. 2023;41(4):528–44.
122. Kaur H, Bruno JG, Kumar A, Sharma TK. Aptamers in the therapeutics and diagnostics pipelines. Theranostics. 2018;8(15):4016.
123. Ruscito A, DeRosa MC. Small-molecule binding aptamers: selection strategies, characterization, and applications. Front Chem. 2016;4:14.

Targeted Cancer Therapy with Aptamers: A Review on the Current State

6

Vishal Chhabra, Sarasa Meenakshi, Santosh Kumar, and Krishna Murti

Abbreviations

EGFR	Epidermal growth factor receptor
HER2/neu	Human epidermal growth factor receptor 2
SELEX	Systematic Evolution of Ligands by Exponential Enrichment
PSMA	Prostate-specific membrane antigen
VEGF	Vascular endothelial growth factor
PDT	Photodynamic therapy
MOF	Metal-organic framework
LNA	Locked nucleic acid
ApDCs	Aptamer–drug conjugates

The original version of the chapter has been revised. A correction to this chapter can be found at https://doi.org/10.1007/978-981-96-8387-1_15

Authors Vishal Chhabra and Sarasa Meenakshi have equally contributed to this chapter.

V. Chhabra
Department of Pharmacology and Toxicology, National Institute of Pharmaceutical Education and Research (NIPER), Hajipur, Bihar, India

S. Meenakshi · K. Murti (✉)
Department of Pharmacy Practice, National Institute of Pharmaceutical Education and Research (NIPER), Hajipur, Bihar, India
e-mail: krishnamurti@niperhajipur.ac.in

S. Kumar
Division of Cardiovascular Medicine, Carver College of Medicine, University of Iowa, Iowa City, IA, USA
e-mail: santosh-kumar@uiowa.edu

S. Srivastava et al. (eds.), *Biosensors and Aptamers*,
https://doi.org/10.1007/978-981-96-8387-1_6

Overview

Cancer is the largest cause of mortality globally, presenting significant hurdles to medical research and healthcare systems. Two classic cancer treatments that usually lack selectivity, damage healthy tissues, and generate notable side effects not meant to be addressed are chemotherapy and radiation treatment. As a result of the distinctive characteristics that they possess in comparison to other conventional targeted therapies, aptamers have got undivided attention in the field of cancer research. They are also referred to as "chemical antibodies," as they can interact with a variety of biomolecules, including proteins. With an eye on their design, mechanisms of action, and uses in both cancer diagnosis and treatment, this chapter investigates the present developments in targeted cancer therapy employing aptamers.

6.1 Introduction

Cancer can spread to different body parts, invade neighboring tissues, and grow metastatically. Epigenetic and genetic abnormalities cause these undesirable alterations, which, in turn, promote cancer by interfering with normal cellular functions like DNA repair on genes that promote tumor growth and off genes that suppress tumor growth [1]. Aptamer–drug conjugates (ApDCs) are meticulously crafted to precisely target cancer cells for drug delivery, thereby improving treatment efficacy and minimizing overall toxicity. Aptamers possess the ability to specifically target markers associated with cancer, including nucleolin and prostate-specific membrane antigen (PSMA). While there is significant promise, challenges including in vivo safety, effective delivery, and tumor heterogeneity need to be resolved prior to considering clinical application. Progress is being made in altering chemicals, developing delivery methods, and employing combination therapies to enhance the safety and compatibility of aptamers in oncology. This will facilitate their application in precision cancer care. Addressing these challenges and fully exploring the potential of aptamer-based therapies in cancer treatment will require further investigation [2].

Targeted therapy is a way to treat cancer that focuses on certain molecules that help the tumor grow and stay alive. It aims to inhibit pathways specific to tumors while reducing toxicity. Aptamers have the capability to specifically target growth factor receptors such as human epidermal growth factor receptor 2 (HER2/neu) and epidermal growth factor receptor (EGFR) [3]. The emergence of innovative targeted therapies such as aptamer and antibody–drug conjugates is significantly transforming the landscape of cancer treatment. Combining immunotherapies strengthens the immune system's ability to fight cancer. Targeting specific genetic alterations or overexpressed proteins, such as breakpoint cluster region (BCR)-ABL (Abelson murine leukemia viral oncogene homolog 1) or HER2, these therapies offer improved precision and decreased toxicity in cancer treatment. Challenges, including diverse tumor types and medication resistance, underscore the need for additional research to improve the effectiveness of these treatments [4, 5].

Short DNA or RNA molecules called aptamers are gaining popularity as cancer treatments. The word "aptamer" comes from "*aptus*" (Latin for "to fit") and "*meros*" (Greek for "part"). Ellington and Szostak (1990) and Tuerk and Gold (1990) found these compounds in the early 1990s [6]. The Systematic Evolution of Ligands by Exponential Enrichment (SELEX) technique is employed to produce these engineered compounds. They are positioned as a prospective therapeutic approach for tumors due to their strong binding affinity and high target specificity. They can be employed in scientific research, diagnostics, and treatment due to their ability to identify a variety of chemical targets [7]. Aptamers demonstrate a reduced likelihood of provoking immunological responses in patients, making them a safer option for repeated use in comparison to antibodies. Their ability to perform chemical synthesis in large quantities with high consistency makes them more economical compared to biologically derived molecules like antibodies. They can serve as tools for therapy, diagnosis, and research. While they have advantages like stability and cost-effectiveness, they also have challenges, such as in vivo nuclease breakdown and inefficient delivery to target regions. With advancements in delivery systems and chemical transformation, aptamers hold great promise, especially in fields like precision medicine and oncology [8].

Aptamers have become extremely useful tools in oncology because of their great specificity and versatility. These artificial nucleic acid molecules provide a focused approach to cancer treatment by enabling targeting of particular molecules within cancer cells [9]. Aptamers have benefits over conventional medications, including better tumor targeting, less systemic toxicity, and the possibility of combination therapies. Additionally, aptamers can target immunological checkpoints such as cytotoxic T-lymphocyte–associated protein 4 (CTLA-4) and programmed cell death protein 1 (PD-1), strengthening the body's defenses against malignancies [10]. Scientists can further improve the medicinal efficacy of aptamers by designing them for valency control and covalent binding. These adaptable chemicals could transform cancer care by offering safer and more individualized alternatives. Kumar et al. (2024) showed that by targeting particular antigens, such as prostate-specific membrane antigen

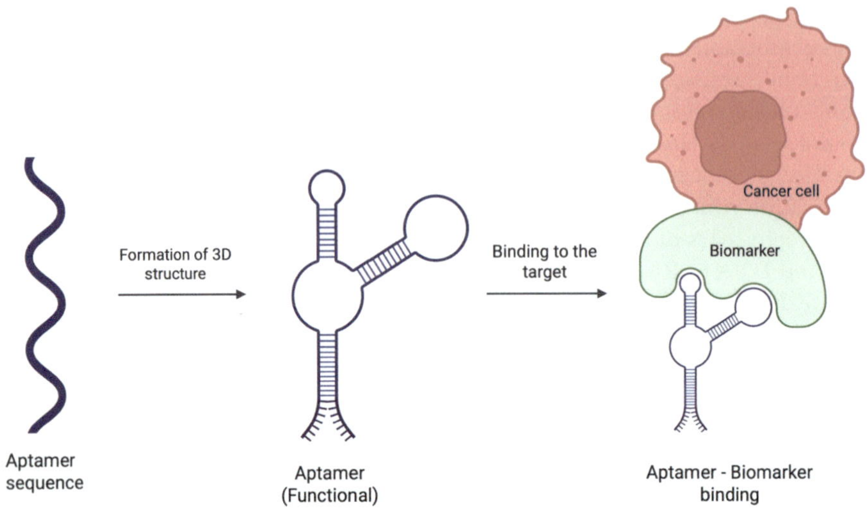

Fig. 6.1 Mechanism of aptamer–biomarker binding and therapeutic applications. This diagram demonstrates the process of aptamer–biomarker interaction, emphasizing the high specificity and affinity of aptamer sequences for their targets. It illustrates the aptamer's ability to recognize and bind to biomarkers overexpressed on diseased cells, enabling applications such as targeted drug delivery, diagnostic sensing, and therapeutic modulation

(PSMA), aptamer-modified nanocarriers can reduce adverse effects and enhance medication delivery [11], as shown in Fig. 6.1.

6.2 Mechanism of Action

6.2.1 Tumor-Selective Targeting and Drug Delivery

Aptamers have the ability to carry chemotherapy medications straight to the tumor cells, enhancing their efficacy and reducing their side effects. By attaching specifically to biomarkers associated with cancer, such as growth factor receptors, signaling proteins, or cell-surface molecules, they enable precision targeting [12]. Because they fold into unique three-dimensional structures including loops, stems, and bulges, they can bind to molecules like EGFR (lung cancer), PSMA (prostate cancer), HER2 (breast cancer), and nucleolin (different malignancies) with high affinity and specificity. Due to their frequent overexpression on the surface of cancer cells, these targets are ideal for tumor-selective targeting [13]. In cancer cells, aptamers can detect overexpressed biomarkers that are either not present or only faintly expressed in healthy cells. By using the Systematic Evolution of Ligands by Exponential Enrichment (SELEX) approach, aptamers that bind to these biomarkers specifically are created [14]. Unlike tiny molecules or antibodies that may interact with nonspecific sites, aptamers decrease off-target interactions by iterative selection and optimization. By preventing vascular endothelial growth factor

(VEGF), which is essential for the blood supply to tumors, pegaptanib and other anti-VEGF aptamers stop angiogenesis [15]. A BET-targeting PROTAC (Proteolysis Targeting Chimera) was coupled to the nucleic acid aptamer AS1411 (AS) via a cleavable linker to create the first aptamer–PROTAC conjugate (APC) [16].

Since cells can absorb a variety of aptamers, medications like doxorubicin, which efficiently destroys tumor cells while reducing side effects, can be administered directly to cells. Targeting receptors involved in signaling cascades, such as EGFR or VEGF, aptamers are naturally internalized. Following their binding and internalization via receptor-mediated endocytosis, aptamers penetrate the cancer cell [17]. Two main processes—macropinocytosis and receptor-mediated endocytosis—are involved in their internalization. The latter may be essential for nuclear uptake and aiding in the escape of cargo molecules from endosomal compartments, as demonstrated by the internalization of nucleolin-binding aptamers that move between the nucleus and cytoplasm. One intriguing strategy to improve the effectiveness of aptamer-based delivery systems is to take advantage of the macropinocytosis route. Optimizing this method increases the usefulness of nucleolin-like aptamers as precise therapeutic delivery tools by enabling their identification and customization for targeted distribution to particular cell types [18]. Aptamers are conjugated to doxorubicin, paclitaxel, or cisplatin for direct delivery to cancer cells. They facilitate the introduction of drugs that inhibit the synthesis of oncogenes by silencing genes in cancer cells [19]. Aptamers specifically kill cancer cells when combined with cytotoxic substances or radioactive isotopes. Environmental signals, such as pH, enzymes, or redox conditions, inside the tumor microenvironment can cause drug release. This method of tailored administration optimizes therapeutic efficacy while minimizing systemic toxicity [20]. They can be attached to drug-encapsulating nanoparticles to improve stability and delivery effectiveness. In order to enable simultaneous diagnosis and therapy, these nanocarriers can be designed to carry both therapeutic drugs and imaging molecules [21], as shown in Fig. 6.2.

6.2.2 Oncogenic Pathway Inhibition

Through their ability to bind selectively to target proteins, aptamers can disrupt tumorigenic processes by blocking their function. The overexpression or mutation of oncoproteins, which control cell growth, survival, and metastasis, is what causes cancers [22]. These oncoproteins are specifically susceptible to aptamer binding, which impairs their functionality and stops tumor growth. This chapter discusses how aptamers interfere with carcinogenic pathways, focusing on immune checkpoint suppression, oncogenic protein targeting, and microRNA (miRNA) activity modulation [13].

Recently, Huang et al. showed how aptamers could improve immune checkpoint blockade treatment. Aptamers can support antitumor immunity and restore T cell activity by targeting immunological checkpoints such as PD-1 and CTLA-4. To avoid immune recognition and continue to grow unchecked, cancer cells frequently take advantage of these immunological checkpoints. Aptamers can aid in

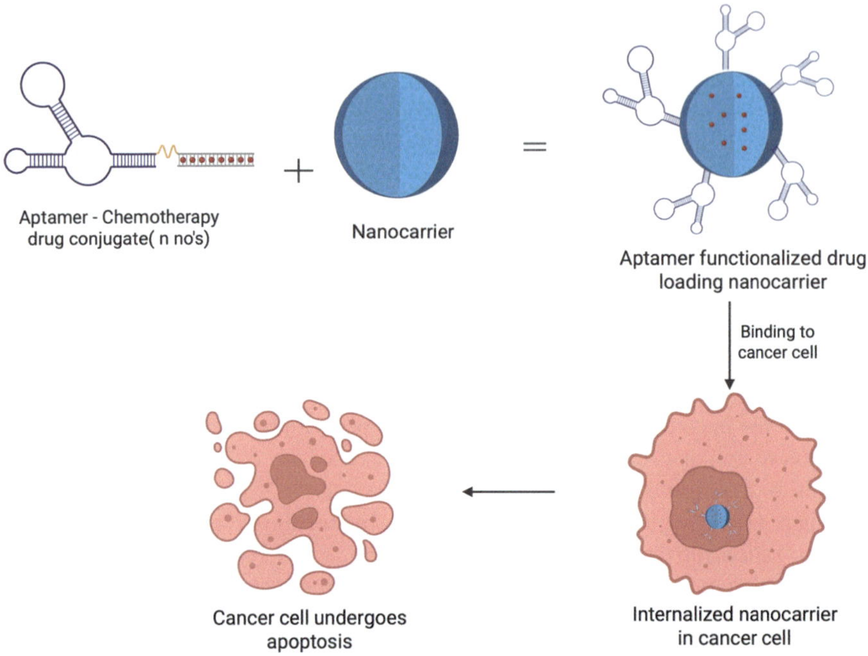

Fig. 6.2 Aptamer-functionalized nanocarrier in targeted cancer therapy. This diagram demonstrates the process of aptamer-functionalized nanocarriers in targeted cancer therapy. Aptamers selectively bind to specific biomarkers on cancer cells, enabling the precise delivery of chemotherapy drugs. The nanocarrier is internalized by the cancer cell, where the drug is released. This targeted approach induces apoptosis in cancer cells, minimizing damage to healthy tissues

reviving the immune system's capacity to identify and combat tumor cells by inhibiting these checkpoints [10]. For example, aptamers that target proteins involved in cell adhesion and motility can limit cancer cells' metastatic potential. Mi et al. evaluated breast cancer models and found that the OPN-R3 aptamer, which targets osteopontin, was effective in reducing cell adhesion, migration, and invasion [23]. Dysregulation of miRNAs, particularly overexpression of oncogenic miRNAs, is a feature of many malignancies. Aptamers can target and block these oncogenic miRNAs by binding to their primary precursors (pri-miRNAs), thereby preventing their processing into precursor forms (pre-miRNAs) and ultimately inhibiting the formation of mature, functional miRNAs, responsible for

Table 6.1 Key features and applications of aptamers in cancer therapy

Aspect	Description	Examples	References
Mechanism	Aptamers selectively bind to biomarkers overexpressed on cancer cells, enabling targeted drug delivery	EGFR (lung cancer), PSMA (prostate cancer), HER2 (breast cancer), nucleolin (various cancers)	[26]
Aptamer structure	Fold into unique 3D structures (loops, stems, and bulges) for high specificity and affinity	SELEX technique for aptamer selection	[27]
Internalization pathways	Receptor-mediated endocytosis and macropinocytosis enable aptamer uptake into cancer cells	EGFR-targeted aptamers, nucleolin-binding aptamers	[28]
Drug conjugation	Aptamers conjugated to drugs like doxorubicin, paclitaxel, or cisplatin for targeted therapy	Aptamer–doxorubicin conjugates	[29]
Stimuli-responsive release	Environmental triggers like pH, enzymes, or redox conditions release drugs in the tumor microenvironment	Stimuli-responsive drug delivery systems	[20]
Nanoparticle integration	Aptamers conjugated to nanoparticles enhance drug stability and delivery efficiency	Gold nanoparticles, liposomes	[30]
Therapeutic applications	Block angiogenesis, deliver cytotoxic agents, or inhibit oncogenic pathways	Anti-VEGF aptamers (e.g., pegaptanib), PROTAC conjugates	[31]

This table outlines the major aspects of aptamers, including their mechanisms, structural characteristics, pathways for cellular internalization, methods for drug conjugation, stimuli-responsive drug release mechanisms, integration with nanoparticles, and diverse therapeutic applications in cancer treatment

oncogenic effects [24]. Subramanian et al. discovered that the pri-miR-17~92 aptamer inhibits the maturation of miRNAs from the carcinogenic miR-17~92 cluster, causing death and cell cycle arrest in retinoblastoma cells [25]. Table 6.1 summarizes the key aspects of tumor-selective targeting and drug delivery using aptamers.

6.3 Aptamer–Nanoparticle Conjugates

Electrochemical biosensors are developed using nanomaterials with unique conducting characteristics. Carbon-based nanomaterials, including graphene, fullerenes, quantum dots, and carbon nanotubes, are especially popular as conductive transducers due to their superior electronic properties. These materials are well known for their high conductivity, which allows them to efficiently carry electrical information [32]. As nanotechnology and aptamer identification technologies progress, they converge to form what is known as aptamer nanotechnology. Aptamer–nanoparticle conjugates represent a significant step forward in targeted medication delivery and cancer treatment. They combine the unique properties of aptamers, which are small, single-stranded nucleic acids that may preferentially bind to specific molecular targets, with the varied activities of nanoparticles [33]. This combination increases therapy efficacy and specificity while decreasing negative effects. The combination of aptamers with nanoparticles allows for multifunctional applications, including drug delivery, biosensing, and bioimaging [34].

Ohno et al. demonstrated an immunosensor utilizing Immunoglobulin E (IgE)-specific aptamers attached onto the graphene surface to detect the IgE protein by creating an electrical signal [35]. To integrate these advantageous electrical qualities with biological systems, Abidian et al. constructed low-impedance, biologically active polymer nanotubes on the surface of a gold electrode, permitting a slow breakdown that allows for the prolonged release of biologically active chemicals [36]. A novel biosensor for the detection of tumor biomarkers, such as carcinoembryonic antigen, was also developed, utilizing gold nanoparticles coupled with aptamers. Combining electroactive nanomaterials with aptamers in diagnostic applications increases their potential, broadens their use, and improves sensitivity, allowing for the detection of targets at lower concentrations [37, 38].

6.3.1 Aptamer Modification and Conjugation Techniques

Aptamers can be easily changed, allowing for their successful assembly on nanoparticle surfaces by covalent conjugation techniques, such as the Au-S linkage, which was created by Mirkin et al. in 2020 [39]. These Au-S covalent bonds are required to form a stable and specific connection between aptamers and nanoparticles, allowing precise control over aptamer orientation on the nanoparticle surface. This configuration increases the stability and efficacy of functionalized nanoparticles [40]. For example, Farokhzad et al. employed nanoparticle and A10 aptamer conjugates to target increased transmembrane proteins in prostate cancer, highlighting the potential of drug-encapsulated nanoparticles. Furthermore, aptamers have shown potential in suppressing autoimmune antibodies, with important implications for treating insulin resistance. These examples highlight the potential of aptamers to pioneer targeted nanotechnology-based therapeutics aimed at altering illness pathways across multiple disorders [41, 42].

6.3.2 Covalent and Non-covalent Conjugation Strategies

Covalent methods are commonly employed to bind aptamers to nanomaterials, as they provide more stability than non-covalent approaches. These covalent coupling chemistries are common in the synthesis of different nanomaterials, giving them distinct surface characteristics and functional groups. Normally, a thiol group is added to the aptamer as a functional entity, which then reacts chemically with complementary groups—like carboxylic acid or aldehyde groups—on the nanoparticle surface or directly with the nanoparticles themselves [43]. Non-covalent approaches can form aptamer–nanomaterial conjugates through interactions such as hydrogen bonding, π-π stacking, van der Waals forces, and electrostatic interactions, although they are often less stable [44]. Encapsulation methods are an effective way to conjugate aptamers with nanomaterials by encapsulating them in protective carriers or matrices. This approach, which uses materials like silica, polymers, or gels, successfully protects aptamers from enzymatic degradation during transport across cell membranes, especially since DNA and RNA molecules are highly susceptible to degradation [45]. Wang et al., for example, created a therapeutic nanosystem using a metal-organic framework (MOF) and chlorin e6–modified DNAzyme for gene therapy and photodynamic treatment (PDT). This method has high pH sensitivity, enabling precise release of the doped DNAzyme into a newly generated ZIF-8 structure. A nanosystem based on MOF and chlorin e6–modified DNAzyme has been developed to combine gene therapy and PDT [46]. This therapeutic DNAzyme revealed the potential for delivery to cancer cells utilizing ZIF-8 nanoparticles without undergoing any degradation [47].

6.3.3 Aptamer-Conjugated Nanodevices

Aptasensors, or fluorescently labeled aptamers, are biosensors that use aptamers as recognition components to detect target molecules [48]. Their chemical alteration and probe engineering design make them ideal for detecting tiny substances. However, the low binding affinity of anti–small-molecule aptamers limits detection sensitivity. Efforts to enhance binding affinity achieved only minor advances [49]. To address this issue, combining aptamers with nanomaterials has emerged as a viable strategy, paving the way for the development of sophisticated biosensors. Such combinations improve the diagnostic and therapeutic potential of aptasensors by taking advantage of the unique features of nanomaterials [50]. Several types of aptasensors, including those based on metallic, magnetic, and carbon nanomaterials, have been developed to improve functionality. These nanomaterial-functionalized aptasensors have potential therapeutic uses for sensing, detecting, and targeting certain chemicals [51].

6.3.4 Aptamer-Functionalized DNA Nanomaterials

When combined with DNA nanotechnology, aptamers show great promise for a variety of applications such as biosensing, drug delivery, and therapeutic treatments. The use of DNA nanotechnology enables the simultaneous display of several aptamers on nanostructures, which boosts their binding affinity and overall efficacy [52]. Research indicates that DNA nanostructures can enhance the target-binding efficacy of aptamers by a factor of 100 via multivalent interactions [53]. These DNA-based nanostructures, like viral capsids or nanoparticles, provide exact self-assembly for targeted drug delivery. DNA hydrogels have exhibited prolonged release of aptamer-based therapeutics, while DNA micelles offer regulated release and stability within biological contexts [54, 55]. Moreover, DNA liposomes augment the encapsulation and targeting of medicinal drugs, thus enhancing their bioavailability. These hybrid nanomaterials exhibit significant potential in cancer diagnostics and therapy, improving the sensitivity of aptamer-based sensors and probes. This nascent discipline integrates DNA nanotechnology with aptamer creation, producing adaptable instruments for clinical and diagnostic purposes [56].

6.4 Clinical Applications

Aptamers have emerged as attractive tools in clinical therapy, notably owing to their distinctive characteristics and adaptability.

6.4.1 Examples of Aptamers in Cancer Therapy

6.4.1.1 FDA-Approved Aptamers

A. **Pegaptanib (Macugen)**
   Pegaptanib, branded as Macugen, is the inaugural aptamer-based medication authorized for the treatment of age-related macular degeneration (AMD). This aptamer suppresses angiogenesis and lowers vascular permeability by targeting vascular endothelial growth factor (VEGF), effectively addressing the root causes of vision loss in neovascular AMD [57].
B. **Nexavar (Sorafenib)**
   Sorafenib, also known as Nexavar, is a small-molecule kinase inhibitor. In clinical investigations, it has been used with aptamers to enhance its anticancer efficacy [58]. Sorafenib is an efficacious therapy for advanced renal cell carcinoma, hepatocellular carcinoma, and thyroid cancer, as it inhibits many protein kinases involved in tumorigenesis and angiogenesis [59].

6.4.1.2 Clinical-Phase Aptamers

A. **AS1411**
   AS1411 specifically targets nucleolin, a protein that is overexpressed on the surface of cancer cells, and demonstrates antiproliferative and proapoptotic actions across multiple malignancies, including liver, kidney, lung, and breast cancers [60]. The overexpression of nucleolin in aggressive tumors correlates with the modulation of angiogenesis and cellular proliferation. AS1411 interacts with nucleolin, impairing its tumor-promoting activities and facilitating apoptosis [61]. Preclinical investigations in breast cancer have exhibited its antimetastatic capabilities. Moreover, phase I and II clinical trials of AS1411 have demonstrated encouraging outcomes regarding safety and therapeutic effectiveness [62, 63].
B. **NOX-A12**
   NOX-A12 is an RNA aptamer specifically engineered to target CXCL12 (stromal cell–derived factor-1 (SDF-1)), a chemokine essential for tumor growth,

angiogenesis, and metastasis [64]. NOX-A12 binds to CXCL12 and inhibits its interaction with CXCR4 and CXCR7 receptors, which are important regulators of tumor cell migration, proliferation, and the development of new blood vessels in the tumor microenvironment. This inhibits the signaling pathways that promote cancer growth and metastasis [65]. Clinical trials of NOX-A12 as a cancer treatment agent have yielded promising findings, indicating that it has the ability to prevent tumor development and metastasis. It has also been investigated in combination with other medicines, like immune checkpoint inhibitors and radiation, to boost antitumor activity [66]. These findings highlight its potential as a unique technique in the treatment of aggressive cancer.

C. **AGRO100 (or ACT-GRO-777)**
AGRO100, also known as ACT-GRO-777, is an aptamer that exclusively targets nucleolin and has demonstrated antiproliferative effects in tumor cells during phase I clinical studies. This chemical displayed a positive safety profile and successfully blocked nucleolin's function in supporting tumor cell development, which contributed to its potential anticancer properties [67].

D. **A10 RNA Aptamer**
Therapeutic medicines are frequently delivered to PSMA-expressing cells with accuracy using the A10 RNA aptamer. For instance, chemotherapy medicines like docetaxel (Dtx) loaded into nanoparticles functionalized with the A10 RNA aptamer displayed enhanced drug uptake and delivery in PSMA-positive cancer cells [68, 69]. These procedures improve medical efficacy, reduce side effects, and increase bioavailability. Studies have demonstrated that using these targeted delivery strategies reduces tumor growth significantly in prostate cancer xenograft animals. Aptamer-conjugated liposomes loaded with radioactive isotopes, for example, specifically target PSMA-expressing cells, giving a unique way of radiation with minimal off-target consequences [70].

6.4.1.3 Target-Specific Aptamers

A. **EpCAM (Epithelial Cell Adhesion Molecule)-Targeting Aptamers**
EpCAM, a significantly expressed marker in epithelial malignancies, is a target for certain aptamers. These aptamers are frequently coupled with nanocarriers to improve their distribution to tumor cells. This conjugation dramatically increases the targeting and uptake of therapeutic drugs directly into cancer cells, enhancing treatment efficacy while reducing unwanted effects on healthy organs [71, 72].

B. **PSMA-Specific Aptamers**
PSMA is a well-known biomarker for prostate cancer. Aptamers that target PSMA enable the targeted delivery of chemotherapeutic drugs to prostate cancer cells. These aptamers improve therapy efficacy while reducing systemic toxicity by concentrating therapeutic chemicals at the tumor site [73].

C. **Tumor Angiogenesis–Suppressing Aptamers**
Vascular endothelial growth factor (VEGF) promotes angiogenesis within malignancies. Aptamers that bind directly to VEGF are being investigated to suppress this mechanism and reduce tumor vascularization. By decreasing

VEGF activity, these aptamers may hinder the formation of new blood vessels that nourish the tumor, thus slowing its growth and progression [15].

D. **Oncogene-Targeting Aptamers**
   HER2 is an oncogene that is frequently overexpressed in particular breast tumors. Aptamers that target HER2 bind exclusively to this protein. These aptamers are commonly used with drug delivery methods to improve therapy outcomes for HER2-positive breast cancer patients. This technique improves treatment precision, maximizes therapeutic impact, and minimizes negative effects [74, 75].
E. **Mucin1 Aptamers**
   Ovarian and breast tumors have high levels of Mucin1 (MUC1). MUC1-targeting aptamers are being studied for drug administration and cancer imaging, which would allow for more precise therapeutic delivery and increased imaging accuracy. This selectivity increases the precision of imaging modalities and the targeting efficiency of medicines, potentially lowering side effects and improving patient outcomes [76].

6.5 Challenges and Barriers to Clinical Translation

6.5.1 Stability in Biological Environments

One of the most significant issues faced by aptamer-based medicines is their vulnerability to degradation in biological systems.

6.5.1.1 Degradation by Nucleases

RNA-based aptamers degrade quickly in the bloodstream by nucleases, limiting their half-life and efficacy in vivo. Despite being more stable than their RNA counterparts, DNA aptamers still require chemical modifications (such as 2′-O-methylation and phosphorothioate couplings) to increase their stability for therapeutic usage [77, 78].

6.5.1.2 Limited Circulation Time

Short systemic circulation periods limit aptamer efficacy by lowering medication bioavailability in target tissues. To address this, improvements such as PEGylation (polyethylene glycol attachment) and locked nucleic acid (LNA) alterations have been demonstrated to improve stability and half-life. However, these advances lead to higher production complexity and costs [33, 79].

6.5.2 Effective Delivery Systems

Delivery remains a significant bottleneck, especially in targeted therapy and intracellular applications.

6.5.2.1 Targeted Delivery

Aptamers must selectively deliver therapeutic payloads to specific tissues or cells while reducing off-target effects. Various delivery methods, including liposomes, nanoparticles, and aptamer–drug conjugates, are being intensively researched for this purpose. However, expanding these delivery systems for clinical use poses major regulatory and manufacturing obstacles [80].

6.5.2.2 Cellular Uptake

Aptamers that target intracellular proteins face considerable obstacles in traversing cell membranes. Although recent advances in conjugating aptamers with nanocarriers like gold nanoparticles and lipid-based nanovesicles are promising, attaining consistent internalization remains a difficult challenge [81, 82].

6.5.3 Immunogenicity and Toxicity

Aptamers often generate a lower immunological response than protein-based therapies such as monoclonal antibodies. However, chemical changes or connection with nanomaterials might occasionally cause immunological reactions. It is critical to thoroughly assess the toxicity profile of each aptamer design. Aptamers with substantial chemical changes or nonbiodegradable carriers may cause unexpected immune responses, emphasizing the necessity for rigorous preclinical safety assessments [83].

6.5.4 Manufacturing Complexity

Large-scale manufacture of therapeutically viable aptamers presents significant logistical and economic challenges, particularly in terms of cost and scalability. Aptamer synthesis requires high accuracy to assure purity and functionality, which is further hampered by the demand for changed nucleotides to improve stability and biological activity [84]. These adjustments, while necessary for therapeutic efficacy, considerably increase production costs. Scalable and cost-effective synthesis techniques are still in development, restricting the possibility of mass manufacturing. Furthermore, maintaining consistent quality across production batches is crucial for clinical success but difficult due to the aptamers' complicated structures and changes. Stringent quality control processes are required to guarantee clinical-grade aptamers that meet regulatory criteria, creating additional barriers to their widespread use [85].

6.5.5 Regulatory Hurdles in the Clinical Development of Aptamers

Aptamer-based pharmaceuticals encounter major regulatory challenges in clinical development because they are relatively new in comparison to established therapeutic modalities, such as monoclonal antibodies and small compounds.

6.5.5.1 Lack of Established Guidelines

Aptamer regulatory frameworks are still emerging, with global regulatory organizations such as the FDA and EMA having more defined standards for other medication categories. The absence of defined rules for evaluating aptamers causes confusion in clinical trial designs and approval processes [86]. While there are defined criteria for pharmacokinetic and immunogenicity testing of antibodies, aptamers require specialized techniques due to their distinct molecular architectures and modes of action. Customized methodologies for preclinical and clinical studies must address challenges like stability, biodistribution, and clearance. The variation in regulatory expectations between regions hinders global commercialization attempts [87].

6.5.5.2 Long Development Timelines

Extensive preclinical study is critical to address concerns about aptamer stability, toxicity, and efficacy, which greatly delays their progression to clinical trials [77]. For example, stability concerns with RNA aptamers require rigorous testing of chemical changes, such as 2'-fluoro or locked nucleic acid (LNA) substitutions, consequently lengthening research and development schedules [88]. Furthermore, because aptamers are frequently conjugated to other therapeutic agents, such as nanoparticles or chemotherapeutic medicines, these combination products require additional levels of regulatory scrutiny, prolonging the licensing process [89].

6.5.6 Challenges with Binding Affinity and Specificity

In contrast to antibodies, which often have dissociation constants in the low nanomolar to picomolar range, many aptamers have lower affinities, particularly against small-molecule targets, limiting their sensitivity in precise applications [84]. The commonly utilized method for developing aptamers frequently fails to produce aptamers with high binding affinity. Modifications introduced after selection, such as multimerization or chemical stabilization, might improve affinity but increase development complexity [90]. Additionally, aptamers that target proteins with conserved or homologous sections, such as receptor families, may exhibit cross-reactivity concerns. Obtaining 100% specificity in these cases necessitates substantial iterative optimization, which raises both development costs and delays [91].

6.5.7 Competition from Antibodies

Monoclonal antibodies dominate the therapeutic sector due to their proven efficacy, extensive production infrastructure, and long clinical track record. Antibodies often have higher binding affinities, frequently in the nanomolar to picomolar range, and longer systemic half-lives than aptamers, providing them a considerable advantage in therapeutic applications [92]. A well-established global manufacturing ecosystem, comprising scalable bioreactor systems and modern purification procedures, supports this high efficacy, ensuring consistent output and supply. Furthermore, monoclonal antibodies have substantial clinical histories and well-documented safety profiles, making them the favored choice among clinicians and regulatory agencies. To effectively compete in the therapeutic market, aptamers must clearly demonstrate their distinct advantages, such as decreased immunogenicity and ease of synthesis, as these aspects collectively provide antibodies with a dominant edge [93]. Combination therapies that use both aptamers and antibodies may pave the path for acceptance in specific niches, exploiting the benefits of both types of medicines [94].

6.5.8 Intellectual Property (IP) Challenges

The patent environment for aptamer technology is extremely clogged, posing significant impediments to research and commercialization. Core SELEX techniques and various aptamer sequences are strongly patented, frequently by only a few companies. This needs costly license agreements for commercial use, limiting entry for new market participants [95]. Patents on aptamer–nanoparticle conjugates and innovative delivery technologies further impede the development of new applications [96]. Overlapping intellectual property claims may result in costly legal battles or less operational freedom. Companies must manage a complex licensing landscape, which can impede product development. While collaborations between academia and industry have the potential to overcome these barriers, they frequently face issues related to intellectual property rights and revenue sharing, adding another layer of complexity to the commercialization of aptamer-based innovations [89, 97].

6.6 Future Perspectives in Aptamer-Based Cancer Therapy

The strategic enhancement of aptamer-based cancer therapy's stability, targeting effectiveness, and adaptability through chemical modifications and integration with cutting-edge technology is critical to its future. Deoxyribose/ribose sugars, nitrogenous bases, and the phosphodiester backbone have all shown promise in increasing aptamer resistance to nuclease degradation and affinity for specific targets [98]. Hydrophobic base substitutions can increase systemic stability by interacting with serum albumin, a protective carrier that facilitates aptamer dissociation near tumor cells [79].

The elimination of aptamers by organs such as the kidney and liver also shortens their lifespan in vivo. Conjugating to bigger nanoparticles is the most common method for increasing the aptamer's lifespan against renal clearance. To reduce the renal clearance rate of the drug delivery system, materials such as proteins, dendrimers, and inorganic nanoparticles were also efficiently coupled with aptamers [99, 100]. Aptamers and nanomaterials have been coupled to create multimodal conjugates with both medicinal and diagnostic functions. These nanostructures are expected to improve treatment outcomes, reduce therapy costs, and address challenges, such as multiple medication resistance [101]. Cyclonization approaches, such as circular and bivalent aptamer–drug conjugates, provide additional structural stability, dual-targeting capabilities, and reduced toxicity to healthy tissues [102].

Aptamers are being developed in immunotherapy for applications such as immune checkpoint inhibition and tumor vaccination. To improve therapy specificity and efficacy, these innovations include functionalizing aptamers for covalent binding, valency management, and nanostructure construction [103]. Investigating molecular processes such as cell–cell communication and glycosylated protein interactions broadens their potential for developing effective immune-based cancer therapeutics [104].

Aptamer–drug conjugates (ApDCs) provide the tailored delivery of cytotoxic agents via chemically diverse linkers, exemplifying precision medicine. Aptamer–T cell therapy and aptamer–PROTAC conjugates represent two innovative approaches that demonstrate potential for personalized treatment of hematologic malignancies [105]. Moreover, stimuli-responsive devices, actuated by light, magnetic fields, or ultrasound, facilitate controlled drug release. These technologies offer synergistic anticancer effects and enhance precision oncology [106, 107].

High-throughput screening technologies are employed to identify aptamers with superior binding properties to expedite clinical translation. By resolving challenges related to biological stability and delivery mechanisms, these platforms ensure that aptamers can realize their complete therapeutic potential [77]. Market-driven research is expected to accelerate the adoption of aptamer-based therapies in academic and industrial environments, fostering the development of novel cancer treatment strategies. Aptamers are anticipated to play a pivotal role in precision medicine as improvements continue, offering expanded therapeutic applications in oncology, diminished toxicity, and improved specificity [108, 109].

6.7 Conclusion

Aptamers represent a significant breakthrough in targeted cancer therapy owing to their exceptional specificity, low immunogenicity, and adaptability. They provide creative ways to address the limitations of existing medicines, including non-specificity, systemic toxicity, and resistance. Chemical changes and the incorporation of modern technologies such as nanomedicine are crucial for improving aptamer stability and therapeutic effectiveness [110]. Promising advancements encompass multimodal aptamer–nanomaterial conjugates, facilitating accurate drug delivery and diagnostic functions. Advancements in aptamer–drug conjugates and stimuli-responsive systems underscore their promise in customized oncology, especially for hematologic malignancies [111]. Their function in immunotherapy, particularly in immune checkpoint inhibition, enhances their therapeutic uses. High-throughput screening systems for aptamer development are essential for expediting clinical translation and addressing issues of biological stability, effective transport, and in vivo efficacy [112].

Problems such as nuclease degradation, inefficient distribution, and complicated manufacturing continue despite their promise. Chemical alterations, distribution systems, and methods of mass manufacture need to be the subject of ongoing investigation in order to resolve these concerns. To help overcome intellectual property restrictions and regulatory roadblocks, academic institutions, businesses, and government agencies must work together to promote clinical adoption [88].

6.8 Future Research

Research in the future should focus on developing new aptamers against unknown disease targets and integrating them with cutting-edge nanomaterials to enhance imaging, biosensing, and therapeutic efficacy [113]. Forecasting aptamer structures, affinities, and potential modifications; optimizing aptamer-based platforms; exploring synergies with other therapeutic modalities; and expanding their applications in cancer immunotherapy and diagnostics will all require computational techniques like artificial intelligence (AI) and machine learning (ML) to maximize performance and speed up the development process. By overcoming these obstacles, aptamers will be able to significantly contribute to precision oncology, which will ultimately benefit patients by enhancing treatment outcomes while decreasing treatment burden [114].

Acknowledgments The authors are thankful to the Department of Pharmaceuticals, Ministry of Chemicals and Fertilizers, Government of India. All the figures are from https://www.biorender.com.

Credit Authorship Contribution Statement **Conceptualization**: Vishal Chhabra, Sarasa Meenakshi **Writing – Original Draft Preparation**: Vishal Chhabra, Sarasa Meenakshi **Visualization and Supervision**: Krishna Murti **Editing – Final Draft**: Santosh Kumar, Krishna Murti

Declaration of Competing Interests The authors declare no competing or financial interest relevant to this chapter.

Consent for Publication None to declare.

References

1. Yadav AK, Desai NS. Cancer stem cells: acquisition, characteristics, therapeutic implications, targeting strategies and future prospects. Stem Cell Rev Rep. 2019;15:331–55.

2. Xia L, Oyang L, Lin J, Tan S, Han Y, Wu N, et al. The cancer metabolic reprogramming and immune response. Mol Cancer. 2021;20:1–21.
3. Anand P, Soni S, Padwad YS. Targeted molecular therapies in cancer; 2021. p. 59–101.
4. Li J, Wang Q, Xia G, Adilijiang N, Li Y, Hou Z, et al. Recent advances in targeted drug delivery strategy for enhancing oncotherapy. 2023;15(9):2233.
5. Ward RA, Fawell S, Floc'h N, Flemington V, Mckerrecher D, Smith PD. Challenges and opportunities in cancer drug resistance. Chem Rev. 2020;121(6):3297–351.
6. Hianik T. Aptamer-based biosensors. 2018. Vol. 7, p. 11–9.
7. Darmostuk M, Rimpelova S, Gbelcova H, Ruml T. Current approaches in SELEX: an update to aptamer selection technology. 2015;33(6):1141–61.
8. Morita Y, Leslie M, Kameyama H, Volk DE, Tanaka TJC. Aptamer therapeutics in cancer: current and future. 2018;10(3):80.
9. Ma H, Liu J, Ali MM, Mahmood MAI, Labanieh L, Lu M, et al. Nucleic acid aptamers in cancer research, diagnosis and therapy. 2015;44(5):1240–56.
10. Huang Y, Lin G, Liu S, Chen M, Yang CY, Song YJC. Aptamer-based immune checkpoint inhibition for cancer immunotherapy:e202400599.
11. Kumar A, Bahadure S, Chilamakuri SN, Dadhale A, Gulbake A. Multifunctional nanocarrier-mediated codelivery for targeting and treatment of prostate cancer. In: Multifunctional nanocomposites for targeted drug delivery in cancer therapy. Elsevier; 2024. p. 81–111.
12. Zhu J, Huang H, Dong S, Ge L, Zhang YJT. Progress in aptamer-mediated drug delivery vehicles for cancer targeting and its implications in addressing chemotherapeutic challenges. 2014;4(9):931.
13. Zhou G, Latchoumanin O, Hebbard L, Duan W, Liddle C, George J, et al. Aptamers as targeting ligands and therapeutic molecules for overcoming drug resistance in cancers. 2018;134:107–21.
14. Yüce M, Kurt H, Hussain B, Budak H. Systematic evolution of ligands by exponential enrichment for aptamer selection. In: Biomedical applications of functionalized nanomaterials. Elsevier; 2018. p. 211–43.
15. Riccardi C, Napolitano E, Platella C, Musumeci D, Melone MA, Montesarchio D. Anti-VEGF DNA-based aptamers in cancer therapeutics and diagnostics. 2021;41(1):464–506.
16. He S, Gao F, Ma J, Ma H, Dong G, Sheng CJAC. Aptamer-protac conjugates (apcs) for tumor-specific targeting in breast cancer. 2021;133(43):23487–93.
17. Yoon S, Rossi JJ. Aptamers: uptake mechanisms and intracellular applications. 2018;134:22–35.
18. Wan L-Y, Yuan W-F, Ai W-B, Ai Y-W, Wang J-J, Chu L-Y, et al. An exploration of aptamer internalization mechanisms and their applications in drug delivery. 2019;16(3):207–18.
19. Xu W, Siddiqui IA, Nihal M, Pilla S, Rosenthal K, Mukhtar H, et al. Aptamer-conjugated and doxorubicin-loaded unimolecular micelles for targeted therapy of prostate cancer. 2013;34(21):5244–53.
20. Park D, Lee SJ, Park JW. Aptamer-based smart targeting and spatial trigger–response drug-delivery systems for anticancer therapy. 2024;12(1):187.
21. Xie S, Ai L, Cui C, Fu T, Cheng X, Qu F, et al. Functional aptamer-embedded nanomaterials for diagnostics and therapeutics. 2021;13(8):9542–60.
22. Zhou G, Wilson G, Hebbard L, Duan W, Liddle C, George J, et al. Aptamers: a promising chemical antibody for cancer therapy. 2016;7(12):13446.
23. Mi Z, Guo H, Russell MB, Liu Y, Sullenger BA, Kuo PC. RNA aptamer blockade of osteopontin inhibits growth and metastasis of MDA-MB231 breast cancer cells. 2009;17(1):153–61.
24. Al Hasan A, Azam AZ. Small RNA-mediated prevention, diagnosis and therapies of cancer. In: Design of nanostructures for theranostics applications. Elsevier; 2018. p. 341–436.
25. Subramanian N, Kanwar JR, Kanwar RK, Krishnakumar S. Blocking the maturation of OncomiRNAs using pri-miRNA-17~ 92 aptamer in retinoblastoma. 2015;25(1):47–52.
26. Akpa PA, Peter IE, Onwuka AM, Obi BC, Akunne MO, Nworu CS, et al. Nanotheranostics: platforms, current applications, and mechanisms of targeting in breast and prostate cancers. 2023;4(3):346–83.

27. Yu H, Zhu J, Shen G, Deng Y, Geng X, Wang L. Improving aptamer performance: key factors and strategies. 2023;190(7):255.
28. Alamudi SH, Kimoto M, Hirao I. Uptake mechanisms of cell-internalizing nucleic acid aptamers for applications as pharmacological agents. 2021;12(10):1640–9.
29. Liu P, Ga L, Aodeng G, Wang Y, Ai J. Aptamer-drug conjugates: new probes for imaging and targeted therapy. 2022;10:100126.
30. Shiao Y-S, Chiu H-H, Wu P-H, Huang Y-F. Aptamer-functionalized gold nanoparticles as photoresponsive nanoplatform for co-drug delivery. 2014;6(24):21832–41.
31. Zhou P, Zhang S, Li L, Zhang R, Guo G, Zhang Y, et al. Targeted degradation of VEGF with bispecific aptamer-based LYTACs ameliorates pathological retinal angiogenesis. 2024;14(13):4983.
32. Kucherenko I, Soldatkin O, Kucherenko DY, Soldatkina O, Dzyadevych SJNA. Advances in nanomaterial application in enzyme-based electrochemical biosensors: a review. 2019;1(12):4560–77.
33. Ghasemii K, Darroudi M, Rahimmanesh I, Ghomi M, Hassanpour M, Sharifi E, et al. Advances in aptamer-based drug delivery vehicles for cancer therapy. 2022;140:213077.
34. Liu M, Wang L, Lo Y, Shiu SC-C, Kinghorn AB, Tanner JA. Aptamer-enabled nanomaterials for therapeutics, drug targeting and imaging. 2022;11(1):159.
35. Ohno Y, Maehashi K, Matsumoto K. Label-free biosensors based on aptamer-modified graphene field-effect transistors. 2010;132(51):18012–3.
36. Abidian MR, Kim DH, Martin DC. Conducting-polymer nanotubes for controlled drug release. 2006;18(4):405–9.
37. Atapour A, Khajehzadeh H, Shafie M, Abbasi M, Mosleh-Shirazi S, Kasaee SR, et al. Gold nanoparticle-based aptasensors: a promising perspective for early-stage detection of cancer biomarkers. 2022;30:103181.
38. Xiang W, Lv Q, Shi H, Xie B, Gao L. Aptamer-based biosensor for detecting carcinoembryonic antigen. 2020;214:120716.
39. Mirkin CA, Letsinger RL, Mucic RC, Storhoff JJ. A DNA-based method for rationally assembling nanoparticles into macroscopic materials. In: Spherical nucleic acids. Jenny Stanford; 2020. p. 3–11.
40. Zhang M, Shao S, Yue H, Wang X, Zhang W, Chen F, et al. High stability au nps: from design to application in nanomedicine. 2021:6067-6094.
41. Farokhzad OC, Jon S, Khademhosseini A, Tran TNT, Lavan DA, Langer R. Nanoparticle-aptamer bioconjugates: a new approach for targeting prostate cancer cells. 2004;64(21):7668–72.
42. Hu J, Ye M, Zhou Z. Aptamers: novel diagnostic and therapeutic tools for diabetes mellitus and metabolic diseases. 2017;95:249–56.
43. Rabiee N, Chen S, Ahmadi S, Veedu RN. Aptamer-engineered (nano)materials for theranostic applications. Theranostics. 2023;13(15):5183–206.
44. Chen Z, Luo H, Gubu A, Yu S, Zhang H, Dai H, et al. Chemically modified aptamers for improving binding affinity to the target proteins via enhanced non-covalent bonding. Front Cell Dev Biol. 2023;11:1091809.
45. Ghasemii K, Darroudi M, Rahimmanesh I, Ghomi M, Hassanpour M, Sharifi E, et al. Advances in aptamer-based drug delivery vehicles for cancer therapy. Biomater Adv. 2022;140:213077.
46. Wang H, Chen Y, Wang H, Liu X, Zhou X, Wang F. DNAzyme-loaded metal-organic frameworks (MOFs) for self-sufficient gene therapy. Angew Chem Int Ed Engl. 2019;58(22):7380–4.
47. Zeng Z, Zhong M, Liao T, Zhou X, Shi L, Zhang X, et al. Nano-fuels-driven self-sacrificed ZIF-8@Apt integrated chip coupled with a DNAzyme system for the isolation and detection of glioblastoma-derived extracellular vesicles. Chem Eng J. 2024;502:157445.
48. Wang RE, Zhang Y, Cai J, Cai W, Gao T. Aptamer-based fluorescent biosensors. 2011;18(27):4175–84.
49. Ning Y, Hu J, Lu FJB. Aptamers used for biosensors and targeted therapy. Pharmacotherapy. 2020;132:110902.

50. Flores-Contreras EA, González-González RB, González-González E, Melchor-Martínez EM, Parra-Saldívar R, Iqbal HM. Detection of emerging pollutants using aptamer-based biosensors: recent advances, challenges, and outlook. 2022;12(12):1078.
51. Heydari-Bafrooei E, Shamszadeh NS. Electrochemical bioassay development for ultrasensitive aptasensing of prostate specific antigen. Bioelectronics. 2017;91:284–92.
52. Huang Z, Qiu L, Zhang T, Tan W. Integrating DNA nanotechnology with aptamers for biological and biomedical applications. 2021;4(2):461–89.
53. Zhao Y-X, Shaw A, Zeng X, Benson E, Nystrom AM, Hogberg BJ. DNA origami delivery system for cancer therapy with tunable release properties. 2012;6(10):8684–91.
54. Agrawal NK, Allen P, Song YH, Wachs RA, Du Y, Ellington AD, et al. Oligonucleotide-functionalized hydrogels for sustained release of small molecule (aptamer) therapeutics. 2020;102:315–25.
55. Liu C, Han J, Pei Y, Du J. Aptamer functionalized DNA hydrogel for wise-stage controlled protein release. 2018;8(10):1941.
56. Plourde K, Derbali RM, Desrosiers A, Dubath C, Vallée-Bélisle A, Leblond J. Aptamer-based liposomes improve specific drug loading and release. 2017;251:82–91.
57. Venkatesan S, Chanda K, Balamurali MM. Recent advancements of aptamers in cancer therapy. ACS Omega. 2023;8(36):32231–43.
58. Wang L, Chen M, Ran X, Tang H, Cao DJP. Sorafenib-based drug delivery systems: applications and perspectives. 2023;15(12):2638.
59. Santarpia G, Carnes E. Therapeutic applications of aptamers. 2024;25:6742.
60. Thongchot S, Aksonnam K, Thuwajit P, Yenchitsomanus P-T, Thuwajit C. Nucleolin-based targeting strategies in cancer treatment: focus on cancer immunotherapy. 2023;52(3):1–14.
61. Reyes-Reyes EM, Šalipur FR, Shams M, Forsthoefel MK, Bates PJ. Mechanistic studies of anticancer aptamer AS1411 reveal a novel role for nucleolin in regulating Rac1 activation. 2015;9(7):1392–405.
62. Rosenberg JE, Bambury RM, Van Allen EM, Drabkin HA, Lara PN, Harzstark AL, et al. A phase II trial of AS1411 (a novel nucleolin-targeted DNA aptamer) in metastatic renal cell carcinoma. 2014;32:178–87.
63. Malik MT, O'Toole MG, Casson LK, Thomas SD, Bardi GT, Reyes-Reyes EM, et al. AS1411-conjugated gold nanospheres and their potential for breast cancer therapy. 2015;6(26):22270.
64. Citro A, Pellegrini S, Dugnani E, Eulberg D, Klussmann S, Piemonti L. CCL2/MCP-1 and CXCL12/SDF-1 blockade by L-aptamers improve pancreatic islet engraftment and survival in mouse. 2019;19(11):3131–8.
65. Portella L, Bello AM, Scala S. CXCL12 signaling in the tumor microenvironment. 2021;1302:51–70.
66. Cerchia L. Aptamers: promising tools for cancer diagnosis and therapy. Cancers (Basel). 2018;10:132.
67. Platella C, Riccardi C, Montesarchio D, Roviello GN, Musumeci D. G-quadruplex-based aptamers against protein targets in therapy and diagnostics. 2017;1861(5):1429–47.
68. Fan X, Guo Y, Wang L, Xiong X, Zhu L, Fang K. Diagnosis of prostate cancer using anti-PSMA aptamer A10-3.2-oriented lipid nanobubbles. 2016;11:3939–50.
69. Nasri N, Saharkhiz S, Dini G, Ghasemvand FJH. In vitro study of a new theranostic smart niosomal nanostructure for direct delivery of docetaxel via anti-PSMA aptamer. 2024;10:17.
70. Meher N, VanBrocklin HF, Wilson DM, Flavell RR. PSMA-Targeted nanotheranostics for imaging and radiotherapy of prostate cancer. 2023;16(2):315.
71. Vandghanooni S, Sanaat Z, Farahzadi R, Eskandani M, Omidian H, Omidi Y. Recent progress in the development of aptasensors for cancer diagnosis: focusing on aptamers against cancer biomarkers. 2021;170:106640.
72. Subramanian N, Kanwar JR, Athalya PK, Janakiraman N, Khetan V, Kanwar RK, et al. EpCAM aptamer mediated cancer cell specific delivery of EpCAM siRNA using polymeric nanocomplex. 2015;22:1–10.
73. Arese M, Mahmoudian M, Bussolino F. RNA aptamer-mediated gene therapy of prostate cancer: lessons from the past and future directions. 2023;20(11):1609–21.

74. Varty K, O'Brien C, Ignaszak AJC. Breast cancer aptamers: current sensing targets, available aptamers, and their evaluation for clinical use in diagnostics. 2021;13(16):3984.
75. Sitia L, Sevieri M, Signati L, Bonizzi A, Chesi A, Mainini F, et al. HER-2-targeted nanoparticles for breast cancer diagnosis and treatment. Cancers. 2022;14(10)
76. Vivo-Llorca G, Candela-Noguera V, Alfonso M, García-Fernández A, Orzáez M, Sancenón F, et al. MUC1 aptamer-capped mesoporous silica nanoparticles for navitoclax resistance overcoming in triple-negative breast cancer. Chemistry. 2020;26(69):16318–27.
77. Zhou J, Rossi JJ. Aptamers as targeted therapeutics: current potential and challenges. 2017;16(3):181–202.
78. Zheng YY, Wu Y, Begley TJ, Sheng J. Sulfur modification in natural RNA and therapeutic oligonucleotides. 2021;2(4):990–1003.
79. Odeh F, Nsairat H, Alshaer W, Ismail MA, Esawi E, Qaqish B, et al. Aptamers chemistry: chemical modifications and conjugation strategies. 2019;25(1):3.
80. Liang C, He Y, Liu Y, Gao Y, Han Y, Li X, et al. Fluoride exposure alters the ultrastructure of sperm flagellum via reducing key protein expressions in testis. Chemosphere. 2020;246:125772.
81. Jia H-R, Zhang Z, Fang X, Jiang M, Chen M, Chen S, et al. Recent advances of cell surface modification based on aptamers. 2022;18:100188.
82. Wan Y, Wang L, Zhu C, Zheng Q, Wang G, Tong J, et al. Aptamer-conjugated extracellular nanovesicles for targeted drug delivery. 2018;78(3):798–808.
83. Palmieri V, Caracciolo G. Tuning the immune system by nanoparticle–biomolecular corona. Nanoscale Adv. 2022;4(16):3300–8.
84. Yoo H, Jo H, Oh SS. Detection and beyond: challenges and advances in aptamer-based biosensors. 2020;1(8):2663–87.
85. McKeague M. DeRosa MC, Challenges and opportunities for small molecule aptamer development. 2012;2012(1):748913.
86. Pimenta C, Bettiol V, Alencar-Silva T, Franco OL, Pogue R, Carvalho JL, et al. Advanced therapies and regulatory framework in different areas of the globe: past, present, and future. 2021;43(5):e103–e38.
87. Bruno JG. Predicting the uncertain future of aptamer-based diagnostics and therapeutics. 2015;20(4):6866–87.
88. Shi Y, Zhen X, Zhang Y, Li Y, Koo S, Saiding Q, et al. Chemically modified platforms for better RNA therapeutics. 2024;124(3):929–1033.
89. Bruno JG. A review of therapeutic aptamer conjugates with emphasis on new approaches. 2013;6(3):340–57.
90. Kohlberger M, Gadermaier G. SELEX: critical factors and optimization strategies for successful aptamer selection. 2022;69(5):1771–92.
91. Ahirwar R, Nahar S, Aggarwal S, Ramachandran S, Maiti S, Nahar P. In silico selection of an aptamer to estrogen receptor alpha using computational docking employing estrogen response elements as aptamer-alike molecules. 2016;6(1):21285.
92. Yüce M, Ullah N, Budak H. Trends in aptamer selection methods and applications. 2015;140(16):5379–99.
93. Yingngam B. Monoclonal antibody. 2024:419.
94. Vandghanooni S, Eskandani M, Barar J, Omidi Y. Bispecific therapeutic aptamers for targeted therapy of cancer: a review on cellular perspective. 2018;96:885–902.
95. Dua P, Kim S, Lee D-K. Patents on SELEX and therapeutic aptamers. 2008;2(3):172–86.
96. Missailidis S, Hardy A. Aptamers as inhibitors of target proteins. 2009;19(8):1073–82.
97. Groff K, Brown J, Clippinger AJ. Modern affinity reagents: recombinant antibodies and aptamers. 2015;33(8):1787–98.
98. Röthlisberger P, Hollenstein M. Aptamer chemistry. 2018;134:3–21.
99. Heo K, Min S-W, Sung HJ, Kim HG, Kim HJ, Kim YH, et al. An aptamer-antibody complex (oligobody) as a novel delivery platform for targeted cancer therapies. J Control Release. 2016;229:1–9.

100. Jin B, Guo Z, Chen Z, Chen H, Li S, Deng Y, et al. Aptamers in cancer therapy: problems and new breakthroughs. 2023;11(8):1609–27.
101. Mir SA, Hamid L, Bader GN, Shoaib A, Rahamathulla M, Alshahrani MY, et al. Role of nanotechnology in overcoming the multidrug resistance in cancer therapy: a review. 2022;27(19):6608.
102. Huang Z, Wang D, Zhang Q, Zhang Y, Peng R, Tan W. Leveraging aptamer-based DNA nanotechnology for bioanalysis and cancer therapeutics. 2024;5(4):438–52.
103. Kejamurthy P, Devi KTR. Immune checkpoint inhibitors and cancer immunotherapy by aptamers: an overview. 2023;41(1):40.
104. Behl T, Kumar A, Sehgal A, Singh S, Sharma N, Yadav S, et al. Understanding the mechanistic pathways and clinical aspects associated with protein and gene based biomarkers in breast cancer. 2023;126595.
105. Ai L, Jiang X, Zhang K, Cui C, Liu B, Tan W. Tools and techniques for the discovery of therapeutic aptamers: recent advances. 2023;18(12):1393–411.
106. Sun L, Liu H, Ye Y, Lei Y, Islam R, Tan S, et al. Smart nanoparticles for cancer therapy. 2023;8(1):418.
107. Peng X, Liu Y, Peng F, Wang T, Cheng Z, Chen Q, et al. Aptamer-controlled stimuli-responsive drug release. 2024;135353
108. McGrath MJ, Scanaill CN. Sensor technologies: healthcare, wellness, and environmental applications. Springer; 2013.
109. Xiang D, Shigdar S, Qiao G, Wang T, Kouzani AZ, Zhou S-F, et al. Nucleic acid aptamer-guided cancer therapeutics and diagnostics: the next generation of cancer medicine. 2015;5(1):23.
110. Hashim AA, Altememy D, Aljeboury MHM. Advancements in aptamer-based nanoparticle bioconjugates for targeted cancer therapy: a comprehensive review. 2024;3(1):104–25.
111. Das S, Gupta A, Vaishnavi T, Walia S, Bhatia D, Chakraborty B. Aptamers functionalized biomolecular nano-vehicles for applications in cancer diagnostics & therapeutics. 2022;2(2):360.
112. Bertrand P. Aptamers targeting the PD-1/PD-L1 axis: a perspective. 2023;66(16):10878–88.
113. Dougherty CA, Cai W, Hong H. Applications of aptamers in targeted imaging: state of the art. 2015;15(12):1138–52.
114. Kumar S, Mohan A, Sharma NR, Kumar A, Girdhar M, Malik T, et al. Computational frontiers in aptamer-based nanomedicine for precision therapeutics: a comprehensive review. 2024;9(25):26838–62.

Aptamer-Based Cancer Diagnosis: Emerging Updates

7

Mithun Singh Rajput and Gopal Natesan

7.1 Introduction

7.1.1 Background on Cancer Diagnosis

To diagnose cancer, which is a complex medical process, a complete and multifaceted approach is needed to assess the malignancy. The process of diagnosing cancer begins with the physical examination of patient's symptoms and initial clinical suspicion and ends with abnormal screening test results [7]. Medical professionals employ a range of sophisticated diagnostic methods to probe for possible malignancy in the tissues. They start with advanced imaging techniques that give greater details of the interior body parts and potential abnormalities. These include X-ray, ultrasound, positron emission tomography (PET) scan, magnetic resonance imaging (MRI), and computed tomography (CT) scan [30]. After images are taken, specialists may ask for MRI examinations, CT scans of the brain, and blood samples to check for processes caused by distant malignancy. The imaging methods can find malignant conditions in the body, but it is also helpful to carry out comprehensive laboratory studies that give important biochemical and genetic information [77]. The biopsy, a conclusive method of obtaining tissue/cell and testing it by a pathologist, is the key to cancer diagnosis. This study reveals a lot of important information about whether the cancer is present, its type, its cellular characteristics, and possible genetic mutations [56]. After the tumor is found, physician staging is done to find the size and location of the tumor, the extent of tissue invasion, whether the lymph node is involved, and whether there is spread of the tumor. Today, diagnostic tests make use of new molecular and genetic studies to better gauge risk and create treatment plans [77].

M. S. Rajput · G. Natesan (✉)
Institute of Pharmacy, Nirma University, Ahmedabad, Gujarat, India
e-mail: mithunsingh.rajput@nirmauni.ac.in; gopal@nirmauni.ac.in

S. Srivastava et al. (eds.), *Biosensors and Aptamers*,
https://doi.org/10.1007/978-981-96-8387-1_7

The diagnostic workup is extremely complex and requires a collaborative approach that unites different medical specialties, technological advances, and analysis techniques. With the most advanced and accurate diagnostic capabilities concerning cancer, new technologies, such as artificial intelligence (AI), liquid biopsy techniques, advanced molecular screening, and advanced imaging technologies, continue to evolve in cancer diagnosis. Physicians realize that these advances do not provide foolproof confirmation with the help of only one test, so a thorough assessment requiring patient variability and various diagnostic modalities is needed [2].

The aim of cancer diagnosis is no longer to simply detect it; rather, it aims to create a complete, precise, and personalized understanding of the peculiarities of the disease. Using this method, different medical teams can create personalized treatments based on the characteristics of the genetic and molecular profiles of the patient's particular disease. Cancer diagnosis precisely refers to the use of technologies, clinical skills, and other disciplines to establish a correct and relevant diagnosis based on the relevant data. It helps doctors in determining the treatment for the patient.

7.1.2 Need for Innovative Diagnostic Tools

Low precision in early cancer diagnostic decision support systems result in more needless biopsies [44]. The attempts to anticipate therapy response and customize treatments have been hampered by the absence of sophisticated imaging techniques. Oncologic imaging advances in recent years have revolutionized cancer diagnosis, treatment planning, and monitoring by giving physicians unprecedented insights into tumor properties and therapy responses across a range of cancer types and treatment phases [78]. For example, dual-modality imaging combines morphological, metabolic, and functional data to provide a more precise disease assessment. Examples of this include PET and single photon emission computed tomography (SPECT), both combined individually with CT and commercialized, respectively, in 2001 and 2004. By enabling more precise tumor localization, staging, and treatment response tracking, these technologies have improved medical imaging and, ultimately, improved patient outcomes, particularly in oncology [74].

Through the visualization of molecular and cellular mechanisms, the recent and continuous advancement of molecular imaging facilitates the early detection of neoplastic conditions, thereby averting metastasis and other critical stages of illness. These technological innovations enable a more profound comprehension of pathophysiological mechanisms, rendering them an essential instrument for the improvement of patient care [75]. In recent times, molecular imaging has aided several important innovations, most of which are not compatible for use in the clinical practice setting. The field of artificial intelligence (AI) has developed rapidly over the last decade and has found specific application in the field of radiation oncology, in which complex methodologies of computation are used to devise individualized therapy plans with improved diagnostic and therapeutic outcomes [60]. The increasing amount of imaging data produced each year and the breakthrough in the methods of machine learning and deep learning are a great help in discovering latent biomarkers and quantitative features in medical images [3]. Therefore, the need for advanced cancer diagnostic technologies, which can complement the current approaches in different fields of oncology, remains acute [78].

7.1.3 Overview of Aptamers in Biomedical Applications

A new class of chemically synthesized single-stranded DNA or RNA species, known as aptamers, has been identified as a useful tool in a number of biological assays. These chemical probes have been identified for several years by the so-called Systematic Evolution of Ligands by Exponential Enrichment (SELEX) beginning in the early 1990s, and it was shown that these reactants have the ability to interact with their target entities at a relatively high affinity and show a high degree of specificity toward proteins, cells, ions, and small molecules [8]. Aptamers have the capability to identify and interact with certain molecular targets; hence, they have been established as potent agents for various applications in the biomedical domain. There is currently just one FDA-approved aptamer medication (Macugen), while many others are in clinical studies [8]. Numerous illnesses, such as those linked to aging, obesity, diabetes, cardiovascular disease, infectious diseases, blood coagulation problems, bone diseases, immunological disorders, and cancer, have been studied in relation to these molecular ligands [8]. Their treatment approach entails identifying molecular targets with precision and modifying biological activity by disrupting diseased processes. This applies to aptamer applications in diagnostics, which show the same potential. Researchers have successfully synthesized aptamer-modified nanoparticles for more selective recognition of specific cell types, for example, leukemia cells [8]. Scientists can design more complex biosensing systems that permit rapid and highly selective identification of numerous biological species by attaching aptamers to nanoparticles. Due to their versatility, aptamers can be incorporated in specific advanced techniques in diagnostics, including surface plasmon resonance, electrochemistry, colorimetry, and fluorescence [84]. The field is evolving rapidly, thanks to continuous advances in chemistry, nanotechnology, biology, and medicine. Due to their synthetic nature, as well as their high specificity and adaptability, aptamers are transformative molecules in biomedical research, offering novel diagnostic, targeted therapeutic, and personalized medicine solutions [51].

The role of this chapter is to provide a thorough review of aptamer-based cancer diagnostics, how it can work, recent advances, and applications. It addresses difficulties in establishing and promoting biosensor technologies and discusses their combination with aptamers. The final section discusses the role of aptamers in enhancing early cancer diagnosis and personalized medicine, as well as exploring potential future research and development opportunities.

7.2 Aptamers: An Overview

7.2.1 Definition and Characteristics of Aptamers

In 1990, researchers established an alternative way of binding specific molecules and thus identified "aptamers," a heterogeneous group of randomly sequenced RNA that have had the ability to bind to unique chemical dyes that were selected from a very large combinatorial library. Aptamers are single-stranded DNA or RNA molecules that can bind to specific targets through conformational changes, without the need for sequence complementarity. Compared to other ligands, aptamers possess several advantages: they are small, easily synthesized, and fully designed; have minimal immunogenicity; and exhibit high chemical stability [25]. These characteristics make aptamers potential candidates for targeted therapy. A large number of aptamers have been assessed and tested and have demonstrated promising results pending their utilization in prognostics, cancer identification, and the treatment of viral and cancerous diseases in humans [40].

7.2.2 Types of Aptamers: DNA- and RNA-Based

Till date, numerous aptamers have been proposed; all of them have been revealed to possess considerable prospects in numerous applications. Currently, there are two principal forms of synthetic oligonucleotide molecules, called DNA and RNA aptamers, that possess unique physicochemical characteristics, which make it feasible to utilize them for ample biological purposes. That is where they are most different—their molecular characteristics, the methods by which people select them, and how strong their structures can be. DNA aptamers have an in vitro plasma half-life of 30–60 min, unlike RNA aptamers, which degrade within seconds. Due in large part to their chemical structure, which includes C–H bonds at the deoxyribose sugar's 2′ position, DNA aptamers are more resistant to nucleases and are chemically firm. However, due to their distinct molecular characteristics, RNA aptamers have more intricate three-dimensional (3D) structures. Also, the number of selection steps in their process is higher as they perform in vitro transcription and reverse transcription in each SELEX round. The major drawback of RNA aptamers is their limited chemical durability, but they offer better adjustment capabilities. This trade-off requires additional modifications to lengthen their survival time in circulation. The specific properties and lower triggered immune responses with potential therapeutic design possibilities represent the key benefits of creating both types of aptamers. DNA or RNA aptamer selection depends on the specific medical requirement, together with the required structural complexity and anticipated stability period [20, 40, 61].

7.2.3 Systematic Evolution of Ligands by Exponential Enrichment (SELEX) Technology

The basic SELEX protocol for synthesizing aptamers starts from 10^{14} to 10^{16} random single-stranded oligonucleotides with binding capability toward their target biomolecules of interest. A basic selection of oligonucleotides from the SELEX library contains between 40 and 100 nucleotides that display common sequences at their ends and use the intermediate region as a variable sequence. Scientists perform target-specific separation of oligonucleotides, separating the ones that exhibit target binding from those displaying no affinity to the target. Polymerase chain reaction (PCR) is then used to perform elution and amplification of the linked DNA oligomers. The DNA sequences of the aptamers that show improved affinity and specificity after several rounds of selection are enriched within the pool and then characterized [5]. The changes in the standard SELEX protocol made with the purpose of improving the procedure or increasing the aptamer perfection can be reflected in the type of binding conditions, the type of selection platform, the type of target molecule, the library design, and finally, the type of immobilization matrix. Moreover, SELEX has also been successfully used in RNA libraries apart from DNA libraries [33]. The methods employed with RNA SELEX are generally different from those of DNA SELEX; thus, it is necessary to take necessary precautions for RNA protection from RNAses, amplification using T7 RNA polymerase, and reverse transcription before PCR. As a result, a promoter specific to T7 RNA polymerase is often incorporated into the 5′-primer used for RNA SELEX (Fig. 7.1) [54].

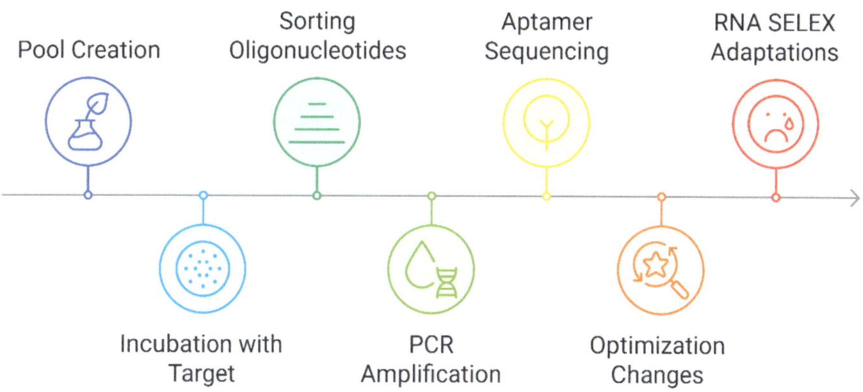

Fig. 7.1 SELEX process for aptamer development

7.3 Mechanism of Aptamer-Based Cancer Diagnostics

7.3.1 Target Identification and Binding Specificity

Effective cancer treatment depends on early detection, and serum cancer biomarker testing (e.g., enzyme-linked immunosorbent assay (ELISA)) is the most prevalent diagnostic technique. Early cancer diagnosis is hampered by the inability to detect low-concentration cancer biomarkers due to complex serum and plasma components. Some processes require a lot of time and effort. Aptamers have thus appeared as a new and potential cancer diagnostic means because of their great sensitivity and selectivity against targets with low concentrations. Aptamers, in contrast to antibodies, undergo conformational changes upon binding to their targets. This conformational shift makes it possible to create novel, switchable aptamer-based probes that antibodies are unable to produce. Aptamers have therefore functioned both as the targeting moiety and the signal transducing moiety in the construction of aptamer-based probes capable of targeting biomolecules associated with cancer. Aptamers are able to distinguish neoplastic and nonneoplastic cells because they can differentiate among proteins that have morphological similarities. Therefore, aptamers show high potential for the detection of all the other sorts of cancer-related metabolites, with distinction between cell and tumor components as well as biomarkers. Under these circumstances, we have summarized detailed information on aptamer-based diagnostic probes relating to different positions of cancer biomarkers (Fig. 7.2) [83].

7.3.1.1 Cancer Surface Membrane Biomarkers

The cell surface membrane is crucial to cellular organization because it functions as an envelope that encloses the generic cellular entity and efficiently divides the two distinct cytoplasmic domains from the external milieu. Proteins with essential, specialized roles make up the majority of the mass of cell surface membranes. These proteins control how cells interact with their surroundings, including chemical signals; the movement of metabolites, ions, or bigger molecules; and the attachment to the extracellular matrix and neighboring cells [57]. Cell surface membrane protein overexpression, deletion, and mutation are linked to a number of cancer pathological conditions. More than half of the licensed medications now target proteins found in cell surface membranes [1].

Some of the significant biomarkers for cancer are cell surface membrane proteins belonging to some groups—epithelial cell adhesion molecules, human epidermal growth factor receptor 2 (HER2), and mucin 1 (MUC1). As a result, many specific aptamers have been developed to bind to cell surface membrane biomarkers for basic physiological and biochemical research and for the identification, diagnosis, and treatment of cancer [83].

A few of them are listed below:

Receptors: The extracellular domain of a receptor binds to its ligand to activate it. After activation, the intracellular pathways are triggered, which leads to a specific response.

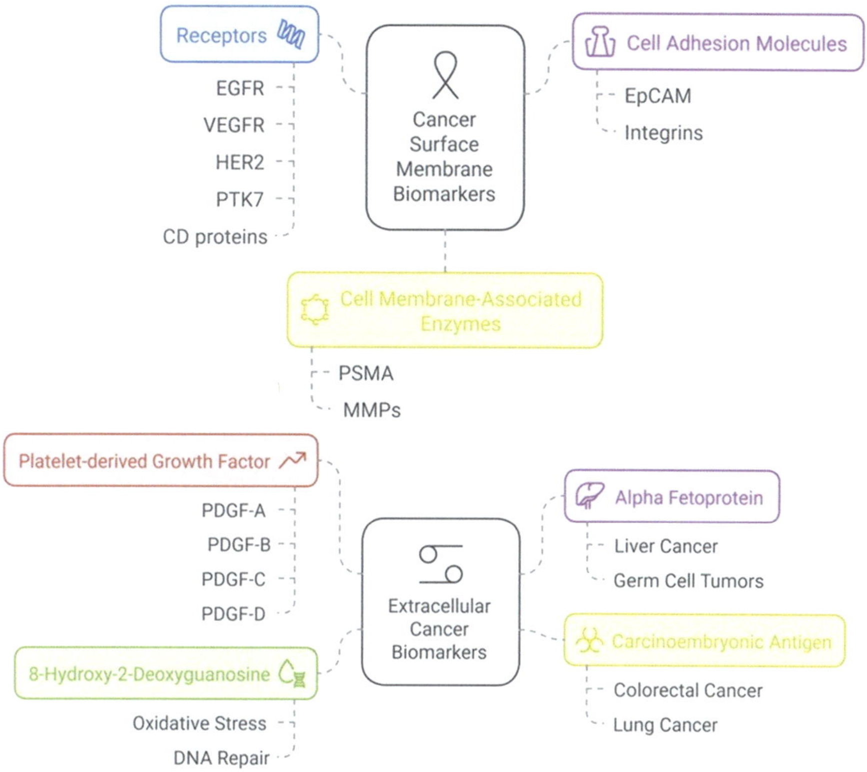

Fig. 7.2 Aptamer-based cancer diagnostics based on the various cancer biomarkers*CD* proteins cluster of differentiation, *EGFR* epidermal growth factor receptor, *EpCAM* epithelial cell adhesion molecule, *HER2* human epidermal growth receptor 2, *MMPs* matrix metalloproteinases, *PDGF* platelet-derived growth factor, *PSMA* prostate-specific membrane antigen, *PTK7* protein tyrosine kinase 7, *VEGF* vascular endothelial growth factor

- Aptamers targeting the epidermal growth factor receptor (EGFR) are among the most well-developed for the diagnosis of relevant tumors. For instance, an electrochemical sandwich immunosensor backed up by aptamers and antibodies with a detection limit of 50 pg/mL was reported by Hoda et al.
- Vascular endothelial growth factor (VEGF) is considered a universal target for nearly all tumor types, as tumor cells largely depend on angiogenesis to supply oxygen and nutrients [19]. For instance, by employing an MRI technique to accurately define the angiogenic vasculature of glioblastoma, an aptamer-functionalized magnetic nanocrystal was developed for the selective recognition of VEGF2 [10].
- Another human receptor within the EGFR family of tyrosine kinase receptors (TKRs) is the human epidermal growth receptor (HER2). It is a preferred drug-selection protein target in breast cancer–targeted therapy because it is synthesized during fetal development, and its overexpression during adulthood is associated with cancer. For instance, an aptamer-based fluorescence sensor for HER2 was constructed, as noted by Manman et al. [52].

- Another membrane receptor protein that greatly assists in carcinogenesis is a catalytically inactive receptor tyrosine kinase known as protein tyrosine kinase 7 (PTK7). It has been reported that many cancers, such as gastric, colon, esophageal, lung, prostate, and breast cancers, overexpress PTK7 [34]. Employing click chemistry reaction, a radiolabeling of PTK7 aptamer Sgc8 with PET tracer isotope 18F was done, and PTK7 expression was quantified in many murine tumor models [59].
- Cell surface receptors, generally termed as cluster of differentiation (CD) proteins, are associated with cellular events like inhibition, adhesion, and activation. The high quantity of CD expressed by these virtually present receptors is used as a major tool for diagnosing several types of cancers. To date, several aptamers selective for CD proteins have been selected. These were the first RNA aptamers for human CD4 to be synthesized [41]. Fluorescein isothiocyanate (FITC) conjugated aptamers were employed to label human peripheral blood mononuclear cells to identify CD4+ T cells. For the enrichment and isolation of cells positive for CD4 expression, Zhou and his team prepared a glass substrate with a specific CD4 RNA aptamer [62].

Cell Adhesion Molecules: The huge and diverse non-holoenzyme membrane protein category that influences morphogenesis is called cell adhesion molecules (CAMs). The definition shown illustrates that the totality of these proteins is involved in actions other than cell–cell or cell–matrix adhesion, notwithstanding their names [83].

- While present at low or moderate levels in many human epithelial tissues, one of the broadly expressed CAMs, epithelial cell adhesion molecule (EpCAM), is overexpressed in approximately 80% of solid tumors and has been identified as an important factor that advances cancer [12]. A forster resonance energy transfer (FRET) biosensor constructed from graphene quantum dot (G-QD)-aptamer and molybdenum disulfide MoS_2 nanosheets was synthesized and used to detect EpCAM, with a detection limit of 450 pM [37].
- Another component of the CAM family is integrin. Cell adhesion molecules known as integrins are heterodimeric receptors that mediate interactions with surrounding cells and the extracellular matrix, playing a key regulatory role in the cell cycle, cell shape, and motility. However, integrin-aptamer-based cancer detection has limited prospects. Positive selection for integrin $\alpha\gamma\beta3$–positive cancer cells was achieved using aptamer-functionalized magnetic nanoparticles, which were potentially visualized using magnetic resonance imaging (MRI) [21].

Cell Membrane–Associated Enzymes: Membrane-associated enzymes represent the best candidates of cancer biomarkers and are implicated in extracellular matrix remodeling, protein uptake, secretion, and proteolytic activities. They modulate the cell-to-cell communication as well as cell and matrix communication to maintain the cell's stability [83].

- Prostate-specific membrane antigen (PSMA), a type II membrane-bound peptidase predominantly expressed in the prostate tissue, is a functional cancer biomarker because of its upregulation on the surface of prostate carcinoma

cells and new vessels of most other solid malignant neoplasms (non-small cell lung, pancreatic, colorectal, breast, renal, ovarian, endometrial, prostate, hepatocellular, gallbladder, and esophagus). The first RNA aptamers targeting PSMA were described to have a detection limit of 2.1 nM. These aptamers were the first to be reported to be selected to bind to tumor-associated membrane antigen and also the first RNA aptamers to be used on prostate cancer cell lines.
- Another invasion-associated protease, which has actually been probed to have an overexpression in a number of cancer types, is matrix metalloproteinase (MMP). Most of the cancer diagnostic aptamer probes have been created utilizing improved membrane-bound or membrane-associated proteolytic enzymes, such as MMP-2, MMP-7, and MMP-9. As it bound with MMP9 preferentially and had the potential to differentiate between MMPs such as MMP-2 and MMP-7, an RNA aptamer containing 20-fluoro pyridine ribonucleosides was chosen.

7.3.1.2 Extracellular Cancer Biomarkers

Tumor and non-tumor tissues are responders to the changes in the extracellular milieu, including the concentration of extracellular cancer biomarkers in the body fluids. Surges or declines in cancer biomarkers in body fluids are employed to assess the reappearance and progression of the disease. Hence, an assiduous diagnosis of cancer often lies in discovering these aberrant alterations.

- As a matter of fact, one of the identified components of the serum is the platelet-derived growth factor (PDGF) that has been reported to advance the formation of arterial smooth muscles [67]. PDGF-BB is a homodimer of PDGF-B, which is well known as a cancer biomarker for cancer diagnosis and detection. According to the color and extinction properties of a specific aptamer and gold nanoparticles (GNPs) due to the aggregation, aptamer-modified gold nanoparticles (Apt-GNPs) were developed to detect the protein PDGF-BB at the sensitivity level as required [14].
- Alpha-fetoprotein (AFP) is an albuminoid protein, which is absent in normal adult human plasma and is released from fetal liver throughout the embryonic period. However, high levels of AFP in adult serum result in a number of diseases, such as liver cancer. Therefore, the potential of AFP to be used for the early detection of cancer requires rapid, sensitive, and targeted analytical techniques. In recent years, some biosensors, which use target-induced aptamer switching mode to detect AFP, have been developed. A similar strategy includes the adsorption of fluorescein amidite (FAM)-labeled aptamers onto gold nanoclusters (AuNCs) [16].
- Carcinoembryonic antigen (CEA) is a tumor-associated antigen that is used in the diagnosis of different clinical diseases, such as gastrointestinal, ovarian, and pancreatic cancers. The MoS_2 nanosheets labeled with fluorophore-tagged CEA aptamer were synthesized for detecting CEA, with a detection range of 34 pg/mL [46].

- The known major end product of DNA oxidative stress damage is a small molecular product called 8-hydroxy-2-deoxyguanosine (8-OHdG). Molecular 8-OHdG levels in human urine reflect several cancers and assess the oxidative DNA damage in the body. Therefore, a clinical diagnosis of cancer is dependent on the concentration of 8-OHdG. A label-free, inexpensive fluorescent biosensor for the detection of 8-OHdG was realized using N-methyl mesoporphyrin IX (NMM) as the fluorescent signal molecule and an 8-OHdG aptamer as the recognition element, with a limit of detection of 1.19 nM [28].

7.3.2 Molecular Recognition and Signaling Mechanisms

Cancer diagnosis, management, and prognosis rely upon the precise identification of malignant cells. Circulating tumor cells (CTCs), which are released into the vasculature from the primary tumor, usually act as a useful indicator for assessing the course of the tumor [58]. However, their capture and isolation still remain a technical challenge due to the very low concentration (1–10 CTCs/mL of the total blood) and significant heterogeneity of circulating tumor cells [48]. Due to their high binding ability and narrow targeting ability toward the surface markers of circulating tumor cells, aptamers have been adopted for use as the targeted ligands to overcome the aforementioned problem [63]. For example, a one-step assay of circulating tumor cells was developed using conjugated aptamers with coupled fluorochrome–quencher molecules to produce a cancer cell–activatable probe [24]. Fluorescence restoration resulted from the specific internalization of an aptamer probe by circulating tumor cells that overexpressed CD30 receptors. The fluorophore–quencher pair experienced separation after undergoing destruction by lysosomal activity. This particular aptamer reporter can accurately quantify circulating tumor cells in the whole blood and bone marrow aspirate from lymphoma–bearing animals. Researchers have developed magnetic nanoparticles having cell membrane–coated surfaces and Ag_2S nanodots functionalized with multivalent aptamers to build a magnetic nanoplatform for improved efficiency in capturing circulating tumor cells and increased sensitivity of detection [11]. As a result of the multifunctional aptamer modification and magnetic separation, this nano-architecture realized target cancer cell recognition and achieved a high cell capture rate of more than 90% with a droplet based system (DBS) sample containing whole blood. Despite the fact that CTCs could be enriched with ease by means of magnetic nanoplatforms, their application was time-consuming and required a large number of blood samples. Microfluidic on-chip systems that enable the manipulation and analysis of small-volume fluids at high throughputs, automation, and multiplexing have been shown to provide a promising methodology for the isolation and identification of circulating tumor cells [9]. When combined in the microfluidic chamber, precisely formulated logical aptamer cocktails were developed that had synergistic actions, making for the creation of a microfluidic assay [47]. The enhancement of circulating tumor cell recovery from patient samples with non-small cell lung cancer (NSCLC) was optimized with the use of silicon

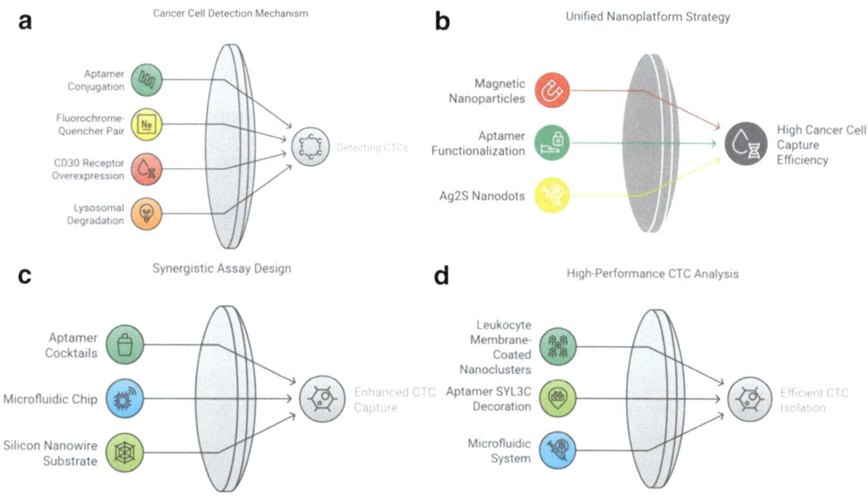

Fig. 7.3 Aptamer-based molecular recognition. (**a**) Conjugated aptamers with paired fluorochrome–quencher molecules [24], (**b**) multivalent aptamer-functionalized Ag_2S nanodots [11], (**c**) aptamer cocktail–based microfluidic assay in combination with silicon nanowire substrate [47], and (**d**) magnetic nanoclusters covered with leukocyte membranes adorned with the aptamer SYL3C [22]

nanowire substrate (SiNS) as well as a microfluidic chip. To address the nonspecific cellular adsorption problem, leukocyte membrane–coated magnetic nanoclusters were synthesized and functionalized with aptamer SYL3C. Consequently, it was possible to load these biomimetic nanoparticles into the microfluidic system, where over 90% of EpCAM-positive cancer cells from a complete blood sample were successfully separated in less than 20 min and counted online using fluorescence imaging. In the context of Fan et al. [22], this carries a strong relation to enhancing the performance of the CTC in complex biological platforms (Fig. 7.3).

7.3.3 Comparison with Antibody-Based Methods

Since the 1990s, immunotherapy has been the most common approach that uses the body's immune system to fight against cancer. It is based on targeting the tumor-associated antigens with monoclonal antibodies (mAbs) to block their carcinogenic function or the immunological checkpoint to modify a precise T cell response to cancer. Still, only a limited number of mAbs have been authorized for clinical use at the present time because of several constraints. Unlike antibodies, oligonucleotide aptamers also have high affinity for their targeted proteins, so they serve as useful tools for active cancer targeting. Aptamers are preferred for therapeutic applications over antibodies due to their size, low or negligible immunogenicity, ease of synthesis as well as solubility, and design versatility to increase stability and therapeutic profile [50].

Aptamers and mAbs can be compared in many aspects:

- First, since aptamers are made by chemical synthesis, they are highly reproducible and may be manufactured without the involvement of animals or cell cultures, which are needed to produce antibodies [50].
- The manufacturing of aptamers is getting ever more economical and efficient as technologies advance [50].
- The three-dimensional shape of the aptamers is complicated, as is that of the antibodies, and possesses high selectivity for the target; their K_D values are typically in the low nanomolar–picomolar range. It was also established that aptamers are exquisite in their ability to recognize proteins that belong to the same family or even the same protein in different conformations [4].
- In their structure, aptamers are very similar to antibodies, but they are molecules that range from 5 to 15 kDa in size. For this reason, they can interact with low-molecular targets or specific, concealed binding sites that are not revealed to large-sized antibodies [73].
- Furthermore, a key characteristic that enables significant tissue penetration—a requirement for cancer treatment—is their reduced size, which is 20–25 times lesser than that of full-sized mAbs. Most significantly, aptamers facilitate a wide range of chemical changes that are essential to overcoming the undeniable restrictions on their clinical use, including rapid renal clearance and uncertain stability [73].
- While mAbs require an immune response, aptamers are reproducible, have fewer side effects, and do not result in immunological rejections [70].
- Finally, modifications of aptamers enable the development of multicomponent therapy by covalent linking of the aptamers with other pharmacological molecules or drugs, enhancing their suitability for usage in clinics [39].

7.4 Emerging Trends and Advances in Aptamer-Based Cancer Diagnosis

7.4.1 Integration with Nanotechnology

On a note of promise, nanotechnology seems to offer an unlikely custom-made substitute for drug delivery systems to deal with the existing problems. It has been recently employed to develop a nanoscale precision-guided platform using aptamers and nanomaterials [45].

To deliver doxorubicin (Dox) to the cancer cells, a DNA nanoscale precision-guided missile (D-PGM) with an impressive loading capacity was created. The self-assembly of three DNA-stranded aptamers produced this nano-carrier, which has a rod-shaped drug carrier and a DNA logic circuit for guidance and control. It was a DNA nanostructure in three dimensions. The self-assembled component may stick to the surface of the cancer cell, function as an initiator, and then dismantle the logical circuit in guidance/control to direct the doxorubicin-loaded warhead toward the target cells during drug transportation. Encoded logic gates into intelligent guidance/control that could change its structure allowed this missile, which contained three aptamers, to perform better than its aptamers [13]. To carry the doxorubicin action directly to the target cell during delivery, these self-assembled components could attach to the cell surface, work as the initiators to disassemble the logical circuit in guidance/control, and help control the delivery direction. In these missile devices, intelligent guidance/control accounted for their shape transformation and, thus, managed to dramatically outperform the other aptamers. Sgc8 can target PTK7 in HeLa and CCRF-CEM cells, and sgC4f (target protein unknown) binds to CEM and Ramos cells, while TC10 (receptor protein unknown) is purported to target several cancer lines. A cytotoxicity profile showed that D-PGM-doxorubicin injection, compared with free doxorubicin, greatly reduced the viability of Ramos and CEM cells [13].

A multifunctional DNA dendrimer nanostructure with nucleic acid vectors was built by a layered muster of functional Y-shaped blocks of DNA. The sgc8 aptamer was specific in its coupling with PTK722 and could spontaneously hybridize with the outer shell building components of the DNA dendrimer. In addition, in a proof-of-concept study, nanostructures were conjugated with fluorophores to form a DNA dendrimer for bioimaging of CCRF-CEM and Ramos cancer cell lines. Here, DNA dendrimer and sgc8 aptamer worked together to allow for the specific identification and uptake of doxorubicin by target cells. At pH 7.4, the multifunctional nanostructure with 666 nM of doxorubicin released less than 7% of the drug after 60 hours, as measured through the doxorubicin fluorescence intensity monitoring. Thus, the Dox payload was stable enough to prevent the drug from leaking during circulation in the bloodstream. The MTS assay showed increased selectivity in CEM-targeted cells, as well as increased cytotoxicity with increasing concentrations of doxorubicin and DNA dendrimers [29]. A light-activable double stranded (dsDNA) aptamer has been developed based on its ability to penetrate tissues considerably with near-infrared (NIR) light used in cancer phototherapy. To hybridize and mask the sgc8 aptamers used in this approach, a matching DNA sequence needs to be coupled to photothermal agents, such as single-walled carbon nanotubes or gold nanorods. Localized photothermal heating of the nano-agent's surface exposed to an NIR laser induces dehybridization of the dsDNA and releases the aptamer sequence, allowing for specific targeting of tumor cells. Single-walled carbon nanotubes loaded with doxorubicin were used as a model system to deliver drugs to cancer cells upon activation with near-infrared light. Binding of sgc8 to PTK7 exhibited high avidity and targeted drug delivery. Upon 808-nm NIR laser irradiation, the nanostructure showed a significant and concentration-dependent photothermal effect [88]. In addition, a rolling circle amplification (RCA)–based poly-aptamer–drug delivery system was synthesized for targeted drug delivery. The RCA process involves DNA polymerase elongation of DNA from a primer sequence by continuously copying a circular DNA template; it results in a single-stranded DNA product that works to carry up to tens of thousands of nucleotides. Besides, a spacer domain was introduced between these aptamers, and this renders the physical aggregation of a chemotherapeutic drug, say, doxorubicin. According to one study, this poly-aptamer had profound cytotoxic activity against leukemia cells and promoted doxorubicin internalization. Its affinity was around 40 times greater than that of its monovalent version [90].

7.4.2 Role of Artificial Intelligence in Aptamer Design

The following are some of the obstacles to SELEX technology: (a) It takes weeks or even months to produce aptamer candidates, (b) aptamer candidate success rates are still poor, and (c) from the next-generation sequencing data, only a few representative aptamer candidates could be synthesized for affinity characterization [91].

Due to its affordability and ease of use, some researchers have recently chosen aptamer candidates by computational methods. These techniques use structural information to predict the aptamer's affinity for targets [6]. For the determination of the secondary and three-dimensional (3D) structures of nucleic acids, numerous web servers, including RNAfold and RNAComposer, have been presented [32]. Similar to other RNAs/DNAs, these web servers could likewise provide the structural details of aptamers. Protein aptamer selection has also demonstrated the suitability of molecular dynamics and molecular docking, which are typically employed in the selection of protein compounds based on structural information [65].

The development of machine learning and deep learning algorithms is spurring a new wave of computational techniques to choose aptamer candidates with high affinity and specificity toward drug development. Several methods using machine/deep learning have shown better performance than a number of conventional methods: binding affinity prediction methods, including molecular docking and virtual screening tools [64]. Computational docking and secondary structure prediction helped refine the initial pool of sequences [86]. Machine learning was used to create a sequence-fitness landscape by training a random forest model on aptamers and their corresponding affinities, albeit the model itself was never used to generate new sequences [15]. Modern neural network approaches have effectively produced sequences across multiple biological domains. Predictive models using experimental data have been exploited to computationally design yeast 5′ untranslated regions (5' UTR) sequences that resulted in improved protein expression [38] and also antibody sequences with a corresponding boost in specificity [43]. Predictive machine learning techniques allow for the directed design of aptamers, where sequences are synthesized and evaluated in silico to drastically cut down the number of sequences that must be screened experimentally [91].

Structure-based drug design is the most frequently applied methodology under the definition of computer-aided drug design. Moreover, advanced machine/deep learning constitutes an intriguing paradigm in drug discovery, as some prediction models have exhibited predictive capability for the binding interaction between ligands and targets. For certain types of drug discovery, this could, therefore, offer a valid and reliable prediction of how aptamers and targets actually interact. The binding prediction of aptamers can be further conducted through additional machine/deep learning techniques. A predictive method for aptamer–target binding affinity can be developed through the combination of structure-based approaches and machine/deep learning, according to Zihao et al. [91].

7.5 Aptamer-Based Biosensors in Cancer Detection

Biosensors of the modern age have upgraded diagnostic performance through new signal amplification technologies, which overcome the shortcomings of traditional methods. The modern biosensors utilize enzyme catalysis with nucleic acid chain reactions, together with biotin-streptavidin interactions, and click chemistry and cascade reactions, combined with nanomaterial applications [23]. Visually represented biological signals through biosensors permit exact protein measurement of tumor cells while detecting very small amounts of proteins precisely. The functional basis of biosensors uses macromolecular elements like enzymes, along with aptamers and antibodies, as biological recognition elements for precise target analyte recognition [79]. Aptamers stand out among recognition elements by demonstrating a great potential for invasive tumor imaging and medical procedures. These diagnostic alternatives also benefit from exceptional characteristics, which include their ability to detect specific targets, economical production costs, and their increased suitability in biological systems. Aptamer-based biosensors have facilitated major progress toward clinical cancer diagnostics by providing superior performance for early disease detection abilities. The combination of sensitive and targeted screening technology within advanced biosensors presents a prospective future for medical diagnosis improvements, along with better healthcare results for patients.

7.5.1 Advantages of Aptamer-Functionalized Biosensors

The key factor for successful cancer prevention and treatment lies in early cancer detection. Various sensor systems created by researchers specialize in detecting cancer-linked proteins, together with tiny chemical indicators and cancerous cells. Antibody–antigen binding constitutes the principle behind traditional devices, where sandwich immunoassay systems identify particular target proteins [27]. The creation of dependable diagnostic sensors proves to be a challenging task. The sandwich detection method requires different types of antibodies to recognize targets, yet it faces natural technical obstacles because of this setup. Sensitive diagnosis remains limited because changes in production-batch antibody-binding capacities lead to inconsistent and less precise results in diagnostic assessments. Qualitative and quantitative requirements highlight why researchers must develop better standardized biomarker detection approaches in cancer medicine, thus emphasizing the value of design innovation for sensors and immunoassays. The strong selective binding between aptamers and cancer-related chemicals and cells makes them excellent candidates for cancer diagnostic tools that transcend current constraints. The ability of aptamers to detect small differences in proteins with related structures leads to their differentiation of malignancies from benign cells on the basis of cell surface characteristics. Aptamer–target interaction causes structural alterations to these molecules, which differ from antibody behavior. The changes in aptamer configuration allow scientists to develop sensors that change states, which traditional antibody-based methods cannot achieve. Aptasensors for cancer biomarkers are developed through the use of aptamers in recognition and signal control units.

7.5.2 Types of Biosensors

7.5.2.1 Optical Aptasensors

Fluorescence-based biosensors represent a strong analytical system that detects cancer cells and biomarkers because of their exceptional sensitivity. Aptasensors, which utilize fluorescent signaling systems, are now prominent in early cancer detection because they specifically identify cancer-related biomarkers. Several optical aptasensor methods specifically for vascular endothelial growth factor (VEGF) detection have been developed through this technological advancement. The innovative detection methods show how fluorescence-enabled aptasensors measure with precision and sensitivity major cancer-related molecular indicators during progression [66]. Fluorescent signaling enables high-resolution molecular process examinations, which reveal new diagnostic possibilities for cancer. The development of aptasensors as cancer cell detectors has received extensive examination through multiple studies. Xiaolan et al. [81] developed an aptamer-coupled FRET silica nanoparticle assay to detect simultaneous cancer cell analysis for multiple samples. The identification of cancer-linked biomarkers became possible through the implementation of colorful and Raman aptasensors, in addition to fluorescent aptasensors. Scientists have developed an aptamer-based colorimetric test for detecting cancerous cells, which employs gold nanoparticles [17].

7.5.2.2 Electrochemical Aptasensors

Due to the high sensitivity, cost-efficiency, and the possibility of using them in clinics, electrochemical sensors were employed together with fluorescent aptasensors for the highly selective detection of cancer-associated biomarkers and cancer cells [49]. Electrochemical aptasensors were generally fabricated by applying one of the two main strategies. The first approach used to recognize cancer cells and biomarkers was the sandwich structure, which closely resembled the structure of antibody-target-antibody [42]. Following the same idea, the conformational change that emerges when aptamers bind to their targets formed the ground for the second one [35]. This conformational change that formed these sensors differed from the initial "signal-on" and "signal-off" aptasensors, as it would translate specific molecules toward or away from the electrode. For example, to detect HER2 and HER2-overexpressing breast cancer cells, the sandwich electrochemical sensor was developed [87].

7.5.2.3 Other Types of Aptasensors

Two methods were used primarily to synthesize the aptasensors, but several other types of aptasensors were also produced for the detection of cancer biomarkers and cancer cells. For example, VEGF aptamers that have been attached to silicon nanowire field effect transistors (SiNW-FETs) were suggested to detect electrical signals of VEGF as anti-VEGF aptamer-modified silicon nanowire field effect transistors (SiNW-FETs) [31]. A sophisticated and adaptable method for detecting cancer cells is chemiluminescence, which does not have autofluorescence interference brought on by photoexcitation in a chemiluminescence reaction [82]. For instance, a chemiluminescence imaging array was created to detect human Burkitt's lymphoma cells, or Ramos cells, by integrating rolling circle amplification, bio-barcode nanotechnology, and cell aptamer identification [68]. Other signals, like MRI, radiologic signals, and ultrasound signals, were also utilized to find cancer cells. However, the majority of these techniques focused on imaging, both in vivo and in vitro. Thus, we include those sections in the subsequent section on cancer imaging.

In general, aptamers were used intensely in the design of several biosensors for the recognition of cancer cells and biomarkers. Furthermore, aptamers can be employed as transducers when target–aptamer binding occurs, simplifying the aptasensor construction.

7.5.3 Choosing Aptasensors

Before deciding on the specificity of detection, it is relevant to consider the peculiar advantages and disadvantages of each type of aptamer sensing. For instance, the electrochemical aptasensor has more specific features, including noninvasiveness, compactness, convenience, and low cost, for the prescreening of tumor markers. The colorimetric aptasensor is the easiest to use and read for differentiating between cancer and normal samples. The fluorescent aptasensor is easier to use for multichannel detection of various tumor cells at the same time than others [79].

7.6 Challenges and Limitations

7.6.1 Stability and Scalability Issues

The main factor that hinders the actual application of aptamers is the short half-life of aptamers, especially RNA aptamers, in biological fluids and blood, in particular due to nuclease activity. In general, the resistance of an oligonucleotide depends on the content and physical confirmation, so the circulation time that it remains in blood can range from a few minutes to many. Several strategies have been pursued to protect aptamers from nuclease degradation because most therapeutic applications cannot tolerate such a limited time span [72].

Aptamers' therapeutic use is complicated by the renal filtration process that removes them from the bloodstream. The majority of aptamers are quickly eliminated by kidneys that can eliminate compounds with a molecular weight of less than 30–50 kDa. Their molecular weights range from 5 to 15 kDa (15 to 50 nucleotides). The most popular remedy for this issue is to conjugate aptamers to polyethylene glycol (PEG) that has a molecular weight of 20 or 40 kDa [72].

Aptamer generation appears to be a very straightforward procedure, but it actually takes a lot of time and effort. Sometimes, a less-than-ideal SELEX process results in the chosen aptamers having the lowest affinity and specificity. These issues can be avoided with automated SELEX, which can produce aptamers with the necessary characteristics in a matter of days [55].

Nevertheless, aptamers and oligonucleotide therapies have drawbacks that hinder their application in clinical settings, specifically toxicity, pharmacodynamics, in vivo stability, and renal clearance [33]. It is simple to modify aptamers to increase their stability in vivo and prevent nuclease degradation.

The quantity of chimera that enters the cytoplasm and acts on a particular target in the target cell is a significant issue that is only associated with aptamer-based chimera molecules. In fact, the cytoplasm only receives 1% of the chimera–aptamer. Although the mechanisms of intracellular processing and endosomal escape remain poorly understood, increasing the chimera's release in the cytoplasm is required to increase the effectiveness of chimera–aptamer compounds. One possible solution to the above issue that has been suggested is the ability to link aptamers to cationic amphipathic peptides or nanomaterials [92].

7.6.2 Off-Target Effects and Specificity Concerns

In general, the development of aptamers requires purified target molecules, which should have high concentrations. Cell culture–expressed protein target molecules are purified by affinity chromatography. The manufacture of equivalent aptamers is delayed by these labor-intensive and time-consuming processes. Furthermore, the chemical characteristics of some proteins make them challenging to purify. Due to the posttranslational modifications, the aptamers formed with target proteins expressed in prokaryotes sometimes do not bind to the same proteins expressed in eukaryotes. The changes in protein synthesis in eukaryotes could mean that aptamers produced against proteins expressed in prokaryotic cells may not be able to bind to the epitopes of eukaryotic proteins [53].

Cancer-causing mutations alter expression patterns initially, followed by changes to cell and tissue architecture. The early stages of cancer cannot be detected by the traditional methods of cancer diagnosis, which mostly concentrate on morphological abnormalities. Cell-SELEX-generated aptamers that identify cancer cells can help with this issue. According to Yuan et al. [89], aptamer microarrays can detect traces of cancer cells in the blood.

7.7 Future Perspectives

7.7.1 Innovations in SELEX Techniques

In the current world of molecular biology and biotechnology techniques, multiple complex techniques have been developed to synthesize more accurate and reliable aptamers. Some of these improvement methods are core to advanced aptamer selection techniques, which are far superior to conventional techniques. The emerging techniques include:

- Atomic Force Microscopy-Based Selection (AFM-SELEX)
- Capture-SELEX
- Cell-SELEX
- Capillary Electrophoresis–SELEX
- Immunoprecipitation-Coupled SELEX (IP-SELEX)
- Artificially Expanded Genetic Information System–SELEX (AEGIS-SELEX)
- Classic Systematic Evolution of Ligands by Exponential Enrichment (SELEX)

These proposed methods all have their strengths in the identification of aptamers with specific binding profile and targeted applications for molecular interactions. They show the continuous advances in nucleic acid selection technologies that allow for better and more specific aptamer selection in a number of scientific and medical applications [85].

7.7.2 Role of Aptamers in Liquid Biopsy and Early Diagnosis

The main advantage of liquid biopsy methods is the identification of total tumor diversity, and clinical applications now facilitate precision medicine approaches. Liquid biopsy serves as an easy procedure to obtain circulating tumor cells, together with cancer-derived extracellular vesicles, through a minimally invasive and reproducible method. Cancer diagnosis and real-time treatment monitoring, along with future options for personalized cancer treatment, can be achieved through these collected samples [18]. The aptamers serve perfectly as identification tools and isolation devices for both extracellular vesicles and circulating tumor cells. Multiple synthesized aptamer derivatives labeled with anti-prostate-specific membrane antigen (PSMA), prostate-specific antigen (PSA), mucin 1 (MUC1), and human epidermal growth factor receptor 2 (HER2) have been utilized for collecting targets from liquid biopsy samples [18]. The generation of specific aptamers for exosome isolation and analysis in complex mixtures depends on the presence of CD63 protein and the extracellular portion of HSP70 as molecular markers located on the vesicle surface [18].

7.7.3 Prospects for Clinical Translation

Aptamer-based probes demonstrate various applications' potential, yet researchers need to address different obstacles to implement them successfully in clinical work. Researcher comprehension of nucleic acid chemistry, tissue distribution, and pharmacokinetics requires improved depth in order to produce such molecular tools [83]. Scientists must acquire superior knowledge about how aptamers function at the molecular level, particularly regarding their complex tertiary structures, alongside their binding principles. Such single-stranded DNA or RNA oligomers have complicated chemical properties, which require advanced analytical methods to ensure reliable performance [83]. The tissue distribution, along with the pharmacokinetic characteristics of aptamers, needs more comprehensive investigation before they can be utilized as tools. The current constraints involve the determination of molecular probe interactions inside biostructures, together with the preservation of their properties across biological surroundings. Specificity is a notable feature of aptamers, yet research continues to create better target molecules that discriminate between cancer cells without reacting with healthy cells. Clinical efficiency depends on the ability to alter binding sites, which exclusively detect high-expression cancer cells [69]. The main difficulty now centers on creating effective drug delivery methods based on aptamers. Studies involving aptamer–drug conjugates exist to overcome internalization, specificity, and target recognition problems [76]. Meeting all the necessary requirements for aptamer translation into clinical use includes maintaining continuous aptamer production, alongside minimizing variances between different production runs. The scientific community needs to standardize chemical stabilization methods and modification techniques to enhance serum efficiency and shelf-life stability [83]. Researchers in the scientific field agree that aptamers require additional development before they can transition to excellent clinical diagnostic solutions [36].

7.8 Conclusion

Research surrounding aptamers provides an innovative method to tackle the most substantial medical challenges that medicine faces today. A comprehensive discussion introduces the promising aptamer technology capability to revolutionize cancer diagnostics and personalized treatment selection. The revolutionary features of nanotechnology, along with artificial intelligence and molecular engineering, make aptamers function better than traditional antibody-based detection methods. The chapter demonstrates how aptamers introduce groundbreaking benefits to cancer diagnostic research. Aptamers have three distinct characteristics, which include high selectivity, minimal immunogenic response, and adaptable molecular organization, that will revolutionize molecular probe–based early cancer detection. SELEX technology demonstrates expanded applications because of its structured combination with state-of-the-art bioengineering techniques. Although stability and off-target effects are concerns, the scientific trajectory of aptamer research is profoundly promising. The convergence of nanotechnology, artificial intelligence, and molecular engineering points to the increased role of aptamers in developing more precise, sensitive, and personalized cancer diagnostic tools. Aptamers possess the potential for earlier intervention and more focused therapeutic approaches because of their excellent sensitivity in identifying a variety of cancer biomarkers. Future studies should concentrate on establishing scalable production techniques, enhancing aptamer stability in intricate biological settings, and improving aptamer design. Aptamers have the potential to revolutionize liquid biopsy techniques into an early cancer detection method, paving the way for a new era in personalized medicine that could significantly improve patient outcomes and survival rates by developing better, less invasive diagnostic techniques. As a result, the chapter concludes by highlighting the fact that aptamers represent a paradigm shift in precision medicine and cancer detection, rather than just a technological advancement.

References

1. Agnes C, Daniel MD, Frédéric D. Methods to identify aptamers against cell surface biomarkers. Pharmaceuticals. 2011;4:1216–35.
2. Akhil P, Anika P, Bilikere SD, Amit V, Rao VP. Technological advancements in cancer diagnostics: improvements and limitations. Cancer Rep. 2023;6(2):e1764.
3. Amelie E, Niklas TR, Titus JB, Tom L, Alexander TP, Jakob NK. Deep learning in cancer pathology: a new generation of clinical biomarkers. Br J Cancer. 2021;124:686–96.
4. Amy DG, Douglas RD, Nebojsa J. Embracing proteins: structural themes in aptamer-protein complexes. Curr Opin Struct Biol. 2016;36:122–32.
5. Andrew DE, Jack WS. In vitro selection of RNA molecules that bind specific ligands. Nature. 1990;346:818–22.
6. Andrey AB, Alexey SV, Anatoly ZV, Boris DZ. Methods and applications of in silico aptamer design and modeling. Int J Mol Sci. 2020;21:8420.
7. Anna NW. Cancer diagnosis in primary care: six steps to reducing the diagnostic interval. Can Fam Physician. 2021;67(4):265–8.
8. Baozhang G, Xingwang Z. Aptamers as versatile ligands for biomedical and pharmaceutical applications. Int J Nanomedicine. 2020;15:1059–71.
9. Bin X, Kangning R, Yiwei S, Yin C, Bo S, Hongkai W. Recent developments in microfluidics for cell studies. Adv Mater. 2014;26(31):5525–32.
10. Bongjune K, Jaemoon Y, Myeonghwan H, Jihye C, Hyun-Ouk K, Eunji J, et al. Aptamer-modified magnetic nanoprobe for molecular MR imaging of VEGFR2 on angiogenic vasculature. Nanoscale Res Lett. 2013;8:399.
11. Caiping D, Cuiling Z, Shasha C, Yuezhong X. Multivalent aptamer-functionalized Ag_2S nanodots/hybrid cell membrane-coated magnetic nanobioprobe for the ultrasensitive isolation and detection of circulating tumor cells. Adv Funct Mater. 2020;30(16):1909781.
12. Carlo P, Roberto MM, Anja KM, Hakan M. Epithelial cell adhesion molecule expression (CD326) in cancer: a short review. Cancer Treat Rev. 2012;38:68–75.
13. Changhe O, Songbai Z, Chang X, Xin Y, Huo X, Zhenmeng W, et al. Precision-guided missile-like DNA nanostructure containing warhead and guidance control for aptamer-based targeted drug delivery into cancer cells in vitro and in vivo. J Am Chem Soc. 2020;142(3):1265–77.
14. Chih-Ching H, Yu-Fen H, Zehui C, Weihong T, Huan-Tsung C. Aptamer-modified gold nanoparticles for colorimetric determination of platelet-derived growth factors and their receptors. Anal Chem. 2005;77:5735–41.

15. Christopher GK, Mark P, William R, David CW, Farid K, Philip JRD, et al. Array-based evolution of DNA aptamers allows modeling of an explicit sequence-fitness landscape. Nucleic Acids Res. 2009;37(1):e6.
16. Chunting L, Dachuan W, Guiyin L. A fluorescence turn-on biosensor based on gold nanoclusters and aptamer for alpha-fetoprotein detection. IOP Conf Ser Earth Environ Sci. 2019;218:012106.
17. Colin DM, Joshua ES, Zhiwen T, Yanrong W, Suwussa B, Weihong T. Gold nanoparticle-based colorimetric assay for the direct detection of cancerous cells. Anal Chem. 2008;80(4):1067–72.
18. Dhruvajyoti R, Andreas P, Mazen AJ, Judith CS. The potential of aptamer-mediated liquid biopsy for early detection of cancer. Int J Mol Sci. 2021;22(11):5601.
19. Eben LR, Jason MW, Esther DB, James PB, Merrill AB, Matthew B. Successful translation of fluorescence navigation during oncologic surgery: a consensus report. J Nucl Med. 2016;57:144–50.
20. Erik WO, Nenad C, Jean G. Delivering cargoes into cancer cells using DNA aptamers targeting internalized surface portals. Biochim Biophys Acta. 2010;1798:2190–200.
21. Eun-Kyung L, Bongjune K, Yuna C, Youngjun R, Eun-Jin C, Jung Hwan L, et al. Aptamer-conjugated magnetic nanoparticles enable efficient targeted detection of integrin $\alpha v\beta 3$ via magnetic resonance imaging. J Biomed Mater Res. 2014;102:49–59.
22. Fan Z, Lili W, Weidong N, Lili H, Jinfeng Z, Feng L, et al. Biomimetic microfluidic system for fast and specific detection of circulating tumor cells. Anal Chem. 2019;91(24):15726–31.
23. Fengchun H, Yingchao Z, Jianhan L, Yuanjie L. Biosensors coupled with signal amplification technology for the detection of pathogenic bacteria: a review. Biosensors. 2021;11(6):190.
24. Fuyin Z, Yao C, Jie W, Jie L, Bin Z, Yuanjin Z, et al. Aptamer-functionalized barcode particles for the capture and detection of multiple types of circulating tumor cells. Adv Mater. 2014;26(43):7333–8.
25. Haitao M, Jinping L, Mohammad MA, Mohammad AIM, Louai L, Mengrou L, et al. Nucleic acid aptamers in cancer research, diagnosis and therapy. Chem Soc Rev. 2015;44:1240–56.
26. Hao H. Matrix metalloproteinase-9 (MMP-9) as a cancer biomarker and MMP-9 biosensors: recent advances. Sensors. 2018;18:3249.
27. Hong YS, Xiaodong Z, Jonathan H, Xiaodi S. Comparative study of random and oriented antibody immobilization as measured by dual polarization interferometry and surface Plasmon resonance spectroscopy. Langmuir. 2012;28(1):997–1004.
28. Hui L, Yong-Sheng W, Xian T, Hui-Xian Y, Si-Han C, Hui Z, et al. A novel fluorescence aptasensor for 8-hydroxy-2′-deoxyguanosine based on the conformational switching of K^+-stabilized G-quadruplex. J Pharm Biomed Anal. 2016;118:177–82.
29. Huimin Z, Yanli M, Yi X, Yuan A, Yishun H, Zhi Z, et al. A controllable aptamer-based self-assembled DNA dendrimer for high affinity targeting, bioimaging and drug delivery. Sci Rep. 2015;5:10099.
30. Huiyi L, Chang L, Linbo H, Xiaobing Z, Guosheng S. Optical–magnetic probe for evaluating cancer therapy. Coord Chem Rev. 2021;441:213978.
31. Hyun-Seung L, Ki SK, Cheol-Joo K, Sei Kwang H, Moon-Ho J. Electrical detection of VEGFs for cancer diagnoses using anti-vascular endothelial growth factor aptamer-modified Si nanowire FETs. Biosens Bioelectron. 2009;24(6):1801–5.
32. Ivo LH. Vienna RNA secondary structure server. Nucleic Acids Res. 2003;31(13):3429–31.
33. Jiehua Z, John R. Aptamers as targeted therapeutics: current potential and challenges. Nat Rev Drug Discov. 2017;16:181–20.
34. Ji-Hee K, Junhye K, Hae Won L, Moon Chul K, Hyeon Joon Y, Seung-Taek L, Jong HP. Protein tyrosine kinase 7 plays a tumor suppressor role by inhibiting ERK and AKT phosphorylation in lung cancer. Oncol Rep. 2014;31:2708–12.
35. Jing Z, Xiaolin H, Bing B, Xinjian L, Yongmei Y, Genxi L. A "signal-on" electrochemical aptasensor for simultaneous detection of two tumor markers. Biosens Bioelectron. 2012;34(1):249–52.
36. Jing H, Liang G, Jinsheng W, Jia W. Application and development of aptamer in cancer: from clinical diagnosis to cancer therapy. J Cancer. 2020;11(23):6902–15.

37. Jingyu S, Jing L, Feng T, Mo Y. A fluorescence turn-on biosensor based on graphene quantum dots (GQDs) and molybdenum disulfide (MoS_2) nanosheets for epithelial cell adhesion molecule (EpCAM) detection. Biosens Bioelectron. 2017;93:182–8.
38. Josh TC, Benjamin G, Anna K, Alexander BR, Nebojsa J, Stanley F, et al. Deep learning of the regulatory grammar of yeast 5′ untranslated regions from 500,000 random sequences. Genome Res. 2017;27(12):2015–24.
39. Justin PD, Paloma HG. Current progress on aptamer-targeted oligonucleotide therapeutics. Ther Deliv. 2013;4:1527–46.
40. Katherine G, Marissa L, Xiaoting Z. RNA aptamers and their therapeutic and diagnostic applications. Int J Biochem Mol Biol. 2013;4:27–40.
41. Kenneth AD, Barnaby A, Yun L, Sumedha DJ. Staining of cell surface human CD4 with 2′-F-pyrimidine-containing RNA aptamers for flow cytometry. Nucleic Acids Res. 1998;26(17):3915–24.
42. Kerstin J, Anton R, Nilsson E, Johan M, György M-V, Hans L, et al. Reverse-phase versus sandwich antibody microarray, technical comparison from a clinical perspective. Anal Chem. 2007;79:5817–25.
43. Kevin M, Eric AS, Steven K, Ling X, Xia T, Dennis M, et al. Machine learning on DNA-encoded libraries: a new paradigm for hit finding. J Med Chem. 2020;63(16):8857–66.
44. Kostas M. The constantly evolving role of medical image processing in oncology: from traditional medical image processing to imaging biomarkers and radiomics. J Imaging. 2021;7(8):124.
45. Kousar G, Mahdieh D, Ilnaz R, Matineh G, Mahnaz H, Esmaeel S, et al. Advances in aptamer-based drug delivery vehicles for cancer therapy. Biomater Adv. 2022;140:213077.
46. Lianjing Z, Ming C, Guannan L, Huiying L, Yuan G, Xu Y, et al. A fluorescent biosensor based on molybdenum disulfide nanosheets and protein aptamer for sensitive detection of carcinoembryonic antigen. Sens Actuators B Chem. 2018;273:185–90.
47. Libo Z, Chuanhao T, Li X, Zhen Z, Xiaoyan L, Haixu H, et al. Enhanced and differential capture of circulating tumor cells from lung cancer patients by microfluidic assays using Aptamer cocktail. Small. 2016;12(8):1072–81.
48. Limei W, Yutong Z, Zhimin W, Yue Z, Jianmei Z, Liping Q. Aptamer-based cancer cell analysis and treatment. ChemistryOpen. 2022;11(10):e202200141.
49. Lingyan F, Yong C, Jinsong R, Xiaogang Q. A graphene functionalized electrochemical aptasensor for selective label-free detection of cancer cells. Biomaterials. 2011;32:2930–7.
50. Lisa A, Simona C, Monica F, Laura C. Aptamers and antibodies: rivals or allies in cancer targeted therapy? Explor Target Antitumor Ther. 2021;2(1):107–21.
51. Luiza IH, Isabel M, Thomas S, Frank JH. Aptamers overview: selection, features and applications. Curr Top Med Chem. 2015;15(12):1066–81.
52. Manman Z, Ge G, Yalin D, Chunyan D, Juan X, Huiyun W. A fluorescent aptasensor for the femtomolar detection of epidermal growth factor receptor-2 based on the proximity of G-rich sequences to Ag nanoclusters. Talanta. 2019;199:238–43.
53. Mao Y, Jun H, Minyuan P, Jing L, Jun L, Huixia L, et al. Generating aptamers by cell-SELEX for applications in molecular medicine. Int J Mol Sci. 2012;13(3):3341–53.
54. Maria AV, Anna SD, Pavel EP, Dmitrii VP, Alya GV. Key aspects of nucleic acid library design for in vitro selection. Int J Mol Sci. 2018;19(2):470.
55. Michael GK, Anthony SF, Richard DW, Charles RB. Gene therapy delivery systems for enhancing viral and nonviral vectors for cardiac diseases: current concepts and future applications. Hum Gene Ther. 2013;24(11):914–27.
56. Ming C, Hongyu Z. Next-generation sequencing in liquid biopsy: cancer screening and early detection. Hum Genomics. 2019;13:34.
57. Muhammed AY, Kwang-Il G, Michael EC, Albert-László B, Marc V. Drug–target network. Nat Biotechnol. 2007;25:1119–26.
58. Nicola A, Aditya B, David TM, Maria CD, Ben SW, Joel AS, et al. Circulating tumor cell clusters are oligoclonal precursors of breast cancer metastasis. Cell. 2014;158(5):1110–22.

59. Orit J, Ido DW, Lu W, Zhe W, Xiangyu Y, Andrew D, et al. 18F-labeled single-stranded DNA aptamer for PET imaging of protein tyrosine kinase-7 expression. J Nucl Med. 2015;56:1780–5.
60. Panagiotis P, Lennart B, Neo CC, Wistan M, Franck V, Laurent G, et al. Artificial intelligence: deep learning in oncological radiomics and challenges of interpretability and data harmonization. Phys Med. 2021;83:108–21.
61. Qinchang Z, Ge L, Masaaki K. DNA aptamers in the diagnosis and treatment of human diseases. Molecules. 2015;20:20979–97.
62. Qing Z, Ying L, Dong-Sik S, Jaime S, Nazgul T, Alexander R. Aptamer-containing surfaces for selective capture of CD4-expressing cells. Langmuir. 2012;28:12544–9.
63. Qinqin H, Yin W, Xingxiang C, Yimeng W, Zhiqiang L, Shiming D, et al. Nanotechnology-based strategies for early cancer diagnosis using circulating tumor cells as a liquid biopsy. Nano. 2018;2(1):21–41.
64. Qurrat UA, Antoniya A, Florian DR, Pedro JB. Machine-learning scoring functions to improve structure-based binding affinity prediction and virtual screening. Wiley Interdiscip Rev Comput Mol Sci. 2015;5:405–24.
65. Rajesh A, Smita N, Shikha A, Srinivasan R, Souvik M, Pradip N. In silico selection of an aptamer to estrogen receptor alpha using computational docking employing estrogen response elements as aptamer-alike molecules. Sci Rep. 2016;6:21285.
66. Ronit F, Julia G, Amily FJ, Ja-an AH, Thomas H, Jens D, Itamar W. Optical aptasensors for the analysis of the vascular endothelial growth factor (VEGF). Anal Chem. 2012;84(14):6192–8.
67. Russell R, John G, Beverly K, Laurence H. A platelet-dependent serum factor that stimulates the proliferation of arterial smooth muscle cells in vitro. Proc Natl Acad Sci USA. 1974;71:1207–12.
68. Sai B, Bin J, Zhipeng Z, Shusheng Z. A chemiluminescence imaging array for the detection of cancer cells by dual-aptamer recognition and bio-bar-code nanoprobe-based rolling circle amplification. Chem Commun. 2013;49:3452–4.
69. Sarah S, Brett S, Paloma HG, Vittorio DF. Aptamers: cutting edge of cancer therapies. Mol Ther. 2021;29(8):2396–411.
70. Shahid MN, Rebekah RW, Richard CB, Bruce AS. Aptamers as therapeutics. Annu Rev Pharmacol Toxicol. 2017;57:61–79.
71. Shawn EL, Brian JH, Yun L, Donald SC. Identification and characterization of nuclease-stabilized RNA molecules that bind human prostate cancer cells via the prostate-specific membrane antigen. Cancer Res. 2002;62:4029–33.
72. Silvia N, Giuseppina R, Alessandra A, Francesco I, Cristina Q, Gerolama C. Potential and challenges of aptamers as specific carriers of therapeutic oligonucleotides for precision medicine in cancer. Cancers (Basel). 2019;11(10):1521.
73. Stella D, Marcel H. Generation of aptamers with an expanded chemical repertoire. Molecules. 2015;20(9):16643–71.
74. Steven PR, Martin GP. Dual-modality imaging: combining anatomy and function. J Nucl Med. 2008;49:938–55.
75. Steven PR, Martin GP. Molecular imaging in oncology: current impact and future directions. CA Cancer J Clin. 2022;72:333–52.
76. Swathi V, Kaushik C, Musuvathi MB. Recent advancements of aptamers in cancer therapy. ACS Omega. 2023;8(36):32231–43.
77. Tanushree B, Jaishriram R, Sandesh S. Molecular methods in cancer diagnostics: a short review. Ann Med. 2024;56(1):2353893.
78. Tianyuan W, Yicheng N, Li L. Innovative imaging techniques for advancing cancer diagnosis and treatment. Cancers. 2024;16(14):2607.
79. Tong M, Xiyu L, Yiqun L, Liping Z, Zhikun Z, Tong L, et al. Aptamer-based biosensors and application in tumor theranostics. Cancer Sci. 2022;113(1):7–16.
80. Ulrich L, Ernst W. Nucleic acid therapeutics using polyplexes: a journey of 50 years (and beyond). Chem Rev. 2015;115(19):11043–78.

81. Xiaolan C, M-Carmen E, Zhi Z, Yu-Fen H, Yan C, Lin W, et al. Using aptamer-conjugated fluorescence resonance energy transfer nanoparticles for multiplexed cancer cell monitoring. Anal Chem. 2009;81:7009–14.
82. Xu H, Huaicheng C, Wei W. Design of ultrasensitive chemiluminescence detection of lysozyme in cancer cells based on nicking endonuclease signal amplification technology. Biosens Bioelectron. 2010;26(1):248–54.
83. Xueqi H, Dongdong Z, Zheng Z, Linjie H, Xiahui L, Shanni H. Aptamer-based probes for cancer diagnostics and treatment. Life (Basel). 2022;12(11):1937.
84. Ya D, Ping W, Chunyan L, Shufeng X, Qi T, Tong W, et al. Design, bioanalytical, and biomedical applications of aptamer-based hydrogels. Front Med. 2020;7:456.
85. Yang Z, Bo SL, Mario J. Recent advances in aptamer discovery and applications. Molecules. 2019;24(5):941.
86. Yaroslav C, Morley OS. In silico selection of RNA aptamers. Nucleic Acids Res. 2009;37(12):e87.
87. Ye Z, Pranjal C, Yoon-Bo S. Ultrasensitive and selective electrochemical diagnosis of breast cancer based on a hydrazine-Au nanoparticle-aptamer bioconjugate. Anal Chem. 2013;85(2):1058–64.
88. Yu Y, Jingjing L, Xiaoqi S, Liangzhu F, Wenwen Z, Zhuang L, et al. Near-infrared light-activated cancer cell targeting and drug delivery with aptamer-modified nanostructures. Nano Res. 2016;9:139–48.
89. Yuan W, Yaling L, Peter BA, Waseem A, Arif IM, Jifu T, et al. Capture, isolation, and release of cancer cells with aptamer-functionalized glass bead array. Lab Chip. 2012;12(22):4693–701.
90. Zhiqing Z, Ali MM, Mark AE, Dong-Ku K, Yih Yang C, Leonard SS. A polyvalent Aptamer system for targeted drug delivery. Biomaterials. 2013;34:9728–35.
91. Zihao C, Long H, Bao-Ting Z, Aiping L, Yaofeng W, Yuanyuan Y, et al. Artificial intelligence in aptamer–target binding prediction. Int J Mol Sci. 2021;22:3605.
92. Lächelt U, Wagner E. Nucleic Acid Therapeutics Using Polyplexes: A Journey of 50 Years (and Beyond). Chem Rev. 2015;115(19):11043–78. https://doi.org/10.1021/cr5006793. Epub 2015 Apr 15. PMID: 25872804.

Designing Aptamers for Cancer Diagnosis Therapy

8

Rahul Kumar, Sakshi Patel, Shriyansh Srivastava, Shaik Abdul Rahaman, Deepika Sharma, Biplab Pal, and Malakapogu Ravindra Babu

8.1 Introduction

8.1.1 Overview of Aptamers

Aptamers are single-stranded, short nucleic acids or peptides that bind with high affinity and specificity to a target. They are bioengineered by a process called Systematic Evolution of Ligands by Exponential Enrichment (SELEX) [1]. This technology enables the identification of aptamers that can selectively bind to a wide range of molecules, such as proteins, small molecules, ions, and cells. Aptamers are sometimes called the nucleic acid counterparts of the antibodies in view of their specificity to bind targets [2]. Aptamers are synthesized chemically, unlike antibodies, and provide the advantages of ease of production, lower cost, and small batch-to-batch variability [3]. Aptamers are a highly useful alternative to small inhibitor molecules because they fold into structurally complex three-dimensional shapes that enable them to bind to targets through a variety of complementary binding sites (hydrogen bonding, van der Waals forces, and electrostatic interactions) [1, 4].

- *High Specificity and Affinity:* Unlike molecules that share a sequence of bases in DNA, aptamers can differentiate between otherwise similar molecules, such as isomers, and have phenomenal specificity.
- *Chemical Stability:* They are more stable under various circumstances than proteins or antibodies, and chemical change can further increase stability.

R. Kumar · S. Patel · S. Srivastava · S. A. Rahaman · D. Sharma · M. Ravindra Babu (✉)
Department of Pharmacy, School of Medical and Allied Sciences, Galgotias University, Greater Noida, Uttar Pradesh, India

B. Pal
School of Pharmaceutical Sciences, Lovely Professional University, Phagwara, Punjab, India

S. Srivastava et al. (eds.), *Biosensors and Aptamers*,
https://doi.org/10.1007/978-981-96-8387-1_8

- *Rapid Synthesis:* Aptamers can be rapidly and efficiently synthesized using well-established chemical techniques, without relying on biological systems.
- *Decreased Immunogenicity:* As nonprotein molecules, aptamers are less prone to immunological reactions in therapeutic settings.

Aptamers have applications across multiple fields. Aptamers act on the drugs as a pathway that a drug should occupy on the target by modulating or blocking specific molecular interactions [2, 5]. For instance, the aptamer used for age-related macular degeneration (AMD) treatment is the FDA-approved Pegaptanib. Molecular recognition elements are biosensor probes used to detect biomarkers associated with disease states, including cancer and infection [5, 6]. Successful delivery of therapeutic agents to diseased tissues or cells by aptamers is selective, sparing non-target tissues and cells from potentially toxic effects [7]. Despite their many advantages, aptamers also have some disadvantages [8]:

- *Susceptibility to Degradation:* The aptamers are also susceptible to degradation by nucleases in biological environments.
- *Cost of SELEX Process:* Producing is cost-intensive, but production is relatively inexpensive.

These challenges are overcome by ongoing research improving stability and bioavailability through chemical modifications [9, 10]. In addition, SELEX techniques continue to develop in automation and chip high-throughput speeds, hopefully making aptamer development more parallelizable [11]. Another route for the aptamers is to integrate them into new technologies, like nanomedicine and artificial intelligence (AI) for aptamer design, among others [12]. In a nutshell, aptamers are a versatile, promising class of molecules whose applications are of great interest in science, medicine, and technology. Their special properties and versatility remain at the vanguard of molecular recognition research and applications.

8.1.2 Importance in Cancer Diagnosis and Therapy

Being exceptional in specificity, versatility, and biocompatibility, aptamers have emerged as powerful tools for cancer diagnosis and therapy [4, 13]. These agents have positioned themselves as powerful agents in the fight against cancer due to their ability to bind with biomarkers and therapeutic targets much more precisely. This section discusses the way aptamers have helped with cancer diagnostics and therapeutics (Fig. 8.1) [14] and provides advantages and opportunities for innovation [14]. In order for cancer to be best managed, it is vitally important to have an accurate and timely diagnosis. Thus, aptamers have several benefits as diagnostic tools because of their selectivity and their ability to bind a variety of cancer biomarkers, such as proteins, nucleic acids, and small molecules [15].

- *Biomarker Detection:* By engineering aptamers to bind to such human tumor-associated antigens as VEGF, PSMA, or HER2, these antigens may now be targeted. These are necessary to give an accurate diagnosis of the kinds and stages

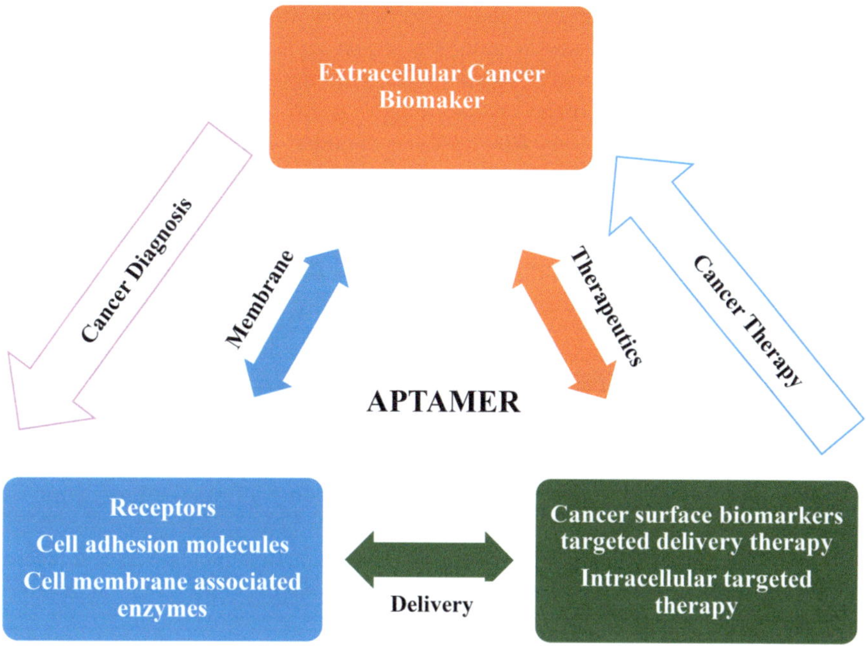

Fig. 8.1 Diagram showing how aptamers have been used to diagnose and treat cancer during the last 10 years

of cancer. Biosensors containing aptamers are used to identify cancer biomarkers. In many cases, they are more sensitive and specific than mainstream diagnostic techniques such as enzyme-linked immunosorbent assay (ELISA). For fast and precise detection, aptamer-based biosensors utilize a colorimetric, electrochemical, or fluorescent method.

- *Imaging Agents:* Imaging agents such as fluorescent dyes, radiolabels, or nanoparticles may be coupled with aptamers to enable targeted imaging of tumors. This approach allows for tumor identification and surveillance using techniques such as PET, MRI, or fluorescence imaging. Aptamers also hold promise for application in cancer treatment.

Aptamers may disrupt molecular pathways essential to the formation of cancer, which is one of the several reasons they have emerged as such potential therapeutic agents in oncology [12, 16]. Aptamers' role in the therapy of cancer. Aptamers, however, are especially appealing as anticancer therapeutic agents because they may interfere with important molecular mechanisms that underlie the onset of cancer.

- *Targeted Therapy:* Aptamers could target cancer cells with precision by attaching to overexpressed receptors on the surface of cancer cells. For example, epidermal growth factor receptor (EGFR) or PD-L1 targeting aptamers may prevent aspects of signaling pathways required for evasion of the immune system and tumor development. Targeted medication delivery systems are ideal candidates for aptamers [16, 17]. However, aptamers can be conjugated to chemotherapeutic medicines to target cancer cells specifically, minimizing systemic toxicity while maximizing treatment efficacy.

- *Delivery of RNA Interference (RNAi):* Thus, aptamers can serve as transporters to get microRNA (miRNA) or small interfering RNA (siRNA) into tumor cells to silence cancer-causing genes.
- *Antiangiogenic Therapy*: Aptamers that recognize angiogenic factors like VEGF may starve cancer cells when they block the development of new blood vessels that feed tumors and do so by preventing the creation of new blood vessels.

Aptamers have several applications in cancer therapy, such as:

- *High Specificity:* This would reduce off-target effects by distinguishing normal from malignant cells.
- *Quick Development:* The in vitro selection procedure allows the production of aptamers for newly discovered cancer targets.
- *Chemical Stability and Modifiability:* Chemical alteration of aptamers to increase their stability and affinity of protein binding confers additional therapeutic potential.
- *Decreased Immunogenicity:* Monoclonal antibodies are more prone to immunological responses; thus, they are relatively unsafe for repeated usage, while aptamers are safer for repeated usage.

Aptamers have much potential and suffer from, for example, nuclease degradability and poor bioavailability, precluding clinical translation [18]. Technologies for cancer diagnosis and therapy integration with nanotechnology, artificial intelligence, and precision medicine strategies are also pursued. Cancer diagnostics and therapeutics using aptamers are a new paradigm. Because of their specificity, adaptability, and ability to function in conjunction with state-of-the-art technologies, they are in the interest of advancing cancer care. Still, on their way, aptamers promise to strengthen cancer patients' chances of success as research continues to perfect their design and application [19].

8.1.3 Historical Development of Aptamer-Based Technologies

Aptamer-based technologies are a testimony to the fast rate of growth in the field of molecular biology and biotechnology in general [20]. After their discovery in the early 1990s, aptamers have developed into versatile tools with significant scientific and clinical implications, being used from their discovery in diagnostics and therapeutics.

(a) *The Early Discoveries and the Origin of SELEX*

Two groups of researchers, Larry Gold and Jack Szostak, independently invented Systematic Evolution of Ligands by Exponential Enrichment (SELEX) in 1990, which formed the basis for aptamer-based technologies [21]. Through this innovative technique, the in vitro selection of nucleic acid molecules (DNA or RNA) capable of high-affinity binding to target molecules was achieved.

This theoretical approach of SELEX allowed the identification of aptamers from large libraries of randomized sequences by enrichment of those sequences exhibiting the highest binding potential in an iterative fashion. The appearance of these studies was a historic milestone in terms of creating new routes of exploration for nucleic acids as functional molecules, not just in genetics [22].

The early 1990s saw the advent of aptamer research in order to determine ways to increase the stability and functionality of aptamers. In biological environments, RNA aptamers were susceptible to degradation by nucleases, and thus unmodified RNA aptamers were effective only in vitro [23]. To address this, chemical modifications were introduced, including:

- 2′-Fluoro and 2′-O-Methyl Modifications: Able to provide enhanced resistance to enzymatic degradation.
- PEGylation: Pharmacokinetics and bioavailability of the aptamers were improved by the addition of polyethylene glycol (PEG).
- Preparation of aptamers for real diagnostics.

This transition occurred at the start of the early 2000s when we exploited aptamers for diagnostics and therapeutics [24]. In 2004, the first FDA-approved aptamer-based drug, Pegaptanib (Macugen), was used in the treatment of age-related macular degeneration (AMD). The results of this milestone validated the capacity of aptamers as therapeutic agents. At the same time, aptamers found use in biosensors and diagnostic assays [25, 27]. Aptamer-based biosensors were developed for the detection of small molecules, proteins, and even whole cells with high specificity and sensitivity and outperformed traditional antibodies in stability and versatility.

(b) *Emerging Technologies Integration*

The 2010s saw the integration of aptamers with cutting-edge technologies, further expanding their applications:

- *Nanotechnology:* Highly sensitive diagnostic tools and targeted drug delivery systems were developed by conjugating nanoparticles with aptamers.
- *CRISPR and Gene Editing:* To control CRISPR systems with more precision during gene editing, we explored using aptamers as regulatory elements.
- *High-Throughput SELEX:* The SELEX process was advanced in automation and computational tools to quickly identify aptamers of a diversity of targets.

Aptamer-based technologies are on the front line of research in precision medicine, biosensing, and nanomedicine today. Some key trends include:

- *Aptamer–Nanoparticle Hybrids:* Transforming cancer diagnostics and therapy, targeted imaging, as well as treatment options, these hybrids are expanding.
- *Real-Time Detection:* We have developed biosensors based on aptamers for point-of-care diagnostics, especially for infectious and chronic diseases.

- *Artificial Intelligence (AI) in SELEX:* Aptamer–target interactions are being predicted using machine learning algorithms to speed up the aptamer discovery process.

However, the development of aptamer-based technologies has not been without a challenge. These issues have prompted the need for continued innovation with respect to SELEX [23, 26]. The lessons learned correspond to technological advancement. The essential part of SELEX and the subsequent incorporation of aptamers into increasingly sophisticated therapeutic and diagnostic platforms make this a true story of SELEX to explore. Aptamers hold promise for assuming an ever more critical role in countering global health challenges and for enabling the next wave of biotechnological innovation [27].

8.2 Aptamers in Cancer Diagnosis

Biomarkers are needed to evaluate therapy effectiveness, allow for early diagnosis, elucidate disease causes, and plan tailored treatments. Due to their sensitivity, specificity, and versatility, they make them both an alternative and a supplement to conventional antibody-based methods in biomarker research. The benefits of aptamers for finding biomarkers are:

- *High Affinity and Specificity:* Often, aptamers can be designed to have a nanomolar to picomolar affinity to attach to certain targets: proteins, tiny compounds, or cells. This accuracy is critical to finding and investigating low-abundance biomarkers.
- *Numerous Target Compatibilities:* Unlike antibodies, aptamers can target acids, proteins, and other molecules.
- Chemical modification of aptamers is performed to enhance their binding capabilities, biostability, and performance in intricate biological samples. They are also stable in a plethora of environments.
- *Rapid Development and Selection:* The SELEX approach allows for the identification of aptamers to new targets without the need to perform animal vaccination to identify antibodies or proteins as biomarkers.
- *Target Identification*: Using aptamers to select against complex mixtures like blood, tissue lysates, or cell surface proteins may reveal new biomarkers for cancer, heart disease, and neurological illness.

For example, acting as sprayers for the surging tumor cells has been used to determine Succar Ferin tumor cells, allowing for diagnostics and prognosis of cancer [28].

Aptamer-based assays (for example, aptamer-linked immunosorbent assays (ALISA) or aptamer-based sensors) are used to analyze biological samples quantitatively and qualitatively to measure biomarkers in biological samples [28, 29]. These approaches are nearly as sensitive or repeatable, if not more so, than conventional procedures. Aptamers enable selective enrichment of uncommon targets in complex samples to detect and characterize rare biomarkers. In particular, this helps to pinpoint metabolites or low-abundance proteins that are essential to the early stages of the disease [30].

- *High-Throughput Screening:* This has been possible due to the combination of SELEX and microarray technologies to allow testing of many possible targets at once. It is useful for identifying biomarker panels that give a good understanding of disease states [31]. The importance of aptamers in the identification of biomarkers aimed at the diagnosis, prognosis, and therapy of cancer has been evidenced.
- *Cardiovascular Diseases:* For example, aptamer-based techniques have aided in the early diagnosis of myocardial infarction as well as inflammation by knowing biomarkers such as troponins and C-reactive protein (CRP).
- *Neurodegenerative Diseases:* Applying aptamers capable of targeting tau and amyloid beta protein biomarkers in research on Alzheimer's disease and other neurodegenerative diseases is advancing.

8.2.1 Obstacles to Aptamer-Based Biomarker Discovery

- *Biological Sample Complexity:* The presence of many proteins and other "compounds" in biological samples can hinder the identification of low abundance.
- *Nuclease Degradation:* Due to their susceptibility to enzymatic degradation, the usefulness of unmodified aptamers in some applications is very limited. However, chemical changes may minimize this problem.
- *Validation and Translation:* Still, the journey is there, but it has strict testing and standardization requirements.

As associated technologies progress, aptamers' relevance in biomarker identification is anticipated to increase [19, 32]:

- Aptamers joined with mass spectrometry permit accurate identification and measurement of biomarkers in complex samples.
- Aptamer–Nanoparticle Conjugates: Through increased sensitivity in detection platforms, these systems enable the discovery of ultralow abundance biomarkers.
- Machine Learning and Artificial Intelligence (AI): AI algorithms are being built to discover the best candidates for biomarker discovery, improve predictions of binding, and speed up aptamer selection.

In conclusion, biomarkers have been identified as such remarkable resources that aptamers have been enlisted to help find them. Because of their special qualities, plus state-of-the-art technical development, they are very useful for disease-specific biomarker location and description [33]. If this is fixed, aptamer-based methods can power biomarker discovery and enable precision medicine and early disease identification [30].

8.3 Techniques for Aptamer-Based Diagnostics

Aptamer-based diagnostics leverage the unique properties of aptamers, including their specificity, affinity, and chemical versatility, to develop innovative tools for disease detection and monitoring [18, 34]. This section explores key techniques employed in aptamer-based diagnostics, focusing on biosensors, assays, imaging technologies, and molecular probes.

8.3.1 Biosensors and Aptamer Assays

Aptamer-based biosensors (apt sensors) and assays are pivotal for detecting and quantifying biomarkers in complex biological samples [35, 32].

(a) *Biosensors*

Apt sensors integrate aptamers as recognition elements in sensor platforms to achieve high sensitivity and specificity. Common types include [27]:

- *Electrochemical Biosensors:* Detect changes in electrical signals upon aptamer–target binding. These sensors are widely used for detecting cancer biomarkers, small molecules, and pathogens.
- *Optical Biosensors:* Utilize interactions. Aptamer-functionalized gold nanoparticles (AuNPs) are frequently employed for signal amplification.
- *Mass-Sensitive Biosensors:* Quartz crystal microbalance (QCM) and other mass-sensitive technologies use aptamers to detect biomarker binding through changes in mass at the sensor surface.

(b) *Aptamer Assays*

Aptamer-linked immunosorbent assays (ALISA) mimic traditional ELISA but employ aptamers as capture agents. These assays provide several advantages [36]:

- *High Specificity:* Effective even for closely related targets.
- *Chemical Stability:* Aptamers withstand extreme conditions, enabling robust assays.
- *Cost-Effectiveness:* Synthetic production reduces costs compared to antibody-based assays.

8.3.2 Imaging and Molecular Probes

Aptamers are now frequently used in imaging and for molecular probes as noninvasive diagnoses, probes, and real-time monitoring [37].

(a) *Imaging Modalities:* By conjugation with imaging agents, such as fluorescent dyes, radioisotopes, or nanoparticles, aptamers can be used for precise imaging of disease sites where specific biomarkers are targeted.

- Fluorescence Imaging: The tumors or other pathological sites are visualized using aptamer–dye conjugates.
- Positron Emission Tomography (PET): Highly sensitive imaging in the detection of cancer or inflammatory diseases is performed with radiolabeled aptamers.
- Magnetic Resonance Imaging (MRI): MRI contrast agents, functionalized with aptamers, enhance MRI signals at disease sites while boosting sensitivity for detection.

(b) *Molecular Probes:* They are molecular probes for real-time analysis of detecting and quantifying biomolecules by aptamers [38]. For example, the fluorescent signal from this sensing is provided by DNA aptamers that have both been functionalized with quantum dots (QDs) and were shown to be able to detect specific cancer biomarkers in a rapid manner [39].

8.3.3 Case Studies of Diagnostic Application

Case Study 8.1: Aptamer-Based Biosensor for Early Breast Cancer Detection [40]

This development of an aptamer-based biosensor for early breast cancer detection is a powerful development in diagnostic technology. As an example, we designed this biosensor to detect HER2, a critical biomarker overexpressed in breast cancer subtypes. Fundamental research and illness diagnostics benefit from the development of extremely sensitive and selective biomarker detection techniques. Here, we developed an electrochemical sandwich-type apt sensor to identify the biomarker for breast cancer cells, human epidermal growth factor receptor P, as signal nanoprobes with tetrahedral DNA nanostructures (TDNs)–aptamer as recognition probes. The TDN–aptamer 1 bio-recognition element was mounted on the gold electrode (GE) surface during the biosensor assembly process in order to capture the biomarker HER2. Aptamer 2 and the natural enzyme HRP connected the Pd-Pt nanozymes that adorned the Mn_3O_4 nanozyme. The biosensor signal was amplified by accelerating the oxidation of hydroquinone (HQ) with hydrogen peroxide (H_2O_2) using the specially constructed Mn_3O_4/Pd@Pt Pd@Pt/HRP nanoprobe (nanoprobe 1). An aptamer–protein–nanoprobe sandwich structure was created on the GE surface after HER2 binding. Finally, to further enhance the signal, a Pd@Pt/HRP/complementary DNA (cDNA) nanoprobe (nanoprobe 2) was added to the surface of nanoprobe 1 by hybridizing aptamer 2 with cDNA to create a dendritic DNA nanostructure. The findings reveal that the apt sensor has a low detection limit of 0.08 ng mL^{-1} and a wide linear response ranging from 0.1 to 100.0 ng mL^{-1}. The developed method has a lot of promise for creating diverse apt sensors for the practical and efficient detection of various biomarkers.

Aptamer-based biosensors had the advantage of being compared to traditional enzyme-linked immunosorbent assay (ELISA) methods. ELISA is a widely used method for biomarker detection; however, ELISA is expensive, requiring multiple washing steps, lengthy incubation times, and expensive antibodies. However, the biosensor based on the aptamer showed faster detection, reduced sample preparation, and lower costs. Furthermore, its potential as a real-time biosensor overbids it in the clinical setting. Aptamer-based biosensors could significantly improve early breast cancer detection and benefit patients, according to this case study.

Case Study 8.2: Applications of Aptamers for Circulating Tumor Cell (CTC) Detection in Liquid Biopsy [41]

Liquid biopsy applications of aptamers that can detect and isolate circulating tumor cells (CTCs), the most important biomarkers in cancer diagnosis, prognosis, and monitoring, have been effectively utilized. A panel of aptamers was developed in this case study to address specific surface markers in CTCs (EpCAM and other tumor markers). On a microfluidic chip, the aptamers were functionalized to capture and identify CTCs in a small volume of patient blood.

Technologies for detecting rare circulating tumor cells (CTCs) can identify as few as a few cells per milliliter of blood. Each technology in the detection of rare CTCs finds as little as a few cells per milliliter of blood. Additionally, the aptamer-based system outperformed conventional antibody-based methods in distinguishing malignant cells from normal blood cells, with fewer false positives than other antibody-based approaches.

The potential of this application for early cancer detection with the purpose of adequate timely intervention and personalized disease progression and therapeutic efficacy through the integration of aptamer technology in liquid biopsy workflows, which represents.

Case Study 8.3: In Vivo Imaging in Colorectal Cancer Using Aptamer-Functionalized Nanoparticles [42]

The integration of aptamer technology with nanotechnology has created in vivo imaging for the management of colorectal cancer. For this case study, aptamers that are specific to carcinoembryonic antigen (CEA), a well-known biomarker for colorectal cancer, were conjugated to nanoparticles, like gold nanoparticles or quantum dots, to make highly targeted imaging agents. Designed to avidly bind to CEA-expressing tumor cells, aptamer-functionalized nanoparticles were created to enhance contrast and resolution in fluorescence imaging and magnetic resonance imaging (MRI).

These aptamer nanocomplexes were extremely biocompatible and stable in vivo with circulation through blood and tumor site accumulation with minimal saturation effects on off-targets. Further exploitation of nanotechnology resulted in signal intensity and detection sensitivity gains, permitting visualization of tumors at earlier stages. This system showed better specificity for colorectal cancer cells than conventional imaging agents, reducing false positives to improve diagnostic accuracy.

In particular, this approach emphasizes the synergy between aptamers and nanotechnology for improving cancer imaging. Aptamer-functionalized nanoparticles provide significant promise for precision oncology applications, enabling noninvasive, real-time visualization of tumors that allows early detection, guides surgical logistics, and monitors treatment efficacy.

Case Study 8.4: Simultaneous Detection of Lung Cancer Biomarkers Using Multiplexed Aptamer Microarray [43]

A multiplexed aptamer microarray provides a major advancement in the ability to assay multiple lung cancer biomarkers at once, thereby drastically reducing the time and cost of diagnostic analysis. A microarray platform was constructed in this case study with a panel of aptamers targeting key lung cancer biomarkers, including epidermal growth factor receptor (EGFR), carcinoembryonic antigen (CEA), and cytokeratin 19 fragments (CYFRA 21-1). This innovative approach allowed us to simultaneously detect these biomarkers in patient serum samples on a single assay.

The multiplexed microarray offered several noteworthy advantages. Most importantly, it significantly reduced diagnostic time by eliminating the need for separate tests for each biomarker. Additionally, its relatively low synthesis and stabilization costs made it suitable for identifying cancer subtypes and stages.

This case study demonstrates that the strengths of aptamers and high-throughput microarray technology can be combined to form a powerful tool for efficient and cost-effective lung cancer diagnosis. In addition to its utility in streamlining the diagnostic workflow, the approach has wider applicability in oncology, where more complete and rapid biomarker profiling is desired within the clinical setting.

8.3.4 Comparative Analysis with Conventional Diagnostic Tools

The features of aptamer-based imaging in cancer detection include their synthetic production method, which differs from that of antibodies and avoids the time and expense required for clinical readiness [44] this synthetic method ensures unique, consistent batch-to-batch production and allows for modification with increased functionality through easy and cheap manipulation [45]. Also, aptamers are much more stable under extreme conditions, such as changing the temperature or pH, and are therefore ideally suited for many diagnostic applications [46].

Aptamer-based platforms show comparable or superior limitations, alongside faster detection times and fewer sample preparation requirements compared to ELISA. Furthermore, aptamer-functionalized agents demonstrate higher target specificity and lower background noise than conventional antibody-based imaging probes in imaging applications [47]. Aptamer-based biosensors are as good as PCR for nucleic acid detection and do not require any complex amplification methods.

Moreover, aptamer-based technology enables multiplexed detection of multiple biomarkers in a single assay, offering greater efficiency. However, in some cases, it may be limited in sensitivity or be more expensive compared to certain conventional methods [48]. Not only does this accelerate diagnostic workflows, but it also uncovers the entire disease profile [49]. Taken together, aptamer-based diagnostics represent an order of magnitude improvement, offering precision, economy, and efficiency all in one compared to traditional models of diagnostics in oncology and beyond [50].

8.4 Aptamers in Cancer Therapy

Thanks to the unique properties of aptamers, aptamers have been developed as versatile tools in cancer therapy [51]. Next, this section reviews the mechanisms by which aptamers exert therapeutic effects, innovative delivery systems, examples of clinical applications and challenges, and opportunities in this exciting field.

8.4.1 Mechanisms of Action in Therapeutic Applications

(a) *Targeting Tumor Cells*

Since they can bind to overexpressed surface markers such as HER2, EGFR, or PSMA, aptamers can target cancer cells directly. By blocking signal transduction pathways responsible for tumor growth and survival, these aptamers provide therapeutic services [52]. Moreover, aptamers can function as targeting ligands for drug delivery systems and selectively deliver cytotoxic agents to cancer cells while sparing healthy tissues.

(b) *Angiogenesis Inhibition*

Cancer therapy is a strategy that inhibits angiogenesis—the formation of new blood vessels. Blocking of angiogenic pathways (starving tumor). This mechanism is useful, particularly in treating cancers that are highly vascularized [53].

(c) *Immune Modulation*

Targeting immune checkpoints, immunomodulatory aptamers can modulate immune responses or activate immune cells. For example, aptamers blocking PD1 or CTLA4 can reverse the field of T cells to restore engagement of the immunocytes and attack the tumor, or aptamers can be engineered to deliver immune-stimulating agents to the tumor microenvironment [54].

8.4.2 Aptamer-Based Therapies Delivery Systems

Aptamer-based therapies are dependent on effective delivery systems. Wide applications of aptamers have been achieved by forming nanoparticles, liposomes, and hydrogels to improve the stability and bioavailability and targeted delivery of aptamers [55]. These systems solve the issue of aptamer enzymatic degradation and improve retention at tumor sites. For example, the conjugation of aptamers to polyethylene glycol (PEG) or other stabilizing agents further extends the half-life of these aptamers in circulation. In addition, many new theranostics are being developed for simultaneous diagnosis and treatment with multifunctional delivery systems capable of therapeutic and imaging [56].

8.4.3 Examples of Aptamers in Clinical Trials

They have advanced several aptamers to clinical trials and shown potential as a therapeutic. The first FDA-approved aptamer, pegaptanib, was originally designed to treat macular degeneration but carries implications for cancer therapy because it has the property of inhibiting VEGF [57]. Aptamer AS1411, targeting nucleoli, is in clinical trials for the treatment of renal and breast cancers. For example, NOX-A12 blocks the tumor microenvironment via its binding to CXCL12 to improve the effect of other treatments. Table 8.1 displays a few examples of aptamers used in clinical studies.

8.4.4 Challenges and Opportunities in Therapeutic Applications

Aptamers hold great promise; however, they also face challenges, including off-target effects. These limitations are being overcome by advances in chemical modifications, including the use of locked nucleic acids (LNAs) and Spiegelmers (mirror image aptamers) [58].

Aptamers can be combined with immunotherapies and personalized medicine approaches, and can also be integrated into advanced technologies such as CRISPR and artificial intelligence to enable optimal treatment design [59]. By moving forward, aptamers are poised to become important building blocks of the treatment regimen for cancer, bringing precision and efficacy in targeting the complexities of the disease.

Table 8.1 Tabular depiction of aptamer instances used in clinical trials [7]

Name of aptamer	Composition	Medical condition	Sponsor	Current phase
AS1411	DNA	Renal cell tumor	Antisoma Research	Phase 2
NOX-A12	L-RNA with 3′PEG	Chronic lymphocytic leukemia	Noxxon Pharma AG	Phase 2
NOX-E36	L-RNA with 3′PEG	Albuminuria and diabetes mellitus type 2	Noxxon Pharma AG	Phase 2 completed
NOX-H94	L-RNA with 5′PEG	Anemia of chronic inflammation	Noxxon Pharma AG	Phase 1 completed
ARC19499	DNA with 3′ inverted dT and 5′PEG	Hemophilia	Baxalta US Inc.	Phase 1 completed
EYE001	RNA with 5′-PEG	Wet age-related macular degeneration	National Eye Institute	Phase 1 completed
E10030	RNA with 3′ inverted dT and 5′PEG	Coronary artery disease	Regado Bioscience	Phase 1 completed

8.5 Engineering and Optimization of Aptamers

A critical requirement for maximizing aptamer efficacy and increasing their applicability in diagnostics, therapeutics, and targeted drug delivery is the engineering and optimization of aptamers [60]. Modification of aptamers through a combo of advanced chemical modifications, structural refinement, and inventive delivery systems allows aptamers to be tailored for improved performance. This section discusses how the key strategies that help to enhance aptamer functionality have been implemented [61].

8.5.1 Enhanced Targeting Strategies

Sufficient targeting is a basic requirement of aptamer performance. Various strategies have been developed to enhance the binding affinity and specificity of aptamers toward their intended targets [62]:

- *SELEX Improvements:* The discovery of an aptamer relies on the use of Systematic Evolution of Ligands by Exponential Enrichment (SELEX). With advances in SELEX, including cell-based SELEX and in vivo SELEX, the identification of aptamers to more complex biological targets, including whole cells and tissues, has resulted in superior targeting in physiological conditions.
- *Multivalent Aptamers:* Multiple aptamer units are engineered to link at multivalent aptamers in order to improve targeting. Consequently, avidity is increased as well as binding to multivalent or subsetted receptors when present on cell surfaces, and this is particularly valuable in tumor targeting applications [63].
- *Chimeric Aptamers:* However, hybrid aptamers, in which more than one sequence combines to target multiple biomarkers, offer broader specificity. Furthermore, the use of dual and metastatic presentation improves.
- *Allosteric Aptamers:* In addition, all of these aptamers undergo conformational change upon target binding, enabling use in switch-like activation. In biosensing applications where binding events must be transduced into detectable signals, this feature is especially useful.

8.5.2 Chemical Modifications for Longevity

A problem with natural aptamers is their ability to be enzymatically degraded and rapidly cleared from the bloodstream. Chemical modifications have been extensively employed to enhance their stability and bioavailability (Fig. 8.2) [64, 65]:

- *Backbone Modifications:* In addition to preventing nuclease resistance, chemical modification of the nucleotides with variation of 2′ hydroxyl group to 2′ fluoro, 2′ amino, or 2′ O methyl RNA improves resistance to nucleases. These modifications do not interfere with aptamer activity and increase the half-life of aptamers in biological systems.

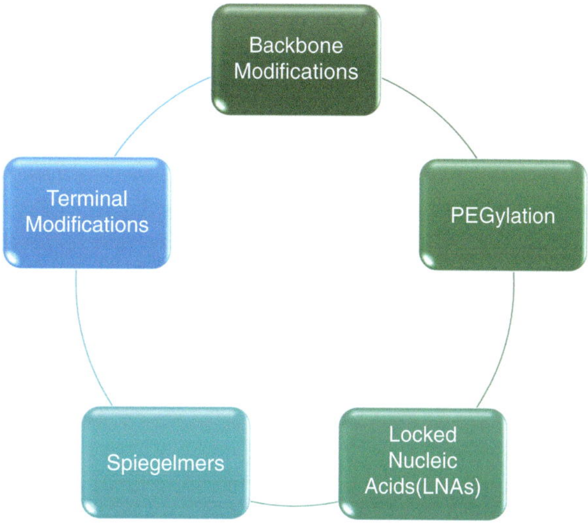

Fig. 8.2 Diagram displaying many chemical changes that have been made to improve their stability and bioavailability

- *PEGylation:* Polyethylene glycol (PEG)-conjugated aptamers increase molecular weight and reduce renal clearance, decreasing aptamer clearance time. Such an approach is of particular advantage for therapeutic applications requiring prolonged systemic exposure.
- *Locked Nucleic Acids (LNAs):* Modifications are used to lock the sugar backbone into a radial conformation, making the binding constant, thermal stability, and resistance to degradation much greater.
- *Spiegelmers:* In each case, these mirrored tides are fully resistant to enzymatic degradation while maintaining specificity.
- *Terminal Modifications:* Most importantly, protecting the 3′ or 5′ ends of aptamers by the addition of protective groups or inverted nucleotides makes the aptamers quite stable, with limited degradation by exonuclease.

8.5.3 Conjugation Nanoparticles and Other Carriers

Conjugation of revolutionizing their application due to nanotechnology. This approach enhances their targeting capabilities and expands their functional roles [66]:

- *Nanoparticle–Aptamer Hybrids:* Aptamers conjugated to nanoparticles like gold nanoparticles (AuNPs), quantum dots (QDs), or magnetic nanoparticles (MNPs) possess both the potential of aptamers to recognize a target and the unique optical, electronic, and/or magnetic properties of the nanoparticles [67]. They are broadly exploited in biosensors, targeted drug delivery, and imaging.
- *Liposome–Aptamer Systems:* Aptamer-guided drug delivery systems are often formed by conjugating the aptamers to liposomes. Therapeutic agents are encapsulated in these systems and delivered only to target cells. As an example,

aptamer-decorated liposomes to target HER2 have been shown to be promising for delivering chemotherapy drugs directly to breast cancer cells [68].

- *Hydrogel Integration:* For sustained-release applications, their aptamers can be embedded into hydrogels. Releasing aptamers at the site of interest in a controlled manner with these hydrogels has applications as a depot for drugs that can enhance therapeutic efficacy and minimize systemic side effects.
- *Multifunctional Carriers:* Multifunctional carriers are also conjugated with aptamers that allow imaging, therapy, and targeting in a single system. They represent "theranostic" platforms, which allow simultaneous diagnosis and treatment, offering a complete answer for precision medicine [69].

8.5.4 Modeling and Computational Tools in Aptamer Design

Computer techniques have sped the use of aptamers for the design and optimization process. These methods facilitate structural modeling.

- *SELEX in Silico:* Computational methods can predict specific aptamer sequences exhibiting high binding affinity and specificity by simulating the SELEX, reducing the need for experimental repetition and associated time and expense [70].
- *Molecular Docking and Dynamics:* Molecular docking methods predict aptamer–target binding interactions. Finally, these models are further improved with molecular dynamics simulations that include the flexibility of the aptamer and the flexibility and conformational shifts of the target molecule.
- *Software for Predicting Structure*: Prediction of secondary and tertiary structures of aptamers can be achieved with the help of the ViennaRNA, RNA structure, and M fold programs, which guess at stable and useful configurations of aptamers.
- *Artificial Intelligence (AI) in Aptamer Design:* Machine learning algorithms are able to reflect their predictions on aptamers by analyzing huge databases of aptamer sequences and how those aptamers bind to their targets [71]. As an added bonus, AI-based systems identify trends and suggest chemical changes to improve performance.
- *Databases for Bioinformatics:* AptaDB is an aptamer database designed to give researchers access to useful information concerning previously discovered aptamers, their sequences, and binding characteristics. These datasets may be used as a starting point for generating new aptamers or as tools used to better refine existing aptamers.

In conclusion, the strategy to achieve aptamer engineering and optimization is multifaceted, requiring unification of computer science, chemistry, and nanotechnology [53, 66]. Chemical changes for stability, improved targeting techniques, nanotechnology for delivery, as well as the use of computational design tools, are leading to increasingly more stable and adaptable aptamers. With this development, these devices also widen their scope of diagnostic and therapeutic applications and address crucial issues of stability and specificity [72]. As research continues, and if the potential is realized, aptamers can revolutionize precision medicine and give solutions developed for the complexities of current healthcare.

8.6 Aptamer Integration and Nanotechnology

Meanwhile, nanotechnology and aptamer science revolutionized the fields of diagnostics, therapeutics, and drug delivery [73]. Consequently, researchers developed highly efficient systems for cancer management by harnessing the specificity of aptamers with the specific physical and chemical properties of nanomaterials. This section discusses the use of nanomaterials in improving aptamer efficacy, hybrid nanomaterial-based systems in cancer applications, and multifunctional nanocarriers for theranostics [74].

8.6.1 Role of Nanomaterials in Expediting Aptamer Ablative Rate

Imperfections of aptamers, such as limited stability, sensitivity, and delivery efficiency, can be overcome using nanomaterials. Encouraged by their unique characteristics, including high surface area-to-volume ratio, tuneable size, and multifunctionality, they allow for enhanced interactions between aptamers and their targets [63].

- *Improved Target Binding:* Immobilization of aptamers onto platforms formed by nanomaterials such as gold nanoparticles (AuNPs), carbon nanotubes (CNTs), and quantum dots (QDs) allows for packaging in orientations that maximize target accessibility. The resulting aptamers have increased binding affinity and specificity.
- *Signal Amplification:* Frequency and nanomaterial amplification are used in biosensing applications. For example, surface plasmon resonance signals under strong resonance conditions can be generated by aptamers with AuNPs, and fluorescence intensity is high in the case of the QD aptamer complex. These properties render diagnostic tools extremely sensitive.
- *Enhanced Stability:* Aptamers are many nanomaterials protected from enzymatic degradation. For instance, encapsulating aptamers into polymeric nanoparticles protects them from nucleases to enhance molecular stability and extend circulation time in biological environments.
- *Controlled Release:* It is specifically aptamers, however, that have proved most useful when released under controlled conditions such as therapeutic applications, which nanomaterials enable. The advantage of this feature is its sustained and localized action, so there are fewer systemic side effects.

The aptamer-based technologies have thus generated nanomaterials as important enablers in translating aptamer-based technologies into clinical and industrial applications.

8.6.2 Hybrid Aptamer–Nanoparticle Systems in Cancer Management

While hybrid systems that combine aptamers and nanoparticles have displayed great potential in cancer diagnostics, imaging, and treatment, their synthetic complexity and extensive post-synthetic processing hinder their commercialization. Both components are exploited to create a synergistic system with superior performance [75].

- *Cancer Diagnostics:* Cancer biomarker detection with aptamer–nanoparticle conjugates is very effective. One example of this is the AuNPs functionalized with aptamers that target prostate-specific antigen (PSA) or HER2, enabling the real-time, label-free detection of cancer biomarkers by means of colorimetry and plasmonic resonance [76]. They achieve picomolar sensitivity for early cancer diagnosis.
- *Imaging:* Aptamer–nanoparticle hybrids have enhanced imaging modalities such as fluorescence, magnetic resonance imaging (MRI), and computed tomography (CT). By utilizing quantum dot (QD) conjugates, highly specific fluorescent signals arising from highly specific cancer tumor localization are attained. Likewise, aptamer-conjugated iron oxide nanoparticles serve as MRI contrast agents and show tumor regions of high resolution [77].
- *Drug Delivery:* Targeted drug delivery in oncology has been revolutionized by using aptamer-guided nanoparticles. These systems achieve this by conjugating drug-loaded nanoparticles with aptamers that are specific to tumor antigens such as EGFR or VEGF, ensuring the delivery of cytotoxic drugs to tumor sites. The combination of these approaches minimizes off-target effects and increases therapeutic efficacy. This includes enhanced targets for breast cancer treatment using aptamer-functionalized doxorubicin-loaded liposomes.
- *Photothermal and Photodynamic Therapy:* The second area of application is hybrid systems for photothermal therapy (PTT) and photodynamic therapy (PDT). In PTT, aptamer-conjugated gold nanorods (AuNRs) are used that selectively bind to tumor cells and are locally heated by site-nanoparticles; pairing of surrounding tissues [78].

Aptamer–nanoparticle hybrids exhibit direct versatility and are valuable tools for comprehensive cancer management.

8.6.3 Multifunctional Nanocarriers for Theranostics

Personalized medicine has come into focus, particularly as theranostics (combining diagnostics and therapy). This innovation includes multifunctional nanocarriers with aptamers, which sense cancer, target therapy, and track the response to treatment at the same time [79].

- *Integrated Diagnostic and Therapeutic Functions:* By functionalization with aptamer, aptamer-function RNA-based drug agents inside a single platform [80]. For example, silica nanoparticles conjugated with aptamers have been created for the delivery of siRNA to cancer cells for fluorescence-based monitoring of drug delivery.
- *Stimuli-Responsive Systems:* Often, multifunctional nanocarriers are designed to release their cargo in response to specific stimuli in the tumor microenvironment, pH, enzymatic, or temperature [81]. As a simple example, pH-sensitive nanoparticles conjugated to aptamers release drugs only in acidic tumor environments, increasing their therapeutic precision.
- *Real-Time Monitoring:* Imaging typically is part of theranostic systems to monitor treatment progress. Conjugation of aptamers to magnetic nanometers enables MRI-based tracking of drug delivery, illustrating drug delivery efficacy and biodistribution.
- *Multimodal Approaches:* Integrating multiple therapeutic modalities, including combining chemotherapy, photothermal therapy, and immunotherapy, is being developed using nanocarriers. These multifunctional systems are guided to tumor sites by aptamers for synergistic effects [82]. For example, aptamer-conjugated gold nanoshells have been employed to facilitate concomitant PTT and immune activation, thereby increasing the percentage of tumors that regress.

Even if the combination of aptamers with nanotechnology has produced innovative outcomes, there are still a number of obstacles to overcome:

- *Scalability and Cost:* However, it is still very expensive to produce nanomaterials and aptamers, let alone to conjugate them on a big scale. Achieving broad clinical acceptance requires resolving these problems.
- *Biocompatibility:* The biocompatibility and safety of the nanomaterial could reduce cell damage and possible toxicities and immunological responses. More work needs to be done on nontoxic, biodegradable nanocarriers.
- *Regulatory Obstacles:* Hybrid aptamer–nanoparticle systems are complicated and thus face considerable regulatory challenges. Standards need to be established for approval, testing, and characterization in uniform processes.

Despite these obstacles, the integration of an aptamer nanophosphine generation theranostic platform development could allow real-time monitoring, tailored therapy, and early detection with a single system, which could change cancer care [83, 84]. In conclusion, due to their ability to engender a nanotechnology system with the malleability of aptamers, cancer treatment has been greatly improved by the combination of aptamer research and nanotechnology. From the enhanced sensitivity of diagnostics to the enabling of complex theranostics, these hybrid systems are creating room for revolution in cancer [85]. With further study and further advancement, aptamer–nanoparticle systems could be a critical part of the future of individualized cancer treatment [86].

8.7 Ethical, Regulatory, and Commercial Aspects

Significant ethical, legal, and business issues are brought up by the creation and use of aptamer-based technologies in cancer research. These elements are necessary to guarantee responsible innovation, standard compliance, and the effective application of research in clinical and business contexts [87]. The commercial potential of medicinal and diagnostic aptamers, regulatory frameworks, and ethical considerations are all covered in this chapter [88].

8.7.1 Ethical Considerations in Aptamer-Based Cancer Research

Aptamer research is shaped by its huge implications on patients, healthcare systems, and society and the ethical aspects involved. Several key considerations need to be addressed to ensure equitable and responsible use of this technology [89]:

- *Patient Consent and Privacy:* Development and testing of aptamer-based diagnostics and therapy often rely on clinical patient-derived samples. It is important to ensure informed consent and to keep patient data private. Rigorous ethical guidelines conceived of in the Declaration of Helsinki should be followed by researchers and clinicians to respect the patient's autonomy and privacy [90].
- *Access and Equity:* Although aptamer technology is advanced, access could be unfair. However, the use of these technologies could be prohibitively expensive, which limits their availability in low-resource settings. To prevent exacerbating healthcare inequities, there must be a focus on addressing disparities and on global access.
- *Animal Testing and Alternative Models:* Moreover, the development of aptamer-based systems is of ethical concern related to issues that exist for many traditional approaches; when feasible, alternative testing methods such as organ-on-a-chip systems and in silico simulations should always be prioritized [91].
- *Dual-Use Concerns:* Misuse of aptamer technologies for nontherapeutic or harmful purposes is possible, including in bioweapons. Critical oversight mechanisms are necessary to prevent dual-use risks; they are to ensure research and development efforts are peaceably and beneficially aligned.
- *Ethical Use of AI in Design:* More and more, that role is being played by computational tools and artificial intelligence (AI). When AI-based approaches are used to make decisions on patient care, it is important to be aware that they are transparent, unbiased, and applied ethically.

Addressing these ethical considerations will help promote public trust and responsible advancement of aptamer-based cancer research, and researchers and stakeholders will benefit from encounters to negotiate these types of ethical questions [92].

8.7.2 Regulatory Framework for Therapeutic and Diagnostic Aptamers

Aptamer-based diagnostics and treatments have a complicated and changing regulatory environment. It includes safety, effectiveness, and quality guidelines, all of which are critical for clinical translation and commercialization [93].

- *Regulatory Classification of Aptamers:* Depending on their intended function, aptamers are categorized differently. Therapeutic aptamers are regarded as biologics or medicines, while diagnostic aptamers may be controlled as in vitro diagnostic (IVD) devices [94]. Specific approval oaths are offered by regulatory bodies such as the FDA (United States), EMA (European Union), and PMDA (Japan).
- *Preclinical and Clinical Trials:* Any aptamer-based product must undergo a great deal of preclinical and clinical testing, just like traditional drugs and diagnostics, before it can be shown to be safe and effective. Such as stability, binding specificity, and toxicity, which are typically the small-scale safety studies and phase III large-scale efficacy trials.
- *Good Manufacturing Practices (GMPs):* The consistency of products, safety, and quality were guaranteed by the need to have produced the aptamer products in the conditions complying with the GMP standards [95]. The aptamers, however, are subject to strong controls on their synthesis, purification, and storage.
- *Harmonization of Regulations:* Differences in regulatory requirements between regions now stand in the way of global commercialization. Firefighting makes those activities easier and eliminates marketplace entry barriers, including the activities targeting the corporate interest of harmonizing market access standards, such as the activities of the International Council for Harmonization of Technical Requirements for Pharmaceuticals for Human Use (ICH).
- *Post-market Surveillance:* Once approved, a product based on the aptamer will need to be monitored constantly. Regulatory agencies require updates on pharmacovigilance programs as well as periodic safety. To avoid losing public safety and confidence in taking aptamer technologies from laboratory to clinic, one must understand the regulatory framework.

8.7.3 Commercialization and Market Potential

The commercialization of aptamer-based diagnostics and therapeutics holds a great opportunity within the global healthcare market [96]. Several factors contribute to the growing interest and market potential of these technologies:

(a) *Market Drivers:*
   - *Unmet Medical Needs*: With the rising incidence of cancer and a need for early and accurate diagnostics, the uptake of new tools such as aptamer-based systems becomes increasingly crucial, offering enhanced specificity, sensitivity, and affordability compared to traditional diagnostic methods.

- *Advancements in Biotechnology:* Modernization of SELEX techniques, chemical modifications, and development of integration with nanotechnology have contributed to the improvement of the operational performance of aptamer-based products, thus improving their commercial attractiveness.
- *Cost-Effectiveness:* Aptamers are less costly cost- and manufacturing-based alternatives for healthcare applications.

(b) *Prominent Applications:*

The global market for aptamer-based technologies includes diagnostics, therapeutics, and drug delivery [97].

- *Diagnostics:* The avidity of the interaction between the aptamer and its target leads to a strong and specific affinity between cancer biomarkers such as PSA (prostate-specific antigen) and HER2 (human epidermal growth factor 2) and aptamers measured using biosensors.
- *Therapeutics:* Pegaptanib and AS1411 have undergone clinical trials with therapeutic aptamers and have shown promise in clinical trials, opening pathways for their broader use in cancer treatment [57, 97].
- *Drug Delivery and Theranostics:* Precision medicine is developed by aptamer-guided nanocarriers for combined diagnostics and therapy in a single platform.

(c) *Market Challenges:*

- *Competition:* Compared with proven technologies, such as monoclonal antibodies with a long history of clinical success, aptamers are facing competition.
- *Production and Scalability:* Aptamers are cheaper to make than antibodies, but scaling up production quality remains difficult.
- *Regulatory Hurdles:* However, delays in commercialization time and a cost blowout can occur when faced with the complex regulatory environment.

(d) *Investment and Industry Trends:*

Aptamer technology is finding investment from start-ups and established biotech companies. Academia and industry partnerships are driving innovation and propelling product development into high gear [62, 98]. The most notable trends are aptamers combined with AI and machine learning for design optimization.

(e) *Market Projections:*

The global market is expected to witness tremendous growth in the future due to high healthcare expenditures, the increasing concern about precision medicine, and technological developments. The compound annual growth rate of the aptamer market is reported to be more than 15%, and the revenue will reach billions in the next decade.

8.8 Future Perspective and Innovations

Now, the field of aptamer technology is still progressing rapidly, and new innovations are on the brink of increasing the application of aptamers in cancer diagnostics and their therapy. In this chapter, we explore next-generation aptamers that include emerging SELEX technologies, aptamer–AI machine learning combinations, and the role aptamers play in personalized medicine [98] [99].

8.8.1 Next-Generation Aptamers

Next-generation aptamers represent a further evolution in both design and function over prior generations, enabling further clinical and research potential above and beyond the abilities attained with earlier aptamer technologies [100].

- *Modified Aptamers for Enhanced Stability:* The addition of chemical modifications, such as 2′-fluoro, 2′-amino, or locked nucleic acids (LNAs), to an aptamer provides increased resistance to nucleases, thereby extending the half-life in biological environments. These modifications increase the applicability of next-generation aptamers in therapeutic applications.
- *Bivalent and Multivalent Aptamers:* Design of aptamers with more than one binding site allows binding affinity and specificity to be enhanced. Moreover, these multivalent aptamers show increased targeting potential of complex tumor microenvironments and diminished off-target effects.
- *Aptamer–RNA Conjugates:* Simultaneous targeting and gene silencing can be performed with aptamers combined with functional RNAs, such as small interfering RNAs (siRNAs) or microRNAs (miRNAs), becoming hybrid constructs. Powerful tools in cancer therapy, these conjugates have emerged.
- *Hybrid Aptamer–Antibody Constructs:* These hybrid systems combine the advantages of aptamers and antibodies and offer simultaneous targeting and therapeutic delivery by improving target binding.
- *Environment-Responsive Aptamers:* Controlled drug release in the tumor microenvironment is being achieved with environment-responsive aptamers that recognize pH, temperature, and specific enzymes [101].

8.8.2 Emerging Technologies in SELEX

The development of aptamers of SELEX technologies is found to be refining the efficiency and precision of aptamer selection [102].

- *Microfluidic SELEX:* Microfluidic platforms are used to incorporate microfluidic platforms for rapid, automated, and high-throughput SELEX aptamer selection. The time and cost of selection are reduced while providing better reproducibility with these systems [103].
- *In Vivo SELEX:* Previous SELEX methods are performed in vitro, which do not necessarily reflect all factors in the tumor microenvironment [104]. Aptamers selected in vivo SELEX are reagents advantaged by being selected directly within living organisms, increasing their relevance and functionality for clinical uses.
- *Cell-SELEX:* The technique of targeting targets has been greatly useful.
- *High-Throughput Sequencing (HTS):* Integration of HTS with SELEX has changed aptamer discovery from an asynchronous approach to a time series of sequence enrichment and binding kinetics. By contrast, HTS facilitates the identification of high-affinity aptamers at unprecedented speeds and accuracies.
- *Photo-SELEX:* Photo-SELEX uses photo crosslinking to stabilize aptamer–target interactions and improve the selection of aptamers with improved binding properties. This is a very useful technique for challenging targets such as membrane proteins.

SELEX technologies will continue to evolve to discover aptamers specific to cancer applications [105].

8.8.3 Artificial Intelligence and Machine Learning Integration

TAs AI and ML are reshaping the aptamer design landscape, giving unprecedented precision and efficiency to this process [71] [106].

- *Predictive Modeling:* The aptamer sequences that can bind to a ligand with high binding affinity and specificity are predictable using the large datasets created through SELEX experiments by using ML algorithms [107]. The models reduce the cycle of selection iterations, saving time and resources.
- *Optimization of Binding Kinetics:* By optimizing aptamer structures with AI tools, aptamers can be optimized for both their binding kinetics and off-target effects [108]. To refine the aptamer–target interactions, molecular dynamics simulations driven by AI are undertaken.
- *Design of Novel Aptamers:* This paves the way for generating entirely novel aptamer sequences with given properties using generative AI (e.g., based on deep learning), thus increasing the repertoire of available aptamers for cancer applications [99, 109].
- *Integration with Multi-omics Data:* Multi-omics data (genomics, proteomics, transcriptomics) can be analyzed to target these biomarkers.
- *Automation in SELEX:* Different stages of the SELEX process are already automated by AI algorithms, from sequence analysis to target validation and high-throughput discovery of functional aptamers.

AI and aptamer science are synergistic in these hopes for accelerating innovation and improving outcomes in cancer diagnostics and therapy [110].

8.8.4 Aptamer-Based Tools for Personalized Medicine

Personalized medicine is an increasingly well-developed area in which treatment is tailored to the specific molecular profile of individual patients. Personalized approaches to cancer management will find aptamer-based tools a good fit [111].

- *Patient-Specific Biomarker Detection:* The ability of aptamer-based diagnostics to identify patient-specific biomarkers and early detection and precise characterization of cancer subtypes enables a more generalized detection of disease for earlier intervention [112]. For instance, aptamer microarrays can read the unique ctDNA or RNA profiles of patients.
- *Targeted Therapies:* You can design aptamers that target patient tumor-specific mutations or overexpressed proteins. Reducing side effects while increasing therapeutic efficacy is the output of this precision [103, 119]. For example, aptamers can develop targeted treatment of lung cancer based on mutant EGFR.
- *Combination Therapies:* Aptamer-based tools allow the combination of multiple therapeutic modalities suited to the patient's disease condition. In particular, aptamer-guided nanoparticles can execute chemotherapeutics and siRNAs concurrently, targeting both primary and secondary tumor pathways [113].
- *Monitoring and Feedback:* Biosensors based on aptamers offer real-time treatment efficacy and disease progression monitoring. Feedback to the patient allows adjustments to therapy that are dynamic and personal and yield better results.
- *Patient-Centric Approaches:* The versatility of aptamers makes them suitable for the development of minimally invasive diagnostic tools, namely, liquid biopsies, that decrease patient pain and provide a comprehensive molecular profile.

Aptamers begin to integrate into personalized medicine strategies that will make cancer care more effective and patient-friendly [95, 114].

8.9 Conclusion

The aptamer story in cancer diagnosis and therapy has increased the awareness of their transformational potential in modern oncology. It turns out that these highly specific, molecularly versatile tools have powered a critical innovation for cancer management, including early diagnosis, targeted treatment, and personalized care, as detailed in this book throughout.

8.9.1 Summary of Key Insights

This book has presented a comprehensive journey into the world of aptamers, beginning with their foundational principles and extending to their applications, engineering, and integration with cutting-edge technologies:

- *Aptamers vs. Conventional Tools:* Traditional antibodies have several disadvantages in comparison: ease of synthesis, stability, and tuneable chemical properties.

- *Diagnostic Applications:* Among their applications are aptamer-based biosensors, imaging probes, and multiplexed assays that improve the sensitivity and specificity of cancer detection. They demonstrated their case studies' utility in breast, lung, and colorectal cancer diagnostics, among others.
- *Therapeutic Applications:* Aptamers possess a multifaceted therapeutic potential, ranging from targeting tumor cells and inhibiting angiogenesis to modulating immune response. Precision therapies are now emerging; delivery systems, such as nanoparticle conjugates, are now finding their potential.
- *Technological Innovations:* The combination of advancements in SELEX, chemical modifications, and nanotechnology integration has, and continues to, fine-tune aptamer designs, making them more efficacious and versatile for clinical use.

8.9.2 Final Thoughts

The development of cancer diagnosis and therapy aptamers is a marriage of biology, chemistry, engineering, and computational science. This convergence of these disciplines has enabled the generation of tools that outperform or, more commonly, match the performance of conventional diagnostic and therapeutic agents. Despite these strides, however, production must be scaled up, regulatory barriers must be conquered, and these innovations need to be made available to broadly impacted populations in an equitable way. To surmount these hurdles, we will need to work with industry, academia, and regulatory bodies. Incredible opportunities remain to fully realize the aptamer's potential that lies ahead on the road. Ongoing work in aptamer research, development, and investment, together with innovation, has the power to create a new oncology landscape and deliver to clinical practice the ability to detect cancer earlier, treat it more effectively, and ultimately better provide for patients. Molecular science holds out a sharp, shining future that is more precise, more personalized, and more accessible than ever to cancer care.

References

1. Pereira RL, Nascimento IC, Santos AP, Ogusuku IEY, Lameu C, Mayer G, et al. Aptamers: novelty tools for cancer biology. Oncotarget. 2018;9(42):26934.
2. Mahmoudian F, Ahmari A, Shabani S, Sadeghi B, Fahimirad S, Fattahi F. Aptamers as an approach to targeted cancer therapy. Cancer Cell Int. 2024;24(1):108.
3. Quazi S. RETRACTED: application of biosensors in cancers, an overview. Front Bioeng Biotechnol. 2023;11:1193493.
4. Khan S, Hussain A, Fahimi H, Aliakbari F, Bloukh SH, Edis Z, et al. A review on the therapeutic applications of aptamers and aptamer-conjugated nanoparticles in cancer, inflammatory and viral diseases. Arab J Chem. 2022;15(2):103626.
5. Liu M, Zaman K, Fortenberry YM. Overview of the therapeutic potential of aptamers targeting coagulation factors. Int J Mol Sci. 2021;22(8):3897.
6. Fu Z, Xiang J. Aptamers, the nucleic acid antibodies, in cancer therapy. Adv Med Biochem Genomics: Physiol Pathol; 2021. p. 143–75.

7. Catuogno S, Esposito CL. Aptamer cell-based selection: overview and advances. Biomedicines. 2017;5(3):49.
8. Szymanowski W, Szymanowska A, Bielawska A, Lopez-Berestein G, Rodriguez-Aguayo C, Amero P. Aptamers as potential therapeutic tools for ovarian cancer: advancements and challenges. Cancers (Basel). 2023;15(21):5300.
9. Vandghanooni S, Sanaat Z, Farahzadi R, Eskandani M, Omidian H, Omidi Y. Recent progress in the development of aptasensors for cancer diagnosis: focusing on aptamers against cancer biomarkers. Microchem J. 2021;170:106640.
10. Cerchia L. Aptamers: promising tools for cancer diagnosis and therapy. Cancers. 2018;10:132.
11. Kejamurthy P, Devi KTR. Immune checkpoint inhibitors and cancer immunotherapy by aptamers: an overview. Med Oncol. 2023;41(1):40.
12. Davodabadi F, Mirinejad S, Fathi-Karkan S, Majidpour M, Ajalli N, Sheervalilou R, et al. Aptamer-functionalized quantum dots as theranostic nanotools against cancer and bacterial infections: a comprehensive overview of recent trends. Biotechnol Prog. 2023;39(5):e3366.
13. Jabir NR, Anwar K, Firoz CK, Oves M, Kamal MA, Tabrez S. An overview on the current status of cancer nanomedicines. Curr Med Res Opin. 2018;34(5):911–21.
14. Varty K, O'Brien C, Ignaszak A. Breast cancer aptamers: current sensing targets, available aptamers, and their evaluation for clinical use in diagnostics. Cancers (Basel). 2021;13(16):3984.
15. Cruz-Hernández CD, Rodríguez-Martínez G, Cortés-Ramírez SA, Morales-Pacheco M, Cruz-Burgos M, Losada-García A, et al. Aptamers as theragnostic tools in prostate cancer. Biomol Ther. 2022;12(8):1056.
16. Kangarshahi BM, Naghib SM. Nanogenosensors based on aptamers and peptides for bioelectrochemical cancer detection: an overview of recent advances in emerging materials and technologies. Discov Appl Sci. 2024;6(2):47.
17. Ning Y, Hu J, Lu F. Aptamers used for biosensors and targeted therapy. Biomed Pharmacother. 2020;132:110902.
18. Pawde DM, Bhattacharya S. Overview of aptamer-based biosensors. In: Aptasensors for point-of-care diagnostics. CRC Press; 2023. p. 1–20.
19. Saraf S, Jain A, Tiwari A, Verma A, Panda PK, Jain SK. Advances in liposomal drug delivery to cancer: an overview. J Drug Deliv Sci Technol. 2020;56:101549.
20. Wang T, Chen C, Larcher LM, Barrero RA, Veedu RN. Three decades of nucleic acid aptamer technologies: lessons learned, progress and opportunities on aptamer development. Biotechnol Adv. 2019;37(1):28–50.
21. Wu D, Gordon CKL, Shin JH, Eisenstein M, Soh HT. Directed evolution of aptamer discovery technologies. Acc Chem Res. 2022;55(5):685–95.
22. Huang J, Chen X, Fu X, Li Z, Huang Y, Liang C. Advances in aptamer-based biomarker discovery. Front Cell Dev Biol. 2021;9:659760.
23. Yan J, Xiong H, Cai S, Wen N, He Q, Liu Y, et al. Advances in aptamer screening technologies. Talanta. 2019;200:124–44.
24. Aslan Y, Atabay M, Chowdhury HK, Göktürk I, Saylan Y, Inci F. Aptamer-based point-of-care devices: emerging technologies and integration of computational methods. Biosensors. 2023;13(5):569.
25. Kanwar JR, Shankaranarayanan JS, Gurudevan S, Kanwar RK. Aptamer-based therapeutics of the past, present and future: from the perspective of eye-related diseases. Drug Discov Today. 2014;19(9):1309–21.
26. Ni S, Zhuo Z, Pan Y, Yu Y, Li F, Liu J, et al. Recent progress in aptamer discoveries and modifications for therapeutic applications. ACS Appl Mater Interfaces. 2020;13(8):9500–19.
27. Wu L, Wang Y, Xu X, Liu Y, Lin B, Zhang M, et al. Aptamer-based detection of circulating targets for precision medicine. Chem Rev. 2021;121(19):12035–105.
28. Zhou W, Huang PJJ, Ding J, Liu J. Aptamer-based biosensors for biomedical diagnostics. Analyst. 2014;139(11):2627–40.

29. Razmi N, Baradaran B, Hejazi M, Hasanzadeh M, Mosafer J, Mokhtarzadeh A, et al. Recent advances on aptamer-based biosensors to detection of platelet-derived growth factor. Biosens Bioelectron. 2018;113:58–71.
30. Cao J, Zhang F, Xiong W. Discovery of aptamers and the acceleration of the development of targeting research in ophthalmology. Int J Nanomedicine. 2023;Volume 18:4421–30.
31. Negahdary M. Aptamers in nanostructure-based electrochemical biosensors for cardiac biomarkers and cancer biomarkers: a review. Biosens Bioelectron. 2020 Mar;152:112018.
32. Khan NI, Song E. Lab-on-a-chip systems for aptamer-based biosensing. Micromachines. 2020;11(2):220.
33. Wu Y, Belmonte I, Sykes KS, Xiao Y, White RJ. Perspective on the future role of aptamers in analytical chemistry. Anal Chem. 2019;91(24):15335–44.
34. Jiang G, Li Y, Liu J, Liu L, Pi F. Progress on aptamer-based SERS sensors for food safety and quality assessment: methodology, current applications and future trends. Crit Rev Food Sci Nutr. 2024;64(3):783–800.
35. Quansah M, Fetter L, Fineran A, Colling HV, Silver K, Rowland TJ, et al. Rapid and quantitative detection of lung cancer biomarker ENOX2 using a novel Aptamer in an electrochemical DNA-based (E-DNA) biosensor. Biosensors. 2023;13(7)
36. Díaz-Fernández A, Ferapontova EE. Electrochemical ELASA: improving early cancer detection and monitoring. Anal Bioanal Chem. 2023;415(18):3831–46.
37. Jolly P, Damborsky P, Madaboosi N, Soares RRG, Chu V, Conde JP, et al. DNA aptamer-based sandwich microfluidic assays for dual quantification and multi-glycan profiling of cancer biomarkers. Biosens Bioelectron. 2016;79:313–9.
38. Norouzi A, Ravan H, Mohammadi A, Hosseinzadeh E, Norouzi M, Fozooni T. Aptamer-integrated DNA nanoassembly: a simple and sensitive DNA framework to detect cancer cells. Anal Chim Acta. 2018;1017:26–33.
39. Kurth T, Witt S, Bolten S, Waniek JJ, Kortmann C, Lavrentieva A, et al. Development of Aptamer-based TID assays using thermophoresis and microarrays. Biosensors. 2019;9(4)
40. Şahin S, Caglayan MO, Üstündağ Z. Recent advances in aptamer-based sensors for breast cancer diagnosis: special cases for nanomaterial-based VEGF, HER2, and MUC1 aptasensors. Microchim Acta. 2020;187(10):549.
41. Wu L, Wang Y, Zhu L, Liu Y, Wang T, Liu D, et al. Aptamer-based liquid biopsy. ACS Appl Bio Mater. 2020;3(5):2743–64.
42. Yavari B, Athari SS, Omidi Y, Jalali A, Najafi R. EpCAM aptamer activated 5-FU-loaded PLGA nanoparticles in CRC treatment in vitro and in vivo study. J Drug Target. 2023;31(3):296–309.
43. Chinnappan R, Mir TA, Alsalameh S, Makhzoum T, Alzhrani A, Alnajjar K, et al. Emerging biosensing methods to monitor lung cancer biomarkers in biological samples: a comprehensive review. Cancers (Basel). 2023;15(13):3414.
44. Blundo A, Cignoni A, Banfi T, Ciuti G. Comparative analysis of diagnostic techniques for melanoma detection: a systematic review of diagnostic test accuracy studies and meta-analysis. Front Med. 2021;8:637069.
45. Cardos AI, Maghiar A, Zaha DC, Pop O, Fritea L, Miere F, et al. Evolution of diagnostic methods for helicobacter pylori infections: from traditional tests to high technology, advanced sensitivity and discrimination tools. Diagnostics. 2022;12(2):508.
46. Dhiman A, Kalra P, Bansal V, Bruno JG, Sharma TK. Aptamer-based point-of-care diagnostic platforms. Sensors Actuators B Chem. 2017;246:535–53.
47. Jarczewska M, Malinowska E. The application of antibody–aptamer hybrid biosensors in clinical diagnostics and environmental analysis. Anal Methods. 2020;12(25):3183–99.
48. Mehmood S, Khan AZ, Bilal M, Sohail A, Iqbal HMN. Aptamer-based biosensors: a novel toolkit for early diagnosis of cancer. Mater Today Chem. 2019;12:353–60.
49. Kelly L, Maier KE, Yan A, Levy M. A comparative analysis of cell surface targeting aptamers. Nat Commun. 2021;12(1):6275.
50. Kaur H, Bruno JG, Kumar A, Sharma TK. Aptamers in the therapeutics and diagnostics pipelines. Theranostics. 2018;8(15):4016.

51. Han J, Gao L, Wang J, Wang J. Application and development of aptamer in cancer: from clinical diagnosis to cancer therapy. J Cancer. 2020;11(23):6902.
52. Ravichandran G, Rengan AK. Aptamer-mediated nanotheranostics for cancer treatment: a review. ACS Appl Nano Mater. 2020;3(10):9542–59.
53. Yang C, Jiang Y, Hao SH, Yan XY, Naranmandura H. Aptamers: an emerging navigation tool of therapeutic agents for targeted cancer therapy. J Mater Chem B. 2022;10(1):20–33.
54. Razlansari M, Jafarinejad S, Rahdar A, Shirvaliloo M, Arshad R, Fathi-Karkan S, et al. Development and classification of RNA aptamers for therapeutic purposes: an updated review with emphasis on cancer. Mol Cell Biochem. 2023;478(7):1573–98.
55. Shigdar S, Schrand B, Giangrande PH, de Franciscis V. Aptamers: cutting edge of cancer therapies. Mol Ther. 2021;29(8):2396–411.
56. He S, Du Y, Tao H, Duan H. Advances in aptamer-mediated targeted delivery system for cancer treatment. Int J Biol Macromol. 2023;238:124173.
57. Van den Avont A, Sharma-Walia N. Anti-nucleolin aptamer AS1411: an advancing therapeutic. Front Mol Biosci. 2023;10:1217769.
58. Gao F, Yin J, Chen Y, Guo C, Hu H, Su J. Recent advances in aptamer-based targeted drug delivery systems for cancer therapy. Front Bioeng Biotechnol. 2022;10:972933.
59. He F, Wen N, Xiao D, Yan J, Xiong H, Cai S, et al. Aptamer-based targeted drug delivery systems: current potential and challenges. Curr Med Chem. 2020;27(13):2189–219.
60. Fan R, Tao X, Zhai X, Zhu Y, Li Y, Chen Y, et al. Application of aptamer-drug delivery system in the therapy of breast cancer. Biomed Pharmacother. 2023;161:114444.
61. Sargazi S, et al. Aptamer-conjugated carbon-based nanomaterials for cancer and bacteria theranostics: a review. Chem Biol Interact. 2022;361:109964.
62. Yin S, Chen Z, Chen D, Yan D. Strategies targeting PD-L1 expression and associated opportunities for cancer combination therapy. Theranostics. 2023;13(5):1520–44.
63. Marangoni K, Menezes R. RNA Aptamer-functionalized polymeric nanoparticles in targeted delivery and cancer therapy: an up-to-date review. Curr Pharm Des. 2022;28(34):2785–94.
64. Venkatesan S, Chanda K, Balamurali MM. Recent advancements of Aptamers in cancer therapy. ACS omega. 2023 Sep;8(36):32231–43.
65. Kim DH, Seo JM, Shin KJ, Yang SG. Design and clinical developments of aptamer-drug conjugates for targeted cancer therapy. Biomater Res. 2021;25(1):42.
66. Morita Y, Leslie M, Kameyama H, Volk DE, Tanaka T. Aptamer therapeutics in cancer: current and future. Cancers (Basel). 2018;10(3)
67. Deng G, Zha H, Luo H, Zhou Y. Aptamer-conjugated gold nanoparticles and their diagnostic and therapeutic roles in cancer. Front Bioeng Biotechnol. 2023;11:1118546.
68. Beals N, Kasibhatla N, Basu S. Efficient delivery of plasmid DNA using incorporated nucleotides for precise conjugation of targeted nanoparticles. ACS Appl Bio Mater. 2019;2(2):717–27.
69. Chakraborty S, Dlie ZY, Mukherjee B, Besra SE, Sengupta S, Sen R, et al. A comparative investigation of the ability of various Aptamer-functionalized drug Nanocarriers to induce selective apoptosis in neoplastic hepatocytes: in vitro and in vivo outcome. AAPS PharmSciTech. 2020;21(3):89.
70. Hamada M. In silico approaches to RNA aptamer design. Biochimie. 2018;145:8–14.
71. Chen Z, Hu L, Zhang BT, Lu A, Wang Y, Yu Y, et al. Artificial intelligence in Aptamer-target binding prediction. Int J Mol Sci. 2021;22(7)
72. Chen L, Zhang B, Wu Z, Liu G, Li W, Tang Y. In Silico discovery of aptamers with an enhanced library design strategy. Comput Struct Biotechnol J. 2023;21:1005–13.
73. Zhu J, Huang H, Dong S, Ge L, Zhang Y. Progress in aptamer-mediated drug delivery vehicles for cancer targeting and its implications in addressing chemotherapeutic challenges. Theranostics. 2014;4(9):931–44.
74. Zheng L, Zhang B, Chu H, Cheng P, Li H, Huang K, et al. Assembly and in vitro assessment of a powerful combination: aptamer-modified exosomes combined with gold nanorods for effective photothermal therapy. Nanotechnology. 2020;31(48):485101.

75. Vázquez-González M, Willner I. Aptamer-functionalized hybrid nanostructures for sensing, drug delivery, catalysis and mechanical applications. Int J Mol Sci. 2021;22(4):1803.
76. Ram TB, Krishnan S, Jeevanandam J, Danquah MK, Thomas S. Emerging biohybrids of aptamer-based nano-biosensing technologies for effective early cancer detection. Mol Diagn Ther. 2024:1–29.
77. Fu Z, Xiang J. Aptamer-functionalized nanoparticles in targeted delivery and cancer therapy. Int J Mol Sci. 2020;21(23):9123.
78. Altalbawy FMA, Ali E, et al. Aptamer-magnetic nanoparticle complexes for powerful biosensing: a comprehensive review. Crit Rev Anal Chem. 2023:1–14.
79. Kandasamy G, Maity D. Multifunctional theranostic nanoparticles for biomedical cancer treatments-a comprehensive review. Mater Sci Eng C. 2021;127:112199.
80. Zhao S, Yu X, Qian Y, Chen W, Shen J. Multifunctional magnetic iron oxide nanoparticles: an advanced platform for cancer theranostics. Theranostics. 2020;10(14):6278.
81. Rahimnia SM, Dehghani S, Saeedi M, Shad A, Yazdian-Robati R. Aptamer-mediated nanotherapy for pancreatic cancer. In: Recent advances in nanocarriers for pancreatic cancer therapy. Elsevier; 2024. p. 375–99.
82. Fernandes DA, Fernandes DD, Malik A, Gomes GNW, Appak-Baskoy S, Berndl E, et al. Multifunctional nanoparticles as theranostic agents for therapy and imaging of breast cancer. J Photochem Photobiol B Biol. 2021;218:112110.
83. Rahiminezhad Z, Tamaddon AM, Borandeh S, Abolmaali SS. Janus nanoparticles: new generation of multifunctional nanocarriers in drug delivery, bioimaging and theranostics. Appl Mater Today. 2020;18:100513.
84. Mi P. Stimuli-responsive nanocarriers for drug delivery, tumor imaging, therapy and theranostics. Theranostics. 2020;10(10):4557.
85. Alshamrani M. Broad-spectrum theranostics and biomedical application of functionalized nanomaterials. Polymers (Basel). 2022;14(6):1221.
86. Altinbasak I, Alp Y, Sanyal R, Sanyal A. Theranostic nanogels: multifunctional agents for simultaneous therapeutic delivery and diagnostic imaging. Nanoscale. 2024;16:14033.
87. Sanjanwala D, Patravale V. Aptamers and nanobodies as alternatives to antibodies for ligand-targeted drug delivery in cancer. Drug Discov Today. 2023;28(5):103550.
88. Kumar S, Mohan A, Sharma NR, Kumar A, Girdhar M, Malik T, et al. Computational frontiers in Aptamer-based nanomedicine for precision therapeutics: a comprehensive review. ACS Omega. 2024;9(25):26838–62.
89. Yan J, Bhadane R, Ran M, Ma X, Li Y, Zheng D, et al. Development of Aptamer-DNAzyme based metal-nucleic acid frameworks for gastric cancer therapy. Nat Commun. 2024;15(1):3684.
90. Thomas BJ, Guldenpfennig C, Daniels MA, Burke DH, Porciani D. Multiplexed in vivo screening using barcoded aptamer technology to identify oligonucleotide-based targeting reagents. Nucleic Acid Ther. 2024;34:109.
91. Chohan DP, Dey B, Tarkunde A, Vyas V, De Sarkar S, Sundara BK. Advancing autonomous nanomedicine: bridging the gap from concept to potential clinical studies. J Clust Sci. 2024;35(8):2607–35.
92. Edison G. Cutting-edge applications of artificial intelligence in healthcare, petroleum fraud detection, and innovative strategies in cancer treatment. Int J Multidiscip Sci Arts. 2024;3(4):103–12.
93. Liu S, Xu Y, Jiang X, Tan H, Ying B. Translation of aptamers toward clinical diagnosis and commercialization. Biosens Bioelectron. 2022;208:114168.
94. Kumar Kulabhusan P, Hussain B, Yüce M. Current perspectives on aptamers as diagnostic tools and therapeutic agents. Pharmaceutics. 2020;12(7):646.
95. Chen J, Fu S, Zhang C, Liu H, Su X. DNA logic circuits for cancer theranostics. Small. 2022;18(20):2108008.
96. Zheng X, Wu Y, Zuo H, Chen W, Wang K. Metal nanoparticles as novel agents for lung cancer diagnosis and therapy. Small. 2023;19(18):2206624.

97. Rabiee N, Chen S, Ahmadi S, Veedu RN. Aptamer-engineered (nano) materials for theranostic applications. Theranostics. 2023;13(15):5183.
98. Wei Z, Zhou Y, Wang R, Wang J, Chen Z. Aptamers as smart ligands for targeted drug delivery in cancer therapy. Pharmaceutics. 2022;14(12):2561.
99. Gholikhani T, Brito BJ, Livingston F, Kumar S. The potential use of aptamers in the process of drug development. Pharm Sci. 2021;27(4):503–10.
100. Zhu L, Zhao J, Guo Z, Liu Y, Chen H, Chen Z, et al. Applications of aptamer-bound nanomaterials in cancer therapy. Biosensors. 2021;11(9):344.
101. Walia S, Chandrasekaran AR, Chakraborty B, Bhatia D. Aptamer-programmed DNA nanodevices for advanced, targeted cancer theranostics. ACS Appl Bio Mater. 2021;4(7):5392–404.
102. Chinchilla-Cárdenas DJ, Cruz-Méndez JS, Petano-Duque JM, García RO, Castro LR, Lobo-Castañón MJ, et al. Current developments of SELEX technologies and prospects in the aptamer selection with clinical applications. J Genet Eng Biotechnol. 2024;22(3):100400.
103. Shigdar S, Agnello L, Fedele M, Camorani S, Cerchia L. Profiling cancer cells by cell-SELEX: use of aptamers for discovery of actionable biomarkers and therapeutic applications thereof. Pharmaceutics. 2021;14(1):28.
104. Li L, Wan J, Wen X, Guo Q, Jiang H, Wang J, et al. Identification of a new DNA aptamer by tissue-SELEX for cancer recognition and imaging. Anal Chem. 2021;93(19):7369–77.
105. Saito S. SELEX-based DNA aptamer selection: a perspective from the advancement of separation techniques. Anal Sci. 2021;37(1):17–26.
106. Adir O, Poley M, Chen G, Froim S, Krinsky N, Shklover J, et al. Integrating artificial intelligence and nanotechnology for precision cancer medicine. Adv Mater. 2020;32(13):1901989.
107. Fallah A, Havaei SA, Sedighian H, Kachuei R, Fooladi AAI. Prediction of aptamer affinity using an artificial intelligence approach. J Mater Chem B. 2024;12(36):8825–42.
108. Emami N, Ferdousi R. AptaNet as a deep learning approach for aptamer–protein interaction prediction. Sci Rep. 2021;11(1):6074.
109. Khan MS, Alshahrani MY, Wahab S, Gupta G, Kesharwani P. Evolution of artificial intelligence as a modern technology in advanced cancer therapy. J Drug Deliv Sci Technol. 2024;98:105892.
110. Taha BA, Kadhim AC, Addie AJ, Haider AJ, Azzahrani AS, Raizada P, et al. Advancing cancer diagnostics through multifaceted optical biosensors supported by nanomaterials and artificial intelligence: a panoramic outlook. Microchem J. 2024;111307:111307.
111. Sousa AP, Rocha AC, Almeida C, Carneiro MCCG, Pais PP, Viana R, et al. Moving towards personalized medicine – the broad use of Aptamers for targeted theranostic. Appl Sci. 2023;13(21):11933.
112. Huang Z, Wang D, Zhang Q, Zhang Y, Peng R, Tan W. Leveraging Aptamer-based DNA nanotechnology for bioanalysis and cancer therapeutics. Acc Mater Res. 2024;5(4):438–52.
113. Girotti A, Escalera-Anzola S, Alonso-Sampedro I, González-Valdivieso J, Arias FJ. Aptamer-functionalized natural protein-based polymers as innovative biomaterials. Pharmaceutics. 2020;12(11):1115.
114. Jiang W, Jones JC, Shankavaram U, Sproull M, Camphausen K, Krauze AV. Analytical considerations of large-scale Aptamer-based datasets for translational applications. Cancers (Basel). 2022;14(9):2227.

9 Aptamer-Based Biosensors for Cancer Biomarker Detection

Ilemobayo Victor Fasogbon, Janarthanan Venkatesan, Patrick Maduabuchi Aja, and Loganathan Rangasamy

9.1 Introduction

Biomarkers play a vital role in providing critical insights into the biological processes that underlie the onset and progression of diseases [1–3]. These indicators, which can range from proteins to small molecules, reflect changes in the body's normal or abnormal biological state. The biomarkers facilitate early diagnosis, treatment monitoring, and prognostic assessments of the various tumor types. Identifying cancer before clinical symptoms appear greatly enhances patient outcomes. For instance, testing prostate-specific antigen (PSA) enables early intervention in cases of prostate cancer [4]. Biomarkers like human epidermal growth factor receptor 2 (HER2) and vascular endothelial growth factor (VEGF) are commonly used to monitor treatment effectiveness in breast and colorectal cancers (Table 9.1) [1, 36, 21, 23, 37]. Similarly, elevated levels of mucin 1 (MUC1) and carcinoembryonic antigen (CEA) are frequently linked to aggressive tumor types, which are associated with poor prognosis [38–40].

I. V. Fasogbon
Department of Biochemistry, Faculty of Biomedical Sciences, Kampala International University, Kampala, Uganda
e-mail: ivfasogbon@kiu.ac.ug

J. Venkatesan · L. Rangasamy (✉)
Drug Discovery Unit (DDU), Centre for Biomaterials, Cellular and Molecular Theranostics (CBCMT), Vellore Institute of Technology, Vellore, Tamil Nadu, India
e-mail: janarthanan.v2022@vitstudent.ac.in; loganathan.r@vit.ac.in

P. M. Aja
Department of Biochemistry, Faculty of Biomedical Sciences, Kampala International University, Kampala, Uganda

Department of Biochemistry, Faculty of Science, Ebonyi State University, Abakaliki, Ebonyi State, Nigeria
e-mail: aja.patrick@kiu.ac.ug

S. Srivastava et al. (eds.), *Biosensors and Aptamers*,
https://doi.org/10.1007/978-981-96-8387-1_9

Table 9.1 Comprehensive table summarizing the list of aptamer-based cancer biomarkers, binding affinities, and target specificities across cancer types

Associated cancer type	Cancer biomarker	Aptamer type	Binding affinity	References
Gastric and non-small-cell lung cancer	Nucleolin	DNA	73 nM	[5, 6]
Breast cancer	Mucin 1	DNA	–	[7–11]
Ovarian, breast, and colorectal cancer	Tenascin	DNA	–	[12]
Prostate cancer	PSA	RNA	–	[13–15]
Tumor progression	MMP-9	RNA	nM-μM range	[16]
Tumor progression	Annexin A2	RNA	nM range	[17]
Tumor progression	MMP-9	RNA	20 nM	[18]
Breast cancer	Osteopontin (OPN)	DNA, RNA	25–100 nM	[19, 20]
Breast cancer	HER2	RNA, DNA	5–50 nM	[21, 22] [23],
Lymphoma—immunoglobulin heavy constant (IGHM)	IGHM	DNA	74.7 nM	[24–26]
Lymphoma—Ramos cells	TE02	DNA	0.76 nM	[24, 27]
Vascular endothelial growth factor 165 (VEGF-165)	VEGF165	RNA	50 nM	[28]
Hepatocellular carcinoma	TLS11a	DNA	7 nM	[29–31]
T cell leukemia	PTK7	DNA	0.8 nM	[32, 33]
41 t aptamer	PDGF	DNA	1 nM	[34]
T cell leukemia	CCRF-CEM cells	DNA	675 nM	[34]
DLD-1 cells—colorectal cancer	KDED 2a-3	DNA	29.2 nM	[25]
HCT 116 cells—colorectal cancer	KCHA10	DNA	21.3 nM	[25]
B cell lymphoma	Sgd5	DNA	70.8 nM	[35]

Traditional diagnostic methods, while foundational to clinical medicine, continue to face a number of constraints that limit their accessibility, cost-effectiveness, and overall efficiency, particularly in resource-constrained environments. Techniques like enzyme-linked immunosorbent assay (ELISA), though widely used, often demand labor-intensive workflows and trained personnel, making them expensive and less practical in decentralized or low-infrastructure settings [41]. Similarly, while polymerase chain reaction (PCR) methods are highly sensitive for detecting nucleic acid biomarkers, they require advanced instrumentation and technical expertise, limiting their application for rapid screening or use outside laboratory environments [42]. Imaging tools such as computed tomography (CT) and magnetic resonance imaging (MRI) are invaluable for visualizing anatomical features, but they typically fall short when it comes to identifying early-stage cancers or detecting subtle molecular changes [42]. Imaging modalities such as magnetic resonance imaging (MRI) and computed tomography (CT) offer insights into crucial anatomical structures; however, they are less effective in detecting early-stage cancers or identifying precise molecular alterations [43, 44]. Traditional methods also face challenges in terms of lower sensitivity, whereas detecting low-abundance biomarkers, more importantly in the early stages of cancer, requires highly sensitive platforms [4, 40, 45]. Another key limitation lies in the sensitivity of traditional platforms. Detecting low-abundance biomarkers, especially those relevant during the early stages of disease, calls for highly refined technologies. Also, cross-reactivity in antibody-based assays often leads to false positives, reducing the reliability of results [46, 47]. High operational costs and the necessity for sophisticated lab environments hinder their widespread adoption in underserved regions, where the cancer burden continues to rise [48, 49]. Many conventional assays also require significant sample volumes, which can be a challenge for vulnerable populations such as pediatric or critically ill patients. Furthermore, time-consuming protocols in techniques like PCR and ELISA may delay the delivery of diagnostic results and slow down treatment decisions [27, 41].

Addressing these limitations, aptamer-based biosensors provide a promising replacement, offering several advantages over traditional systems. Aptamers, short, single-stranded oligonucleotides are engineered to present high binding specificity and strong affinity for several kinds of targets [50–52]. Unlike antibodies, they are produced chemically, which not only improves consistency between batches but also lowers production costs [53]. Aptamers have a wide range of thermal stability, enhancing their utility in diverse clinical settings. Moreover, aptamers could be modified chemically to improve their binding affinity, stability, and detection capabilities. Their exceptional versatility permits them to bind to a diverse array of targets, including proteins, antigens, small molecules, and entire cells, due to their possibility of folding into complex three-dimensional structures that enable highly specific interactions with target biomarkers, rivaling or exceeding the performance of traditional antibodies [42]. When incorporated into biosensors, aptamers serve as recognition elements that pair with different signal transduction mechanisms to detect specific biomarkers [36, 39, 53, 54]. As illustrated in Fig. 9.1, these aptamer-based platforms can be tailored for tumor imaging and therapy. Detection methods range from optical systems such as fluorescence and colorimetric sensors to electrochemical setups that register electrical changes upon target binding. Another highly sensitive method includes Surface-Enhanced Raman Scattering (SERS), which amplifies Raman signals to detect molecular interactions at extremely low concentrations [2, 21, 55]. These technologies have demonstrated impressive sensitivity, often achieving femtomolar detection levels for biomarkers like VEGF and PSA [56]. Their compact design and adaptability further make them well-suited for point-of-care applications, fulfilling the need for fast and accurate cancer diagnostics in both clinical and remote settings.

This chapter explores the expanding role of aptamer-based biosensors in oncology, outlining their design principles, classification, and technological progress. Drawing from recent advancements, it examines how these systems address the shortcomings of conventional diagnostics. Special attention is given to innovations such as nanomaterial conjugation and AI-assisted signal processing. The chapter also delves into current limitations, including challenges in real-world sample analysis, and provides insights into future directions, particularly the integration of

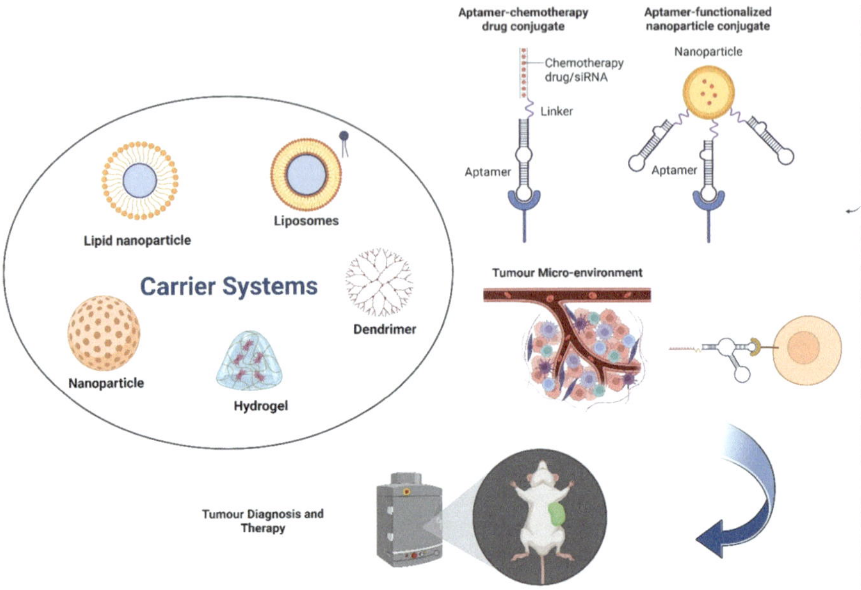

Fig. 9.1 Mechanism of aptasensors for tumor imaging and therapy. (Created by using Biorender)

wearable biosensors and their significance in personalized healthcare. Ultimately, this discussion presents the transforming potential of aptamer-based platforms in reshaping the landscape of cancer detection and management.

9.2 Significance of Cancer Biomarkers

Cancer biomarkers facilitate early detection, prognosis assessment, and cancer monitoring, enabling timely interventions, personalized treatment strategies, and improved therapeutic outcomes [3, 57, 58]. These molecular indicators, comprising proteins, nucleic acids, metabolites, and even whole cells, reflect the physiological and pathological processes associated with tumor development and progression [1, 3, 59]. The ability to detect cancer biomarkers accurately and efficiently can transform patient outcomes by facilitating timely diagnosis, tailoring therapeutic interventions, and improving long-term survival rates [57, 60, 61]. The multifaceted significance of cancer biomarkers underscores their contributions to cancer diagnostics and management. These include:

9.2.1 Early Diagnosis

Early cancer detection is paramount to improving survival rates, as treatment is often more effective at localized stages. Carcinoembryonic antigen (CEA), PSA, CA 15–3, and other biomarkers enable the identification of cancers long before clinical symptoms manifest.

- *PSA for Prostate Cancer*: PSA is broadly recognized for prostate cancer. Elevated PSA levels in the bloodstream signal the presence of prostate abnormalities, including early-stage malignancies [56, 62]. Traditional diagnostic methods, such as immunoassays, detect PSA but often lack sensitivity in distinguishing between malignant and benign conditions. Biosensors that utilize aptamers offer a significant improvement in specificity and have demonstrated the capability to detect prostate-specific antigen (PSA) at extremely low concentrations—even in the femtomolar range. This heightened sensitivity allows for more accurate and earlier diagnosis compared to traditional methods [62].
- *CEA for Colorectal Cancer*: CEA is a glycoprotein frequently elevated in colorectal and other gastrointestinal cancers, and plays an important role in both early detection and disease monitoring. Identifying CEA levels can help spot precancerous changes and assess how the disease is progressing. Recent developments in biosensor technology, particularly those using aptamers for target recognition, have made it possible to detect CEA with impressive sensitivity—down to as little as 0.02 ng/mL. This level of accuracy makes aptamer-based biosensors highly promising for early diagnosis and ongoing evaluation of cancer [40, 63].
- *VEGF and miRNAs in Breast and Lung Cancers*: VEGF is important in the formation of blood vessels and supports tumor development, making it an important indicator for detecting cancers such as breast and lung at an early stage. Biosensors that use aptamers along with advanced nanomaterials such as gold nanoparticles (AuNPs) and graphene, have shown the possibility of detecting VEGF at extremely low concentrations, often in the picomolar range. These platforms offer a noticeable improvement in sensitivity compared to traditional diagnostic approaches [37, 56–58]. Similarly, short noncoding RNAs and miRNAs involved in gene regulation are emerging biomarkers for multiple cancers. Aptamer-integrated microfluidic platforms enable the multiplexed detection of miRNAs with high precision, aiding early diagnosis [64].

9.2.2 Prognostic Assessment

Prognostic biomarkers provide insights into tumor aggressiveness, likelihood of metastasis, and overall patient outcomes. Biomarkers such as HER2, VEGF, and MUC1 are valuable for stratifying patients and guiding treatment choices.

- *HER2 Overexpression in Breast Cancer*: Between 20% and 30% of the cases of breast cancer always present overexpression of HER2 which depicts the aggressiveness of disease progression and poor prognosis. Monitoring HER2 levels aids in risk stratification and helps identify patients eligible for targeted therapies like trastuzumab. Dual-aptamer fluorescence biosensors have shown remarkable sensitivity in HER2 detection, achieving detection limits as low as 0.08 ng/mL, facilitating accurate prognosis and personalized treatment approaches [65].
- *VEGF as a Prognostic Indicator*: VEGF overexpression promotes angiogenesis, which is essential for tumor growth and metastasis. Elevated VEGF levels cor-

relate with poorer outcomes in cancers such as colorectal and lung cancer. Aptamer-based biosensors integrated with plasmonic metasurfaces and SERS platforms provide quantitative assessments of VEGF levels, enhancing prognostic accuracy [60, 61, 66].

- *MUC1 in Aggressive Tumors*: MUC1, a glycoprotein biomarker, is overexpressed in several aggressive cancers, including ovarian and pancreatic cancers. Electrochemical aptasensors targeting MUC1 have been able to detect this biomarker at concentrations below the picomolar level. This level of sensitivity supports timely clinical intervention and helps in making more accurate prognostic assessments [39, 67].

9.2.3 Monitoring Treatment Efficacy

- Fluctuations in biomarker levels during treatment offer valuable insight into how well a therapy is working, allowing healthcare providers to adjust strategies early and monitor for signs of relapse.
- *VEGF and Treatment Monitoring*: Targeting VEGF levels throughout antiangiogenic therapy is essential for assessing the effectiveness of the treatment and making necessary dosage modifications. VEGF has been detected at femtomolar concentrations using aptamer-based biosensors, offering the sensitivity needed to support personalized therapy decisions and improve clinical outcomes [4, 58].
- *Alpha-Fetoprotein (AFP) in Liver Cancer Therapy*: AFP is a key biomarker for hepatocellular carcinoma (HCC), commonly used to track disease recurrence after surgery or treatment. Electrochemical aptasensors, incorporating nanomaterials such as gold nanoparticles, have enabled real-time monitoring of AFP levels with exceptional precision, offering a highly accurate method for patient surveillance [2, 37].
- *Circulating Tumor Cells (CTCs)*: CTCs offer valuable information about metastasis and therapy resistance. Aptamer-functionalized biosensors have been designed to isolate and quantify CTCs, allowing for continuous monitoring of disease progression and assessing the effectiveness of treatments [64].

9.3 Challenges That Need to Be Addressed in Existing Diagnostic Methods

Although notable progress has been made in cancer diagnostics, identifying biomarkers continues to face several obstacles that limit its broad clinical use and overall effectiveness. These difficulties arise from the constraints of conventional diagnostic techniques, the complex nature of biological fluids, and limited access to reliable testing in underserved areas. In this context, aptamer-based biosensors offer a promising solution to overcome these issues in the following ways:

9.3.1 Immunoassays and Antibody Instability

Immunoassays such as ELISA are commonly utilized to detect cancer biomarkers such as PSA, HER2, and CEA. Despite their widespread use, these techniques face limitations due to the inherent instability of antibodies, which can lose their structural integrity and functionality when exposed to fluctuations in temperature or pH. This sensitivity reduces the reliability and shelf life of the assays, particularly in settings where controlled storage and handling conditions are difficult to maintain. Antibody cross-reactivity with nontarget molecules further compromises assay specificity, leading to false positives and erroneous diagnoses [3, 37]. Additionally, antibody production involves high costs, and batch-to-batch variability, making it unsuitable for large-scale, low-cost diagnostics (Table 9.2) [42].

Table 9.2 Comparison with antibodies

Feature	Aptamers	Antibodies
Selection process	Systematic Evolution of Ligands by Exponential Enrichment (SELEX), a chemical synthesis process	Generated through the immune response, involving the maturation of B cells
Generation time	Requires a few months	It takes several months for the generation
Molecular weight	5–15 kDa	150–170 kDa
Production variability	Lower variability due to synthetic processes	Higher variability due to reliance on biological systems
Production scalability	Highly scalable	Limited scalability because of dependence on animal or cell culture production
Shelf life	Long shelf life; can be lyophilized and stored without degradation	Short shelf life; prone to degradation under improper storage
Modifications	Easily modifiable with functional groups or chemical tags	Limited options for modifications
Stability	Highly stable under diverse pH, temperature, and pressure conditions	Sensitive to pH change. Also to pressure and temperature; prone to denaturation
Cost	Cost-effective production enabled by chemical synthesis	High production costs due to animal-derived processes
Nuclease susceptibility	Susceptible to degradation by nucleases, but chemical modifications can enhance stability	Not susceptible to nucleases
Target binding range	Able to bind a range of targets, including ions, small molecules, and large biomolecules	Primarily binds to larger biomolecules and specific proteins
Immunogenicity	Non-immunogenic; does not trigger immune responses	Potentially immunogenic; may cause immune reactions in vivo
Reusability	Reusable after regeneration with no loss in function	Not reusable after certain conditions or extended usage

9.3.2 Limited Utility in Imaging Techniques

Imaging techniques like CT and MRI are pivotal in cancer diagnosis and staging. However, these methods have limited utility in detecting molecular biomarkers at early stages. Imaging techniques are expensive, require sophisticated infrastructure, and expose patients to potentially harmful radiation [2, 66]. This limits their application in routine screenings, particularly in low-resource settings.

9.3.3 Low Sensitivity in Traditional Methods

Traditional methods often struggle to detect biomarkers at low concentrations, particularly in the early stages of cancer. For instance, CTCs and miRNAs, critical early indicators, are often below the detection threshold of conventional assays like ELISA and PCR [39]. The inability to detect such low-abundance biomarkers reliably results in missed diagnoses or delayed treatment.

9.3.4 Complexity of Biological Samples

Biological fluids like blood, serum, saliva, and urine present a significant challenge for diagnostic applications due to their complex composition. These fluids comprise different interfering substances, such as proteins, nucleic acids, and lipids that can mask or compete with target biomarkers, complicating accurate detection. In such matrices, nonspecific interactions between detection probes and unrelated molecules often result in background noise, thereby reducing both the sensitivity and precision of the analysis [56, 64]. This issue is especially evident in immunoassays, where antibodies can sometimes bind nontarget molecules due to structural similarities, leading to false readings [51]. Additionally, traditional diagnostic approaches typically require labor-intensive preprocessing steps, including centrifugation, filtration, or dilution for the isolation of relevant biomarkers. These procedures not only demand larger sample volumes but also increase the overall time and cost of testing, limiting their suitability for rapid or large-scale screening. Moreover, individual differences in biological fluid composition, such as those shaped by factors like age, diet, medications, and existing health conditions, can influence biomarker expression levels, making it difficult to establish consistent and reliable diagnostic thresholds [52, 68]. Interindividual variability in the composition of biological fluids adds another layer of complexity. Factors like diet, age, medication, and underlying conditions can influence biomarker levels, complicating the establishment of standardized detection thresholds [1, 4].

9.3.5 Barriers to Accessibility

Access to cancer diagnostics remains a major challenge, especially in regions with limited resources where cancer rates are steadily increasing but medical infrastructure is lacking. Conventional methods such as ELISA and PCR are often too expensive, relying on costly reagents, specialized equipment, and skilled technicians. In many cases, the price of a single ELISA test for markers like HER2 or VEGF exceeds what is feasible for healthcare systems in developing nations [61]. Advanced diagnostic techniques, including imaging and molecular testing, also require infrastructure like imaging facilities or thermal cyclers resources that are typically unavailable in rural or remote areas. As a result, early detection efforts are largely confined to urban centers equipped with specialized healthcare services [42]. Furthermore, traditional diagnostic equipment tends to be large and unsuitable for mobile or point-of-care use. For instance, PCR systems are fixed and depend on controlled lab conditions, limiting their application in decentralized healthcare environments [52].

9.3.6 How Aptamer-Based Biosensors Address These Challenges

Cancer biomarkers are indispensable for early diagnosis, prognosis, and monitoring treatment efficacy. Aptasensors have the potential to redefine the biomarker detection landscape, providing unparalleled specificity, sensitivity, and real-time abilities. By addressing traditional diagnostic tools' limitations, these platforms can revolutionize cancer diagnosis, improving patient outcomes globally. Aptamer-based biosensors promise enhanced sensitivity and limit of detection in the femtomolar range for PSA, VEGF, and HER2 to ensure reliable identification of low-abundance biomarkers [23, 36, 56]. It also promises high specificity, exhibiting minimal cross-reactivity due to their precise three-dimensional binding structures, hence reducing false positives [3, 42, 53, 69]. Unlike antibodies, aptamers are chemically synthesized, significantly reducing production costs. Portable platforms, such as paper-based biosensors and microfluidic devices, are being developed to facilitate low-cost, on-site cancer diagnostics [57, 68]. Aptamer-based biosensors are compatible with minimally processed biological samples, such as whole blood or saliva. Hydrogel-protected aptamer platforms, for instance, prevent biofouling and enable direct detection of biomarkers like doxorubicin (Dox) in whole blood samples [38, 70]. The aptamers' thermal stability and compatibility with simple detection systems (colorimetric or electrochemical readouts) also make them ideal for use in low-resource settings. Aptamer-based lateral flow assays (LFAs) have demonstrated their utility in decentralized cancer diagnostics, providing rapid and reliable results for biomarkers like VEGF and PSA [71]. Additionally, rapid turnaround is an attractive prospect for aptamer-based biosensors. Real-time and point-of-care capabilities of the platforms promise faster clinical decision-making, particularly in resource-limited settings [61, 68]. Aptamer-based biosensors are, therefore, emerging as game-changing solutions to the challenges associated with traditional cancer diagnostics. By enabling minimally invasive and portable diagnostic platforms, aptamer-based biosensors are promising to revolutionize cancer diagnostics and enhance global healthcare equity [72–74, 54].

9.4 Overview of Aptasensors

Aptasensors combine the binding affinity and specificity of aptamers with advanced signal transduction technologies. These biosensors are engineered to detect a broad spectrum of cancer biomarkers with exceptional specificity, sensitivity, and cost-effectiveness. By overcoming the limitations of antibody-based systems, aptasensors provide a versatile and scalable platform for cancer diagnostics. Unlike antibody-based approaches, aptasensors present distinct advantages, as outlined in Table 9.2.

The core components of aptamer-based biosensors include: biorecognition elements (Enzymes, Antibodies, or metabolites), transducers, and signal output systems.

9.4.1 Biorecognition Elements

Aptamers are highly versatile recognition elements that can fold into complex three-dimensional structures that enable their target binding with high specificity and strong affinity. Their binding strength, often expressed as dissociation constants (Kd), mostly falls within the pM to nM range, matching or even exceeding that of antibodies. For instance, aptamers targeting prostate-specific antigen (PSA) have achieved a Kd of 1.5 nM, supporting early detection efforts in prostate cancer. They have been successfully used to detect CTCs and miRNAs, both vital indicators in the early stages of cancer diagnosis [4, 75]. Additionally, aptamers offer superior thermal stability and resistance to denaturation, making them suitable for use under various clinical and environmental conditions. This robustness contributes to consistent sensor performance over time, addressing a common drawback of antibody-based systems [39, 64]. A notable example is an aptasensor developed for HER2 detection in breast cancer, which achieved 0.08 ng/mL as the limit of detection—surpassing traditional immunoassays in both sensitivity and reliability [42, 65].

9.4.2 Transducers

They are in aptamer-based biosensors as they translate the binding event between the target and the aptamer into a measurable signal. Depending on the sensor's design and intended use, different transduction methods, such as electrochemical, optical, or piezoelectric—may be employed to achieve accurate and sensitive detection.

9.4.2.1 Optical Transducers

The choice of transduction mechanism ranges from optical and electrochemical to piezoelectric techniques, which is determined by the requirements for the design of the biosensor and the nature of the application, directly influencing the sensitivity and precision of the detection process. Fluorescence-based biosensors utilize the specific binding between aptamers and target molecules to generate detectable light signals. These sensors typically work by changes in fluorescence intensity, either through quenching or enhancement, depending on the presence of the target. This method has proven effective in identifying several cancer biomarkers. The high sensitivity of this platform allowed for fast and noninvasive detection of breast cancer, providing improved diagnostic performance compared to conventional immunoassay techniques [3, 38, 64]. Dual-aptamer fluorescence sensors for HER2 and VEGF have achieved detection limits in the sub-picomolar range, providing high sensitivity for early cancer diagnosis [57, 58, 76].

SERS biosensors amplify Raman signals using aptamer-functionalized nanoprobes, enabling ultrasensitive detection of cancer biomarkers. SERS biosensors are chiefly effective for the early detection of breast, gastric, and ovarian cancers, where traditional methods often fail to achieve sufficient sensitivity. A SERS biosensor employing aptamer-functionalized gold nanoparticles detected VEGF and thrombin in gastric cancer with a detection limit as low as 0.5 pg/mL. This system demonstrated high specificity, even in complex serum samples [45, 58, 71, 77].

9.4.2.2 Electrochemical Transducers

Electrochemical biosensors quantify variations in electrical properties, including potential difference, current, or impedance, resulting from aptamer-target interactions. These biosensors (Fig. 9.2) have been utilized to detect PSA and TNF-α and assess drug efficacy, offering a highly sensitive and reliable diagnostic approach [2, 31, 56, 79, 80]. These biosensors are favored for their high sensitivity, portability, and low-cost manufacturing.

- *Field-Effect Transistor (FET)-Based Biosensors*: Graphene-based FET biosensors are highly sensitive platforms that integrate aptamers on graphene sheets to

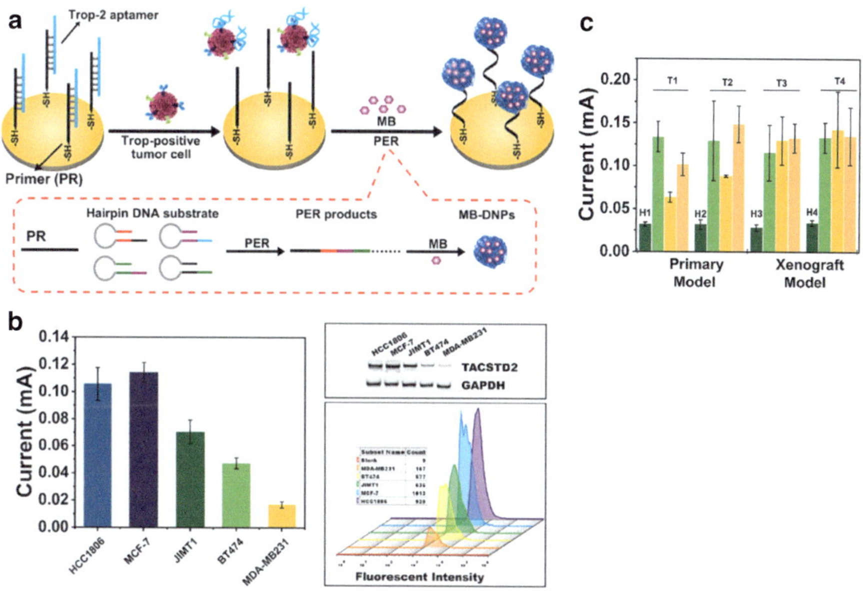

Fig. 9.2 (**a**) A conceptual representation of the electrochemical biosensor designed for the detection of Trop-2-positive breast cancer cells. (**b**) Square wave voltammetry (SWV) profiles across various tumor cell lines, alongside RT-PCR analysis for Trop-2 mRNA expression and flow cytometry assessment of FAM-labeled aptamer binding. (**c**) Comparative SWV peak currents were recorded for Trop-2-expressing tumor tissues versus normal somatic tissues. (Adapted with permission from [57, 78])

detect cancer biomarkers. A graphene-based FET biosensor achieved a 0.13 pM detection limit for cervical cancer biomarkers like TNF-α. This biosensor demonstrated excellent performance in minimally processed biological samples, highlighting its potential for real-time diagnostics [4, 68, 78].

- *Hydrogel-Protected Electrochemical Biosensors*: These systems use hydrogel coatings to prevent biofouling and enhance sensor stability. A hydrogel-protected electrochemical aptasensor was developed for doxorubicin detection in whole blood, achieving high sensitivity with minimal interference from nonspecific molecules (Fig. 9.3). This biosensor is ideal for therapeutic monitoring [70].

9.4.2.3 Nanomaterial-Enhanced Transducers

Nanomaterial-enhanced biosensors integrate nanostructures, like graphene, gold nanoparticles, and quantum dots, as transducers to enhance sensitivity, specificity, and amplification of signal. Nanomaterial-enhanced biosensors effectively detect multiplexed biomarkers in serum, urine, and saliva.

- *Gold Nanoparticles*: Gold nanoparticles (AuNPs) increase the surface area for aptamer binding, significantly enhancing detection limits. A g-C3N4/Fe3O4 nanoparticle-based aptasensor detected CA 15-3 at 0.2 U/mL, enabling highly sensitive breast cancer diagnostics (Fig. 9.4). Incorporating nanomaterials improved the biosensor's performance in serum samples [57].
- *Graphene Oxide*: Graphene oxide (GO) enhances fluorescence quenching efficiency, making it an essential component in optical biosensors. A GO-based biosensor was developed for multiplex detection of miRNAs and VEGF, providing simultaneous and precise quantification of ovarian cancer biomarkers [64].

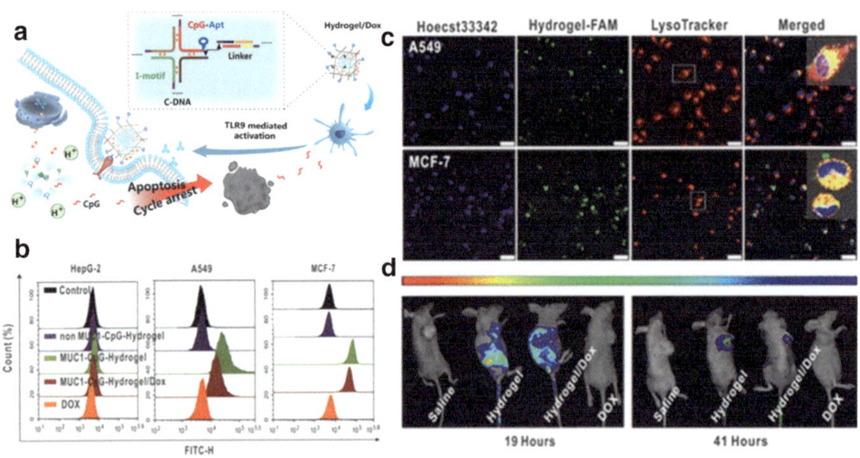

Fig. 9.3 (**a**) Diagrammatic overview of the CpG-MUC1 hydrogel system loaded with doxorubicin (Dox). (**b**) Binding interaction of FAM-labeled MUC1-CpG hydrogels with MCF-7, A549, and HepG-2 cell lines. (**c**) Confocal laser scanning microscopy (CLSM) showing co-localization of MUC1-CpG-hydrogel-FAM with lysosomes. (**d**) In vivo fluorescence imaging of mice following intravenous administration of saline, Cy5-labeled hydrogel, Cy5-hydrogel/Dox, and free Dox. (Adapted with permission from Ref. [81] Copyright © 2019, American Chemical Society)

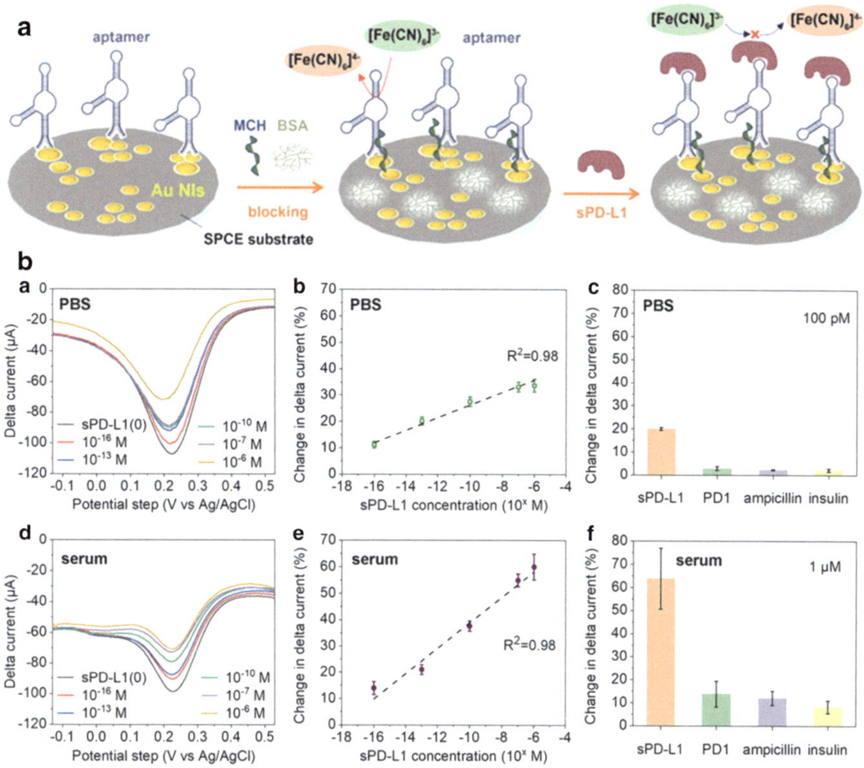

Fig. 9.4 (**a**) Schematic illustration of the biosensor layout for sPD-L1 detection: Au NIs/SPCE surface with ss-DNA aptamer. (**b**) Differential pulse voltammetry response of aptasensor as a function of sPD-L1 and selectivity for sPD-L1 against PD1, ampicillin, and insulin. (Reproduced with permission from [82]. © 2024 The Author(s). Small Science published by Wiley-VCH GmbH)

9.4.2.4 Microfluidic Transducers

Microfluidic-based biosensors integrate aptamer-based systems into compact, portable devices for high-throughput analysis. Microfluidic biosensors are being applied in early cancer detection and monitoring, particularly in underserved regions. These platforms are ideal for point-of-care applications and in resource-limited settings.

- *High-Throughput Biomarker Detection*: Microfluidic biosensors enable rapid screening of multiple biomarkers using small sample volumes. A microfluidic biosensor detected VEGF and miRNAs in ovarian cancer with high sensitivity. The system demonstrated excellent reproducibility and portability, which makes it appropriate in point-of-care diagnostics (Fig. 9.5) [60, 61].
- *Portable Diagnostics*: These biosensors are designed for decentralized healthcare settings, reducing dependence on centralized laboratory infrastructure. A

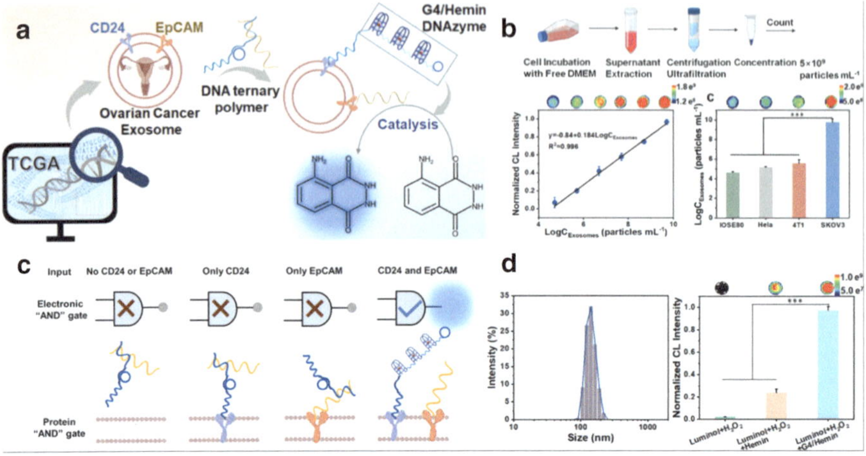

Fig. 9.5 (**a**) Schematic representation of ternary polymer response to ovarian cancer exosome-specific logic gate. (**b**) Chemiluminescence signal data of exosomes with different concentrations are recognized by DNA ternary polymer and the number of exosomes in different cells. (**c**) Schematic diagram of logic gate calculation. (**d**) Particle size of exosomes and feasibility analysis of the biosensor to realize signal amplification. (Adapted with permission from [83]. Copyright © 2024, American Chemical Society)

paper-based microfluidic biosensor employed aptamer-functionalized silver nanoparticles to detect PDGF in ovarian cancer, achieving a detection limit of 0.01 μg/mL [84].

9.4.2.5 Piezoelectric Transducers

Piezoelectric biosensors measure changes in mass or mechanical vibrations upon biomarker binding. Microcantilever-based systems for PSA detection demonstrated label-free and real-time detection capabilities, achieving unparalleled accuracy in prostate cancer diagnostics [42, 85].

9.5 Signal Amplification

Signal amplification techniques are integral to enhancing the sensitivity of aptamer-based biosensors, particularly for detecting low-abundance biomarkers in complex biological samples. These techniques include:

(a) *Rolling Circle Amplification (RCA)*

RCA is a powerful technique for amplifying DNA signals. RCA systems have been employed to detect miRNAs and VEGF in liquid biopsies, achieving detection limits in the femtomolar range [3, 60, 61].

(b) *Nanomaterial-Based Amplification*

Nanomaterials like gold nanoparticles, graphene, and quantum dots enhance signal strength and stability. Gold nanoparticles increase the surface area for aptamer binding, amplifying signals in optical and electrochemical systems. A gold nanoparticle–enhanced biosensor for MUC1 detected ovarian cancer biomarkers with sub-picomolar sensitivity [36, 67]. Graphene oxide was integrated into microfluidic platforms to improve fluorescence quenching efficiency, enabling multiplexed biomarker detection [64].

(c) *Catalytic Amplification*

Enzyme-linked catalytic amplification systems improve sensitivity by producing multiple signals from a single aptamer-target interaction. For instance, horseradish peroxidase (HRP)-linked systems have been employed for the detection of VEGF and HER2 via colorimetric, enhancing signal visibility in low-resource settings (Fig. 9.6) [39].

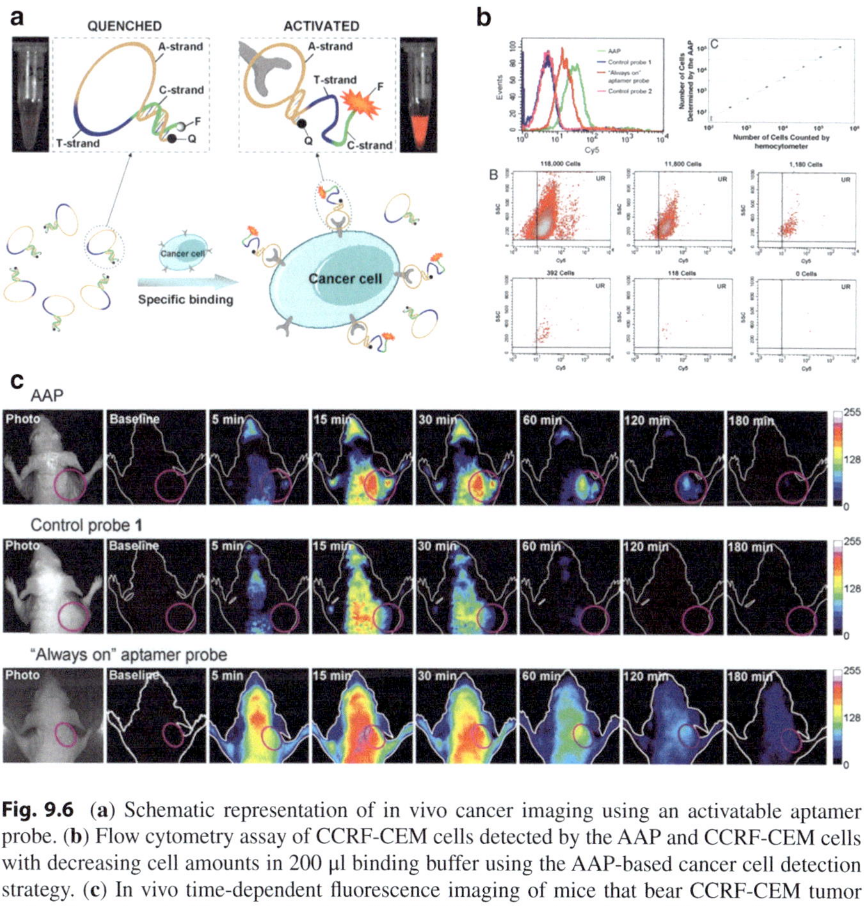

Fig. 9.6 (**a**) Schematic representation of in vivo cancer imaging using an activatable aptamer probe. (**b**) Flow cytometry assay of CCRF-CEM cells detected by the AAP and CCRF-CEM cells with decreasing cell amounts in 200 μl binding buffer using the AAP-based cancer cell detection strategy. (**c**) In vivo time-dependent fluorescence imaging of mice that bear CCRF-CEM tumor nude. (Reproduced with permission from [32].©2011, National Academy of Sciences)

9.6 Challenges and Limitations of Biosensors for Detecting Cancer Biomarkers

Although aptamer-based biosensors hold great promise for advancing cancer diagnostics, their broader implementation is hindered by various obstacles. Key among these are the difficulties in consistently synthesizing aptamers and the intricate nature of biological samples, both of which can adversely affect the accuracy and dependability of the sensors.

9.6.1 Reproducibility

Ensuring consistency in aptamer-based biosensors is critical for their effectiveness in diagnostics. However, achieving this consistency is often hindered by variations in the procedures used for aptamer selection and functionalization. These inconsistencies can lead to unpredictable sensor behavior, affecting their accuracy and performance. To overcome these challenges, it is crucial to refine the processes involved in aptamer development and sensor assembly. Fine-tuning these steps can help reduce variability, thereby enhancing the reliability and precision of the biosensor in detecting targeted analytes.

Variability in SELEX Processes: SELEX is the conventional technique used for selecting aptamers, requiring several repetitive steps to identify those with high affinity. Despite its widespread use, the method is inherently complex and susceptible to variations, which can result in inconsistent binding affinities and specificities [19, 50, 53]. Small changes in experimental conditions, like variations in target concentration or stringency of selection, can lead to aptamers with distinct properties, making it challenging to standardize the process.

Functionalization of Sensor Surfaces: Immobilization of aptamers on sensor surfaces is critical in biosensor fabrication, i.e., the process of attaching aptamers onto sensor surfaces plays a crucial role in developing effective biosensors. Differences in surface modification techniques—such as employing thiol linkers with gold nanoparticles or using covalent bonding methods on graphene oxide can lead to inconsistent aptamer placement, which in turn disrupts signal transmission. A notable instance involves graphene-based field-effect transistor (FET) sensors, where irregular functionalization has been shown to compromise the reliability of detecting cervical cancer biomarkers [57, 68]. Functionalization of graphene-based FET sensors has been reported to affect the reproducibility for detecting biomarkers of cervical cancer [48, 71].

Strengthening quality control during the development and functionalization of aptamers can help address many current limitations [58]. In addition, exploring alternative strategies—such as computationally guided aptamer design and enzymatic generation techniques beyond traditional SELEX—may improve reproducibility and broaden the scope of aptamer selection [50, 53], as well as non-SELEX-based enzymatic generation aptamers [86–88]. The applications of aptasensors of various types in cancer diagnosis and therapy have been summarized in Table 9.3.

Table 9.3 Applications of aptasensors in cancer diagnosis and therapy

Category	Delivery method/sensor type	Model/detection	Marker	Therapeutic agent/ detection target	Application	References
Nanoparticle-based Aptasensor	MUC-1 aptamer/AuNPs and ATP aptamer/QDs nanocomplex	MCF-7	MUC-1, ATP	–	Fluorescent imaging of cancer cells	[38]
	EpCAM aptamer-conjugated silica-coated Gd-Zn-Cu-In-S/ZnS QDs	4 T1, MCF-7	EpCAM	Doxorubicin (Dox)	Tumor-targeted delivery	[89]
	AS141 aptamer-conjugated Fe3O4@UiO-66-NH2 MOF/DOX/CDs	MDA-MB-231	Nucleolin	Dox	Tumor-targeted delivery	[90]
	SERS-based biosensors utilizing Au@Ag nanoparticles on graphene oxide have been developed, incorporating aptamers specifically targeting EpCAM and HER2 proteins. This innovative platform enhances signal amplification, enabling highly sensitive cancer biomarker detection	MCF-7 cells	EpCAM and HER2		High sensitivity, detecting as few as 150 particles/mL, with potential for early cancer diagnosis and differentiation of cancer types in clinical samples	[91]
	HER2 aptamer-conjugated gold nanoclusters	BT-474, MDA-MB-231, mouse xenograft	HER2	Mertansine (DM1)	Imaging and therapy	[92]
Liposomal formulations	Encapsulation of aptamer-Dox in liposomes	Human breast tumor (MCF-7/Adr cells)	Nucleolin	Dox	Enhanced drug stability and delivery	[93]
	Covalent bonding of paclitaxel (PTX) to AS1411 aptamer	SKOV3, OVCAR3	Nucleolin and cathepsin	Paclitaxel (PTX)	Tumor-specific therapy	[94]

(continued)

Table 9.3 (continued)

Category	Delivery method/sensor type	Model/detection	Marker	Therapeutic agent/ detection target	Application	References
Polymer-based systems	AS141 aptamer-conjugated Pluronic F127/PEG-block copolymers	MCF-7, female BALB/c nude mice	Nucleolin	Dox	Targeted delivery	[95]
Self-assembled systems		MCF-7	MUC1	Dox	Targeted drug delivery	[96]
	DNA nanohydrogel formed with CpG-MUC1	A549, MCF-7, HepG2, female BALB/c mice	MUC1	Dox	Drug delivery and immune modulation	[81]
Electrochemical sensors	Label-free electrochemical sensor with MUC1 aptamer	Detection of MUC1 in serum	MUC1	–	Breast cancer biomarker detection	[97]
	The use of HepG2-derived cellular exosomes for electrochemical detection of exosomes	HepG2 cells	CD63 aptamer		TME-associated exosomes can be detected through c63 binding aptamers for the early detection of tumors	[98]
	Electrochemical biosensor made by assembling methylene blue-assisted DNA nanoparticles for targeting Trop-2 of breast cancer cells	Human trophoblast surface cell antigen 2 (Trop-2)	Trop-2		Trop-2-expressing breast cancer cells HCC-1806, with the LOD of 1 cell/mL, could be detected	[55]
	Electrochemical aptasensor for detecting the sPD-L1 protein	Detection of the sPD-L1 protein	sPD-L1 aptamer		An efficient LOD of 0.76 aM, which offers a broad linear detection range from 100 aM to 1 μM, ensuring high sensitivity and precision in biomarker analysis	[82]
	Graphene-modified gold electrodes-based electrochemical aptasensor	Detection of cancer cells	MUC1	–	Early cancer diagnosis	[78]

Photodynamic therapy	Aptamer-functionalized superparamagnetic iron oxide nanoparticles (SPIONs)	C26, A549	Nucleolin	TMPyP (photosensitizer)	Photodynamic therapy	[99]
	Photosensitizer conjugated with AS1411 aptamer	MCF7, Hella	Nucleolin	Protoporphyrin IX (ROS generator)	Photodynamic tumor therapy	[100]
RNA interference (siRNA and miRNA)	EpCAM aptamer-conjugated SWNT with siRNA	MCF-7	EpCAM	siRNA targeting BCL9l	Gene silencing and targeted therapy	[101]
	Gold nanoparticles functionalized with FAM-modified EpCAM aptamer	PD-L1	EpCAM	A lateral flow assay (LFA) detected miRNA and exosomes, ensuring the noninvasive diagnosis of liver cancer	Detecting liver cancer-associated miRNA and exosomes	[102]
	HER2 aptamer that is siRNA-conjugated to target Bcl-2	N202.1A	HER2	siRNAs targeting Bcl-2	Gene therapy	[103]
Diagnostics	Smartphone-based aptasensor	MUC1	MUC1	–	Detection of cancer cells	[104]
	DNA polymer with aptamers for EpCAM and CD24 binds ovarian cancer exosomes, triggering a strong sensitivity and a wide detection range	SKOV3 cells	EpCAM and CD24		Detection of ovarian cancer exosomes through a logic gate response with chemiluminescent signals	[83]
	CRISPR/Cas12a-based aptamer biosensor	ctDNA EGFR L858R	EGFR	–	Detection of mutations	[105]

9.6.2 Sample Complexity

Detection of the biomarkers using aptamer-based biosensors in the clinical biological samples such as blood, serum, saliva, and urine presents a challenging environment due to the complex and intricate composition of these fluids. The presence of nontarget molecules can interfere with target recognition and signal transduction and compromise the reliability of signal output, affecting biosensor sensitivity and specificity.

Nonspecific adsorption of biomolecules onto sensor surfaces is a significant issue in real-world applications. For example, proteins in blood or serum can bind to aptamer-functionalized surfaces, resulting in elevated background signals and reduced analytical accuracy. This concern is especially notable in electrochemical platforms, where such interactions can alter current flow or impedance, complicating data interpretation [64, 70]. This issue is particularly pronounced in electrochemical biosensors, where nonspecific interactions can alter electrical properties, complicating signal interpretation [2]. A hydrogel-protected electrochemical aptasensor for doxorubicin detection in whole blood demonstrated reduced interference from nonspecific molecules due to its hydrogel coating, highlighting the importance of antifouling strategies in real-world applications [70]. Low-abundance biomarkers, such as CTCs or specific miRNAs, are difficult to detect in complex samples due to their dilution within the higher concentrations of the interfering molecules. Moreover, identifying biomarkers that occur in very low concentrations, such as CTCs or specific miRNAs, remains a formidable task due to signal suppression from the surrounding biological matrix [3, 61]. Utilizing microfluidic systems in aptamer-based biosensors for sample preprocessing and target enrichment, which enables high-throughput analysis in complex matrices [60].

9.7 Future Perspectives

Rapidly advancing areas such as biomarker discovery and wearable biosensor technology are set to significantly enhance the progress of aptamer-based diagnosis. Identifying novel, disease-specific biomarkers would improve the selectivity and diagnostic value of aptamer platforms, enabling earlier detection for more personalized treatment strategies. At the same time, integrating aptamers into wearable and point-of-care devices presents an opportunity to bring real-time cancer monitoring closer to clinical and even home settings. These portable systems can facilitate continuous health tracking, enhance patient compliance, and lessen the reliance on centralized laboratory testing. Moreover, advancements in material science and microfluidics are anticipated to boost the sensitivity, stability, and user-friendliness of these devices. Together, these innovations will help overcome many limitations of current cancer diagnostic methods, aligning with the increasing demand for accessible, noninvasive, and rapid testing options.

9.7.1 Biomarker Discovery: Expanding Aptamer Libraries for Rare Cancers

The discovery of new biomarkers plays a vital role in improving the accuracy and reach of cancer diagnostics. Rare cancers, comprising roughly one-fifth of global cancer cases, often go undetected early due to a shortage of disease-specific markers and dependable screening tools [42]. Developing aptamer libraries tailored to these cancers could open new avenues for timely diagnosis and better clinical outcomes.

Advancing SELEX Techniques: The SELEX technique, widely used for selecting aptamers with high affinity and selectivity, has undergone significant refinements in recent years. Emerging approaches like cell-SELEX and integration with high-throughput sequencing have greatly improved the efficiency of aptamer discovery, particularly for complex and rare cancer biomarkers. Developing customized aptamer libraries for cancers such as sarcomas, mesothelioma, and medullary thyroid carcinoma is becoming increasingly important. These rare malignancies often lack reliable diagnostic tools, and aptamer-based biosensors offer a promising solution by combining sensitivity with cost-effectiveness. For example, a microfluidic biosensor incorporating an aptamer against CD44, a marker found in several rare cancers, have shown strong clinical performance during validation studies [61].

Targeting Emerging Biomarkers: Novel cancer biomarkers such as exosomal proteins, long noncoding RNAs (lncRNAs), and metabolites are gaining attention for their diagnostic and prognostic potential. Aptamer-based biosensors have demonstrated the capability to detect these unconventional targets, like exosomal proteins, with high sensitivity [66]. Aptamers targeting metabolites associated with metabolic reprogramming in cancer cells, such as lactate and glutamine, are developing to provide insights into tumor microenvironments [2]. Developing universal SELEX platforms that identify aptamers for diverse cancer biomarkers in a single workflow may represent future advancement in aptamer-based biosensors.

9.7.2 Biosensor-Enabled Wearables for Continuous Health Monitoring

Incorporating aptasensors into wearable devices marks a groundbreaking advancement in cancer diagnostics and patient care. These wearable sensors facilitate continuous, real-time monitoring of biomarker levels, allowing for early disease progression detection and treatment efficacy assessment, ultimately enhancing personalized healthcare. This method aligns with the advancing prominence of personalized medicine and preventive healthcare. Wearable biosensors integrate flexible, biocompatible materials with aptamer-based sensing platforms, ensuring comfort and usability. Key design features are:

- *Flexibility and Durability*: Materials such as graphene and conductive polymers enable the fabrication of lightweight, stretchable sensors that can conform to the skin or clothing [68].
- *Real-Time Signal Transmission*: Wireless communication technologies, including Bluetooth and near-field communication (NFC), facilitate the seamless transmission of data to healthcare providers for remote monitoring [2].

Wearable sensors can empower patients to actively manage their health, facilitating timely interventions based on real-time biomarker levels. Wearable sensors improve resource allocation in healthcare systems by reducing the need for frequent hospital visits and laboratory tests. Wearable sensors equipped with aptamer-based biosensors have the potential for monitoring biomarkers associated with therapy response and disease recurrence:

- *Therapeutic Monitoring*: A wearable electrochemical aptasensor for VEGF has been developed to monitor angiogenesis inhibitors in cancer therapy, providing real-time feedback on drug efficacy [58].
- *Detection of Recurrence*: Wearable sensors detecting biomarkers like PSA and CEA offer continuous surveillance, enabling the early detection of cancer recurrence [4].

Several innovative wearable devices integrating aptamer-based biosensors are under development. Examples include sweat-based biosensors that detect cancer biomarkers such as exosomal proteins and metabolites in sweat, offering a noninvasive diagnostic option [71], and skin-adhesive sensors. Aptamer-functionalized patches that detect circulating tumor biomarkers in interstitial fluid are being tested for breast and ovarian cancers [70]. Enhancing the durability of wearable devices to withstand prolonged use in varying environmental conditions remains a focus of research [66].

9.8 Conclusion

The future of aptamer-based biosensors lies in discovering novel biomarkers and their integration into wearable devices for real-time monitoring. Expanding aptamer libraries through advancements in SELEX and high-throughput technologies will enable the detection of rare and emerging cancer biomarkers, addressing critical gaps in oncology. Simultaneously, wearable sensors equipped with aptamer-based platforms offer the potential for continuous, noninvasive cancer monitoring, revolutionizing personalized medicine and preventive care. By overcoming current challenges and leveraging technological advancements, these innovations will significantly enhance the impact of aptamer-based biosensors in cancer diagnostics.

References

1. Ahirwar R, Khan N, Kumar S. Aptamer-based sensing of breast cancer biomarkers: a comprehensive review of analytical figures of merit. Expert Rev Mol Diagn. 2021;21(7):703–21. https://doi.org/10.1080/14737159.2021.1920397.
2. Negahdary M. Aptamers in nanostructure-based electrochemical biosensors for cardiac biomarkers and cancer biomarkers: a review. Biosens Bioelectron. 2020;152:112018. https://doi.org/10.1016/j.bios.2020.112018.
3. Zhao X, et al. Aptamer-based fluorescent sensors for the detection of cancer biomarkers. Spectrochim Acta A Mol Biomol Spectrosc. 2021;247:119038. https://doi.org/10.1016/j.saa.2020.119038.
4. Saeidi Tabar F, et al. Ultrasensitive aptamer-based electrochemical nanobiosensor in diagnosis of prostate cancer using 2D:2D reduced graphene oxide/graphitic carbon nitride decorated with Au nanoparticles. Eur J Med Chem Rep. 2024;12:100192. https://doi.org/10.1016/j.ejmcr.2024.100192.
5. Tumor targeting with a 99mTc-labeled AS1411 aptamer in prostate tumor cells. J Drug Targeting 23(6). Accessed 19 Jan 2025. [Online]. Available: https://www.tandfonline.com/doi/abs/10.3109/1061186X.2015.1009075.
6. A nucleolin-activated polyvalent aptamer nanoprobe for the detection of cancer cells. Anal Bioanal Chem. Accessed 19 Jan 2025 [Online]. Available: https://link.springer.com/article/10.1007/s00216-023-04629-3.
7. MUC1 Aptamer-based near-infrared fluorescence probes for tumor imaging. Mol Imaging Biol. Accessed 19 Jan 2025. [Online]. Available: https://link.springer.com/article/10.1007/s11307-014-0763-y.
8. Wen W, Hu R, Bao T, Zhang X, Wang S. An insertion approach electrochemical aptasensor for mucin 1 detection based on exonuclease-assisted target recycling. Biosens Bioelectron. 2015;71:13–7. https://doi.org/10.1016/j.bios.2015.04.001.
9. Aptamer-based detection of epithelial tumor marker mucin 1 with quantum dot-based fluorescence readout. Anal Chem. Accessed 19 Jan 2025. [Online]. Available: https://pubs.acs.org/doi/abs/10.1021/ac901223q.
10. Chen P, et al. Homogeneous visual and fluorescence detection of circulating tumor cells in clinical samples via selective recognition reaction and enzyme-free amplification. ACS Nano. 2021;15(7):11634–43. https://doi.org/10.1021/acsnano.1c02080.
11. Microfluidic paper-based analytical device for sensitive detection of peptides based on specific recognition of aptamer and amplification strategy of hybridization chain reaction – Ma – 2017 – ChemElectroChem – Wiley Online Library. Accessed 19 Jan 2025 [Online]. Available: https://chemistry-europe.onlinelibrary.wiley.com/doi/full/10.1002/celc.201600824.
12. PET imaging of tenascin-C with a radiolabeled single-stranded DNA aptamer. J Nucl Med. Accessed 19 Jan 2025. [Online]. Available: https://jnm.snmjournals.org/content/56/4/616.short.
13. Aptamer-targeted gold nanoparticles as molecular-specific contrast agents for reflectance imaging. Bioconjugate Chem. Accessed 19 Jan 2025 [Online]. Available: https://pubs.acs.org/doi/full/10.1021/bc8001248.
14. Jolly P, Formisano N, Tkáč J, Kasák P, Frost CG, Estrela P. Label-free impedimetric aptasensor with antifouling surface chemistry: a prostate specific antigen case study. Sens Actuators B Chem. 2015;209:306–12. https://doi.org/10.1016/j.snb.2014.11.083.
15. Liu B, Lu L, Hua E, Jiang S, Xie G. Detection of the human prostate-specific antigen using an aptasensor with gold nanoparticles encapsulated by graphitized mesoporous carbon. Microchim Acta. 2012;178(1):163–70. https://doi.org/10.1007/s00604-012-0822-5.

16. Ex vivo and in vivo imaging and biodistribution of aptamers targeting the human matrix MetalloProtease-9 in melanomas. PLOS ONE. Accessed 19 Jan 2025. [Online]. Available: https://journals.plos.org/plosone/article?id=10.1371/journal.pone.0149387.
17. From ugly duckling to swan: unexpected identification from cell-SELEX of an anti-annexin A2 aptamer targeting tumors. PLOS ONE. Accessed 19 Jan 2025. [Online]. Available: https://journals.plos.org/plosone/article?id=10.1371/journal.pone.0087002.
18. Da Rocha Gomes S, et al. 99mTc-MAG3-Aptamer for imaging human tumors associated with high level of matrix metalloprotease-9. Bioconjug Chem. 2012;23(11):2192–200. https://doi.org/10.1021/bc300146c.
19. Meirinho SG, Dias LG, Peres AM, Rodrigues LR. Electrochemical aptasensor for human osteopontin detection using a DNA aptamer selected by SELEX. Anal Chim Acta. 2017;987:25–37. https://doi.org/10.1016/j.aca.2017.07.071.
20. Development of an electrochemical RNA-aptasensor to detect human osteopontin. ScienceDirect. Accessed 19 Jan 2025 [Online]. Available: https://www.sciencedirect.com/science/article/abs/pii/S0956566315300555?via%3Dihub.
21. Bezerra G, et al. Electrochemical aptasensor for the detection of HER2 in human serum to assist in the diagnosis of early stage breast cancer. Anal Bioanal Chem. 2019;411(25):6667–76. https://doi.org/10.1007/s00216-019-02040-5.
22. Self-assembled DNA generated electric current biosensor for HER2 analysis | analytical chemistry. Accessed 19 Jan 2025 [Online]. Available: https://pubs.acs.org/doi/abs/10.1021/acs.analchem.7b01747.
23. Ranganathan V, Srinivasan S, Singh A, DeRosa MC. An aptamer-based colorimetric lateral flow assay for the detection of human epidermal growth factor receptor 2 (HER2). Anal Biochem. 2020;588:113471. https://doi.org/10.1016/j.ab.2019.113471.
24. Liu G, Mao X, Phillips JA, Xu H, Tan W, Zeng L. Aptamer−nanoparticle strip biosensor for sensitive detection of cancer cells. Anal Chem. 2009;81(24):10013–8. https://doi.org/10.1021/ac901889s.
25. Pattern recognition of cancer cells using aptamer-conjugated magnetic nanoparticles. ACS Nano. Accessed 19 Jan 2025 [Online]. Available: https://pubs.acs.org/doi/10.1021/nn3002328.
26. In vivo fluorescence imaging of tumors using molecular aptamers generated by cell-SELEX – Shi – 2010. Chem Asian J. Wiley Online Library. Accessed 19 Jan 2025 [Online]. Available: https://aces.onlinelibrary.wiley.com/doi/10.1002/asia.201000242.
27. Tang Z, et al. Selection of aptamers for molecular recognition and characterization of cancer cells. Anal Chem. 2007;79(13):4900–7. https://doi.org/10.1021/ac070189y.
28. Molecular magnetic resonance probe targeting VEGF165: preparation and in vitro and in vivo evaluation. https://doi.org/10.1002/cmmi.1584.
29. Aptamer combined with fluorescent silica nanoparticles for detection of hepatoma cells. Discover Nano. Accessed 19 Jan 2025 [Online]. Available: https://link.springer.com/article/10.1186/s11671-017-1890-6.
30. An 'activatable' aptamer-based fluorescence probe for the detection of HepG2 cells. Accessed 19 Jan 2025 [Online]. Available: https://www.spandidos-publications.com/10.3892/or.2017.5527.
31. Wei Z, et al. Multifunctional nanoprobe for cancer cell targeting and simultaneous fluorescence/magnetic resonance imaging. Anal Chim Acta. 2016;938:156–64. https://doi.org/10.1016/j.aca.2016.07.037.
32. Activatable aptamer probe for contrast-enhanced in vivo cancer imaging based on cell membrane protein-triggered conformation alteration. PNAS. Accessed 19 Jan 2025 [Online]. Available: https://www.pnas.org/doi/full/10.1073/pnas.1016197108.
33. Tumor cell capture patterns around aptamer-immobilized microposts in microfluidic devices. Biomicrofluidics. AIP Publishing. Accessed 19 Jan 2025 [Online]. Available: https://pubs.aip.org/aip/bmf/article-abstract/11/5/054110/385490/Tumor-cell-capture-patterns-around-aptamer?redirectedFrom=fulltext.

34. A logic-gated nanorobot for targeted transport of molecular payloads. Science. Accessed 19 Jan 2025 [Online]. Available: https://www.science.org/doi/10.1126/science.1214081.
35. Aptamer-based microfluidic device for enrichment, sorting, and detection of multiple cancer cells. Anal Chem. Accessed 19 Jan 2025. [Online]. Available: https://pubs.acs.org/doi/10.1021/ac9012072.
36. Nourizad A, Golmohammadi S, Aghanejad A, Tohidkia MR. Recent trends in aptamer-based nanobiosensors for detection of vascular endothelial growth factors (VEGFs) biomarker: a review. Environ Res. 2023;236:116726. https://doi.org/10.1016/j.envres.2023.116726.
37. Dehghani S, et al. Aptamer-based biosensors and nanosensors for the detection of vascular endothelial growth factor (VEGF): a review. Biosens Bioelectron. 2018;110:23–37. https://doi.org/10.1016/j.bios.2018.03.037.
38. Ranjbar-Navazi Z, Fathi M, Abdolahinia ED, Omidi Y, Davaran S. MUC-1 aptamer conjugated InP/ZnS quantum dots/nanohydrogel fluorescent composite for mitochondria-mediated apoptosis in MCF-7 cells. Mater Sci Eng C. 2021;118:111469. https://doi.org/10.1016/j.msec.2020.111469.
39. Rajabi R, Afrashteh F, Maddah F. Application of aptamer-based biosensors in early diagnosis of gastric cancer: a promising method for early detection. Explor Res Hypothesis Med. 2023;8(3):229–35. https://doi.org/10.14218/ERHM.2022.00125.
40. Xu Z, Wang C, Ma R, Sha Z, Liang F, Sun S. Aptamer-based biosensing through the mapping of encoding upconversion nanoparticles for sensitive CEA detection. Analyst. 2022;147(14):3350–9. https://doi.org/10.1039/D2AN00669C.
41. Ahirwar R, Bhattacharya A, Kumar S. Unveiling the underpinnings of various non-conventional ELISA variants: a review article. Expert Rev Mol Diagn. 2022;22(7):761–74.
42. Sousa DA, Carneiro M, Ferreira D, Moreira FTC, Sales MGF, Rodrigues LR. Recent advances in the selection of cancer-specific aptamers for the development of biosensors. Curr Med Chem. 2022;29(37):5850–80. https://doi.org/10.2174/0929867329666220224155037.
43. Hussain S, et al. Modern diagnostic imaging technique applications and risk factors in the medical field: a review. Biomed Res Int. 2022;2022(1):5164970.
44. Hussain T, Nguyen QT. Molecular imaging for cancer diagnosis and surgery. Adv Drug Deliv Rev. 2014;66:90–100.
45. Hu Z, et al. Aptamer-based novel ag-coated magnetic recognition and SERS nanotags with interior nanogap biosensor for ultrasensitive detection of protein biomarker. Sens Actuators B Chem. 2021;334:129640. https://doi.org/10.1016/j.snb.2021.129640.
46. Juncker D, Bergeron S, Laforte V, Li H. Cross-reactivity in antibody microarrays and multiplexed sandwich assays: shedding light on the dark side of multiplexing. Curr Opin Chem Biol. 2014;18:29–37.
47. Sotnikov DV, Zherdev AV, Zvereva EA, Eremin SA, Dzantiev BB. Changing cross-reactivity for different immunoassays using the same antibodies: theoretical description and experimental confirmation. Appl Sci. 2021;11(14):6581.
48. Kundrod KA, Smith CA, Hunt B, Schwarz RA, Schmeler K, Richards-Kortum R. Advances in technologies for cervical cancer detection in low-resource settings. Expert Rev Mol Diagn. 2019;19(8):695–714.
49. Pearlman PC, et al. The National Institutes of Health Affordable Cancer Technologies program: improving access to resource-appropriate technologies for cancer detection, diagnosis, monitoring, and treatment in low-and middle-income countries. IEEE J Transl Eng Health Med. 2016;4:1–8.
50. Fasogbon I, Yakubu M, Adam M, Obi C, Nuhu T, Alegbe S. Non-selex-based in-silico modeled aptamers against SARS-COV-2 proteins: a systematic review. KIU J Health Sci. 2022;2(1):69–79.
51. Fasogbon IV, et al. UCP-LF and other assay methods for schistosome circulating anodic antigen between 1978 and 2022. Biol Methods Protoc. 2023;8, no. 1:bpad006. https://doi.org/10.1093/biomethods/bpad006.
52. Fasogbon IV, Ondari EN, Deusdedit T, Rangasamy L, Krishnan S, Aja PM. Point-of-care potentials of lateral flow-based field screening for *mycoplasma bovis* infections: a litera-

ture review. Biol Methods Protoc. 2024;9(1):bpae034. https://doi.org/10.1093/biomethods/bpae034.
53. Fasogbon IV, et al. Recent focus in non-SELEX-computational approach for de novo aptamer design: a mini review. Anal Biochem. 2025;699:115756. https://doi.org/10.1016/j.ab.2024.115756.
54. Sequeira-Antunes B, Ferreira HA. Nucleic acid aptamer-based biosensors: a review. Biomedicines. 2023;11(12):Art. no. 12. https://doi.org/10.3390/biomedicines11123201.
55. Yang J, Liang Q, Zhou Q, Sha L, Shi H, Li G. An electrochemical biosensor to assay Trop-2 of breast cancer cells fabricated by methylene blue-assisted assembly of DNA nanoparticles. Biosens Bioelectron. 2024;246:115907. https://doi.org/10.1016/j.bios.2023.115907.
56. Crulhas BP, Karpik AE, Delella FK, Castro GR, Pedrosa VA. Electrochemical aptamer-based biosensor developed to monitor PSA and VEGF released by prostate cancer cells. Anal Bioanal Chem. 2017;409(29):6771–80. https://doi.org/10.1007/s00216-017-0630-1.
57. Pourmadadi M, et al. Construction of aptamer-based nanobiosensor for breast cancer biomarkers detection utilizing g-C3N4/magnetic nano-structure. Biosensors. 2022;12(11):921. https://doi.org/10.3390/bios12110921.
58. Shao P, et al. Aptamer-based functionalized SERS biosensor for rapid and ultrasensitive detection of gastric cancer-related biomarkers. Int J Nanomedicine. 2023;18:7523–32. https://doi.org/10.2147/IJN.S434854.
59. Mikuła E, Kaczmarek H. Aptamer-based biosensors for biomarkers detection (part II). Curr Med Chem. 2023;30(8):893–4. https://doi.org/10.2174/0929867330082212151111423.
60. Vandghanooni S, Sanaat Z, Barar J, Adibkia K, Eskandani M, Omidi Y. Recent advances in aptamer-based nanosystems and microfluidics devices for the detection of ovarian cancer biomarkers. TrAC Trends Anal Chem. 2021;143:116343. https://doi.org/10.1016/j.trac.2021.116343.
61. Vandghanooni S, Sanaat Z, Farahzadi R, Eskandani M, Omidian H, Omidi Y. Recent progress in the development of aptasensors for cancer diagnosis: focusing on aptamers against cancer biomarkers. Microchem J. 2021;170:106640. https://doi.org/10.1016/j.microc.2021.106640.
62. Díaz-Fernández A, Miranda-Castro R, de-los-Santos-Álvarez N, Lobo-Castañón MJ, Estrela P. Impedimetric aptamer-based glycan PSA score for discrimination of prostate cancer from other prostate diseases. Biosens Bioelectron. 2021;175:112872. https://doi.org/10.1016/j.bios.2020.112872.
63. Xiang W, Lv Q, Shi H, Xie B, Gao L. Aptamer-based biosensor for detecting carcinoembryonic antigen. Talanta. 2020;214:120716. https://doi.org/10.1016/j.talanta.2020.120716.
64. Liang L, et al. Aptamer-based fluorescent and visual biosensor for multiplexed monitoring of cancer cells in microfluidic paper-based analytical devices. Sens Actuators B Chem. 2016;229:347–54. https://doi.org/10.1016/j.snb.2016.01.137.
65. Ou D, Sun D, Lin X, Liang Z, Zhong Y, Chen Z. A dual-aptamer-based biosensor for specific detection of breast cancer biomarker HER2 *via* flower-like nanozymes and DNA nanostructures. J Mater Chem B. 2019;7(23):3661–9. https://doi.org/10.1039/C9TB00472F.
66. Hu R, et al. Exploring aptamer-based metasurfaces for label-free plasmonic biosensing of breast tumor-derived exosomes. Adv Opt Mater. 2024;12(28):2401180. https://doi.org/10.1002/adom.202401180.
67. Karpik AE, Crulhas BP, Rodrigues CB, Castro GR, Pedrosa VA. Aptamer-based biosensor developed to monitor MUC1 released by prostate cancer cells. Electroanalysis. 2017;29(10):2246–53. https://doi.org/10.1002/elan.201700318.
68. Wang Z, et al. Aptamer-based graphene biosensor for biomarker detection in undiluted physiological media towards cervical carcinoma diagnosis. SSRN. 2024; https://doi.org/10.2139/ssrn.4821120.
69. Fasogbon IV. Non-SELEX-based in-SILICO modeled APTAMERS against SARS-COV-2 proteins: a systematic review. KIU J Health Sci. 2021;1(1):69–79. https://doi.org/10.59568/KJHS-2022-2-1-007.

70. Luo S, Wu Q, Wang L, Qu H, Zheng L. Direct detection of doxorubicin in whole blood using a hydrogel-protected electrochemical aptamer-based biosensor. Talanta. 2025;285:127289. https://doi.org/10.1016/j.talanta.2024.127289.
71. Li Z, et al. An aptamer-based SERS–LFA biosensor with multiple channels for the ultrasensitive simultaneous detection of serum VEGF and osteopontin in cervical cancer patients. New J Chem. 2022;46(43):20629–42. https://doi.org/10.1039/D2NJ03567G.
72. Recent developments in aptasensors for diagnostic applications. ACS Appl Mater Interfaces. Accessed 19 Jan 2025 [Online]. Available: https://pubs.acs.org/doi/abs/10.1021/acsami.0c14788.
73. Thiviyanathan V, Gorenstein DG. Aptamers and the next generation of diagnostic reagents. PROTEOMICS Clin Appl. 2012;6(11–12):563–73. https://doi.org/10.1002/prca.201200042.
74. Ali MH, Elsherbiny ME, Emara M. Updates on aptamer research. Int J Mol Sci. 2019;20(10):Art. no. 10. https://doi.org/10.3390/ijms20102511.
75. Pan C, Guo M, Nie Z, Xiao X, Yao S. Aptamer-based electrochemical sensor for label-free recognition and detection of cancer cells. Electroanalysis. 2009;21(11):1321–6. https://doi.org/10.1002/elan.200804563.
76. Şahin S, Caglayan MO, Üstündağ Z. Recent advances in aptamer-based sensors for breast cancer diagnosis: special cases for nanomaterial-based VEGF, HER2, and MUC1 aptasensors. Microchim Acta. 2020;187(10):549. https://doi.org/10.1007/s00604-020-04526-x.
77. Ghazi MN, Husain B, Heydaryan K, Mehmandoust S, Kadhim SA, Eskandari V. A review of aptamer-based surface-enhanced Raman scattering (SERS) platforms for cancer diagnosis applications. BioNanoScience. 2025;15(1):44. https://doi.org/10.1007/s12668-024-01673-w.
78. Gupta P, Bharti A, Kaur N, Singh S, Prabhakar N. An electrochemical aptasensor based on gold nanoparticles and graphene oxide doped poly(3,4-ethylenedioxythiophene) nanocomposite for detection of MUC1. J Electroanal Chem. 2018;813:102–8. https://doi.org/10.1016/j.jelechem.2018.02.014.
79. Hianik T. Advances in electrochemical and acoustic aptamer-based biosensors and immunosensors in diagnostics of leukemia. Biosensors. 2021;11(6):177. https://doi.org/10.3390/bios11060177.
80. İnce B, Kavacık M, Sezgintürk MK. Electrochemical aptamer-based biosensors for disease biomarkers. Essent Chem. 2024;1(1):1–23. https://doi.org/10.1080/28378083.2024.2386517
.
81. One-step self-assembly of multifunctional DNA nanohydrogels: an enhanced and harmless strategy for guiding combined antitumor therapy. ACS Appl Mater Interfaces. Accessed 19 Jan 2025 [Online]. Available: https://pubs.acs.org/doi/abs/10.1021/acsami.9b15874.
82. Lotfibakalani Z, et al. Optimal biofunctionalization of gold nanoislands for electrochemical detection of soluble programmed death ligand 1. Small Sci. 2025;5(1):2400411. https://doi.org/10.1002/smsc.202400411.
83. Zhao M, et al. Dual-aptamer recognition of DNA logic gate sensor-based specific exosomal proteins for ovarian cancer diagnosis. ACS Sens. 2024;9(5):2540–9. https://doi.org/10.1021/acssensors.4c00270.
84. Sharma P, et al. Aptamer-based silver nanoparticle decorated paper platform for electrochemical detection ovarian cancer biomarker PDGF. Mater Chem Phys. 2023;306:128114. https://doi.org/10.1016/j.matchemphys.2023.128114.
85. Gao F, et al. Aptamer-based microcantilever biosensors for label-free PSA detection. IEEE Sensors J. 2025;25(1):266–73. https://doi.org/10.1109/JSEN.2024.3496092.
86. Ashley J, et al. Terminal deoxynucleotidyl transferase-mediated formation of protein binding polynucleotides. Nucleic Acids Res. 2021;49(2):1065–74.
87. Ashley J, Potts IM, Olorunniji FJ. Applications of terminal deoxynucleotidyl transferase enzyme in biotechnology. Chembiochem. 2023;24(5):e202200510.
88. Vacacela J, et al. The protein-templated synthesis of enzyme-generated aptamers. Angew Chem. 2022;134(17):e202201061.

89. Akbarzadeh M, et al. Hybrid silica-coated Gd-Zn-Cu-In-S/ZnS bimodal quantum dots as an epithelial cell adhesion molecule targeted drug delivery and imaging system. Int J Pharm. 2019;570:118645. https://doi.org/10.1016/j.ijpharm.2019.118645.
90. Alijani H, Noori A, Faridi N, Bathaie SZ, Mousavi MF. Aptamer-functionalized Fe3O4@ MOF nanocarrier for targeted drug delivery and fluorescence imaging of the triple-negative MDA-MB-231 breast cancer cells. J Solid State Chem. 2020;292:121680. https://doi.org/10.1016/j.jssc.2020.121680.
91. Zhang Q, Ma R, Zhang Y, Zhao J, Wang Y, Xu Z. Dual-aptamer-assisted ratiometric SERS biosensor for ultrasensitive and precise identification of breast cancer exosomes. ACS Sens. 2023;8(2):875–83. https://doi.org/10.1021/acssensors.2c02587.
92. Wang Y, Chen J, Irudayaraj J. Nuclear targeting dynamics of gold nanoclusters for enhanced therapy of HER2+ breast cancer. ACS Nano. 2011;5(12):9718–25. https://doi.org/10.1021/nn2032177.
93. Plourde K, Derbali RM, Desrosiers A, Dubath C, Vallée-Bélisle A, Leblond J. Aptamer-based liposomes improve specific drug loading and release. J Control Release. 2017;251:82–91. https://doi.org/10.1016/j.jconrel.2017.02.026.
94. Li J, et al. AS1411 aptamer-modified theranostic liposomes co-encapsulating manganese oxide nano-contrast agent and paclitaxel for MRI and therapy of cancer. RSC Adv. 2019;9(60):34837–46. https://doi.org/10.1039/c9ra06878c.
95. Li X, Yu Y, Ji Q, Qiu L. Targeted delivery of anticancer drugs by aptamer AS1411 mediated Pluronic F127/cyclodextrin-linked polymer composite micelles. Nanomed Nanotechnol Biol Med. 2015;11(1):175–84. https://doi.org/10.1016/j.nano.2014.08.013.
96. Aptamer-conjugated DNA icosahedral nanoparticles as a carrier of doxorubicin for cancer therapy. ACS Nano Accessed 19 Jan 2025 [Online]. Available: https://pubs.acs.org/doi/abs/10.1021/nn200693a.
97. Florea A, Taleat Z, Cristea C, Mazloum-Ardakani M, Săndulescu R. Label free MUC1 aptasensors based on electrodeposition of gold nanoparticles on screen printed electrodes. Electrochem Commun. 2013;33:127–30. https://doi.org/10.1016/j.elecom.2013.05.008.
98. Cao Y, Li L, Han B, Wang Y, Dai Y, Zhao J. A catalytic molecule machine-driven biosensing method for amplified electrochemical detection of exosomes. Biosens Bioelectron. 2019;141:111397. https://doi.org/10.1016/j.bios.2019.111397.
99. Aptamer-assisted superparamagnetic iron oxide nanoparticles as multifunctional drug delivery platform for chemo-photodynamic combination therapy. J Mater Sci Mater Med. Accessed 19 Jan 2025. [Online]. Available: https://link.springer.com/article/10.1007/s10856-019-6278-y.
100. Lin H-C, et al. Aptamer-guided upconversion nanoplatform for targeted drug delivery and near-infrared light-triggered photodynamic therapy. J Biomater Appl. 2020;34(6):875–88. https://doi.org/10.1177/0885328219882152.
101. Mohammadi M, Salmasi Z, Hashemi M, Mosaffa F, Abnous K, Ramezani M. Single-walled carbon nanotubes functionalized with aptamer and piperazine–polyethylenimine derivative for targeted siRNA delivery into breast cancer cells. Int J Pharm. 2015;485(1):50–60. https://doi.org/10.1016/j.ijpharm.2015.02.031.
102. Wei R, et al. A lateral flow assay strip for simultaneous detection of miRNA and exosomes in liver cancer. Chem Commun. 2024;60(58):7491–4. https://doi.org/10.1039/D4CC02559H.
103. Delivery of chemo-sensitizing siRNAs to HER2+-breast cancer cells using RNA aptamers. Nucleic Acids Res. Oxford Academic. Accessed 19 Jan 2025. [Online]. Available: https://academic.oup.com/nar/article/40/13/6319/1020565.
104. Sanati A, et al. Smartphone-assisted lab-in-a-tube device using gold nanocluster-based aptasensor for detection of MUC1-overexpressed tumor cells. Anal Chim Acta. 2023;1252:341017. https://doi.org/10.1016/j.aca.2023.341017.
105. Liu F, et al. Electrochemical detection of ctDNA mutation in non-small cell lung cancer based on CRISPR/Cas12a system. Sens Actuators B Chem. 2022;362:131807. https://doi.org/10.1016/j.snb.2022.131807.

Aptamer-Based Biosensors for Cancer Imaging

10

Manju Jakhar, Nidhi Rani, and Thakur Gurjeet Singh

10.1 Introduction

Cancer continues to be among the leading causes of mortality globally, and improving patient outcomes for its associated morbidity requires an emphasis on early diagnosis. Traditional methods of diagnosis, like biopsy and imaging, suffer from invasiveness, high costs, and delays in detection. There is thus a pressing need for noninvasive, cost-effective, highly sensitive alternatives [1, 2].

Cancer diagnosis aptasensors have gained rapidly growing interest as powerful biosensors employing aptamers, defined here as very short, single-stranded nucleic acids (either DNA or RNA) that possess an extremely high affinity and specificity for cancer biomarkers. When combined with other biosensing technologies, aptasensors can offer sensitive, real-time, and accurate cancer imaging and diagnosis [3, 4].

Aptamers have the possibility of binding selectively to proteins, small molecules, and full cells considered markers of cancer—as they fold into a three-dimensional structure. Some of the advantages that selective binding provides over traditional diagnostic methods are:

- *Specificity and Affinity*: Aptamers allow precise binding to their target, minimizing false positives [5, 6].
- *Ease of Synthesis and Modification*: Synthesis of the chemically synthesized aptamers is fairly straightforward, and they are easily modified to enhance stability and functionality [7].

M. Jakhar
School of Pharmacy and Emerging Sciences, Baddi University of Emerging Sciences & Technology, Baddi, Himachal Pradesh, India

N. Rani (✉) · T. G. Singh
Chitkara College of Pharmacy, Chitkara University, Rajpura, Punjab, India

S. Srivastava et al. (eds.), *Biosensors and Aptamers*,
https://doi.org/10.1007/978-981-96-8387-1_10

- *Economics of Production*: Aptamers are cheaper than antibodies; hence, they are truly fit for high-scale usage [6, 7].
- *Non-immunogenicity*: The possibility of the aptamers causing an immune response is very low; hence, they are safer for multiple injections in vivo [6, 7].

10.2 Fundamentals of Aptamers

10.2.1 What Are Aptamers?

Aptamers are short sequences of nucleic acids, typically DNA or RNA, that can bind specifically to a variety of target molecules, including proteins, small compounds, and even entire cells. These molecules are created through a synthetic in vitro selection process, allowing them to take on distinct three-dimensional shapes that enable strong binding to their targets, acting like antibodies while also providing a range of unique benefits, as highlighted in Table 10.1 [7–9].

Aptamers are particular in contrast to antibodies in several characteristics that make them useful in biosensing and diagnostic applications:

These advantages make aptamers ideal candidates for noninvasive cancer diagnostics, as they are characterized by high specificity, stability, and cost-effectiveness [12, 13].

10.2.2 Selection of Aptamers or SELEX Technology

Aptamers selected by the SELEX approach, an acronym for Systematic Evolution of Ligands by Exponential Enrichment, are optimized to identify nucleic acid ligands with high affinity and specific binding to a wide range of target molecules. By repeated selective enrichment of specifically binding aptamers to biomarkers of cancer and other target molecules, SELEX generates strongly specific aptamers for a wide range of applications, from cancer imaging and diagnostics to drug delivery and therapeutic applications [14–16]. Various SELEX approaches have typical strengths, as shown in Table 10.2.

10.2.2.1 Process of SELEX

The SELEX process allows ligands to be methodically developed through exponential enrichment. This method allows for the selection of nucleic acid ligands that can

Table 10.1 Comparison of key features of aptamers and antibodies

Feature	Aptamers	Antibodies	References
Size	Small (10–50 kDa)	Larger (150 kDa)	[10, 11]
Stability	High, even in harsh conditions	Sensitive to temperature and pH	
Production	Chemically synthesized	Derived from animals	
Cost	Lower production cost	Higher production cost	

Table 10.2 SELEX techniques and their advantages

SELEX technique	Description	Advantages	References
Traditional SELEX	Aptamers are selected by binding to target molecules	Simple, effective	[17–19]
Magnetic SELEX	Magnetic beads are used to facilitate the selection process	Faster, higher yield	
Capillary SELEX	Involves capillary electrophoresis for aptamer isolation	More accurate, specific	

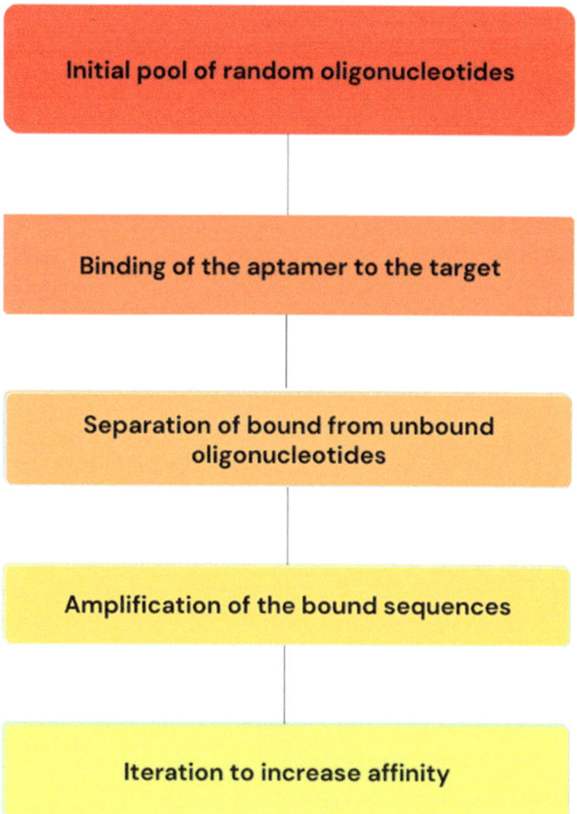

Fig. 10.1 Process of SELEX

bind to target molecules with high affinity. Figure 10.1 shows the sequential SELEX procedure, which demonstrates its ability to optimize aptamers for specific cancer biomarker identification.

SELEX-optimized aptamers have the exact binding characteristics needed to identify cancer biomarkers. Aptamers may perhaps 1 day be employed in extremely sensitive biosensors for cancer imaging [20–22].

10.3 Mechanisms of Aptamer-Based Detection

A biosensor that utilizes aptamers can detect cancer biomarkers through different mechanisms, including electrochemical, optical, and whole-cell. Each mechanism has its advantages in a specific clinical application, and in particular, the sensitivity, in vivo results, and noninvasive characteristics make aptasensors particularly effective for early diagnosis and monitoring of cancer [23, 24].

10.3.1 Electrochemical Detection

Electrochemical aptasensors are extremely sensitive in the detection of biomarkers in cancer patients. Their results can even be directly obtained in real time. The detection mechanism is based on finding changes in electrical characteristics such as current, voltage, or resistance upon binding between the target molecule and the aptamer. Their sensitivity and rapid response make them of significant interest as point-of-care (POC) diagnostics. They can be made, for example, in electrochemical aptasensors that will sense prostate-specific antigens (PSAs) through the use of gold nanoparticles (AuNPs). Such an electrochemical sensor has achieved successful detection even at the femtomolar level, and hence, it is extremely useful in detecting prostate cancer even at an early stage. The sensor is highly sensitive to detect PSA at low concentrations, so it can offer sensitive detection and early intervention. This is summarized in Table 10.3, emphasizing their utility in early prostate cancer diagnostics [25–27].

10.3.2 Optical Detection

Optical aptasensors operate by taking advantage of the interaction of aptamers with light to detect cancer biomarkers. These sensors find application in measuring changes in fluorescence, colorimetric changes, or surface plasmon resonance when an aptamer binds to its target. The optical changes therefore provide a visual or measurable output that makes optical aptasensors ideal for the noninvasive, real-time imaging of cancer biomarkers for accuracy and practicability [31–34].

Table 10.3 Features of electrochemical aptasensors

Feature	Electrochemical aptasensors	References
Detection range	Femto to nanomolar concentrations	[28–30]
Sensitivity	High sensitivity for real-time detection	
Application example	Prostate-specific antigen (PSA) detection	
Advantages	Real-time, high sensitivity, cost-effective	

Table 10.4 Key characteristics of optical aptasensors

Feature	Optical aptasensors	References
Detection principle	Changes in light (fluorescence, colorimetry, SPR)	[37–47]
Application example	Detection of microRNA-21 as a cancer biomarker	
Advantages	Noninvasive, real-time imaging, high sensitivity	

For example, aptamer-conjugated quantum dots (QDs) have been employed to detect circulating miR-21 as a cancer biomarker for breast and liver cancers by optical aptasensors even at low concentrations. Quantum dots, which were nanoparticle probes emitting fluorescent light upon excitation, show drastically improved sensitivity and specificity of the aptasensor for cancer imaging, as summarized in Table 10.4 [35, 36].

10.3.3 Whole-Cell Detection

Whole-cell detection techniques with aptamer-target binding to specifically cancer cell surface markers, enabling direct tumor cell detection in patient samples. The method proves useful in detecting circulating tumor cells (CTCs), which are present in the blood of cancer patients. Aptamers that have been engineered to detect whole cells can identify particular markers on the exterior of such cancer cells, which allows for CTC identification and separation without resorting to invasive biopsies [41–44].

One of the most striking examples of this technology is the targeting of epithelial cell adhesion molecule (EpCAM)-positive circulating tumor cells (CTCs), which are most often linked to metastatic cancers. Aptamers can specifically bind to epithelial cell adhesion molecule (EpCAM), a cell surface marker that is predominantly located on epithelial cancer cells. The detection of CTCs in blood samples is a promising field for noninvasive cancer diagnosis and monitoring of metastatic progression [45–47]. This is given in Table 10.5.

Table 10.5 Whole-cell detection using aptamer-based sensors

Feature	Whole-cell detection aptasensors	References
Detection principle	Binding to surface markers of cancer cells	[48–51]
Application example	Detection of EpCAM-positive CTCs	
Advantages	Noninvasive, detection of metastasis	

10.4 Aptamer-Based Biosensors Design and Principles

Aptamers are distinguished by their special ability of specific binding to their target. Based on this idea, aptamer-based biosensors can be constructed for application using various possible mechanisms of detection. The design and principles involved in these biosensors differ based on the techniques used in the detection process, which include optical, electrochemical, or fluorescence-based methods. Each kind of biosensor offers different merits based on the clinical application [52–54].

10.4.1 Types of Biosensors

Aptamer-based biosensors can be classified broadly based on the detection mode [55]. Significant types are:

- *Optical Biosensors*: These biosensors generally rely on light-based methodologies, including fluorescence, absorbance, or surface plasmon resonance (SPR), to detect the interaction of a target [56].
- *Electrochemical Biosensors*: These sensors measure changes in electrical signals, like current or impedance, during aptamer binding with its target [57].
- *Fluorescence-Based Biosensors*: These biosensors are activated by fluorescent molecules attached to aptamers, emitting light when they bind to a target for its detection [58].

Each of these types of biosensors possesses unique advantages, making each of them more suited to certain diagnostic applications for cancer, as summarized in Table 10.6, such as quick detection and noninvasive imaging [59].

10.4.2 Components of Aptamer-Based Biosensors

Aptamer-based biosensors comprise three primary components:

- *Target Molecule (Cancer Biomarker)*: The cancer cell–specific molecule for which the aptamer is designed to detect. This could be PSA, HER2, or CEA, among others [63].

Table 10.6 Types of aptamer-based biosensors and detection mechanisms

Biosensor type	Detection mechanism	Examples	References
Optical biosensors	Interaction between aptamers and light	Fluorescence, SPR, absorbance	[60–62]
Electrochemical biosensors	Change in electrical signals (current, impedance)	Prostate cancer detection	
Fluorescence-based biosensors	Fluorescent emission upon aptamer-target binding	MicroRNA-21 detection in blood	

- *Aptamer (Recognition Element)*: The aptamer directly binds to the target molecule for detection [64].
- *Transducer (Signal Conversion Element)*: The interaction between the target and the aptamer is converted by the transducer to a measurable signal, optical, electrochemical, or of another type depending on the design of the biosensor [65].

All these components are important to ensure the sensitivity and specificity of the biosensor to detect cancer biomarkers [66–68]. Table 10.7 summarizes the crucial function of each component to guarantee the functioning of the biosensor.

10.4.3 Working Mechanism of an Aptamer-Based Biosensor

The function of an aptamer-based biosensor is based on the binding of an aptamer to a target molecule. The binding causes a conformational change that produces a measurable signal upon the aptamer binding to the target, such as a cancer biomarker. This signal is then captured by the transducer, which converts it into an observable output, allowing one to monitor patient samples in real time for the presence of cancer biomarkers [71, 72].

Table 10.7 Components of aptamer-based biosensors

Component	Role in biosensor	References
Target molecule	Cancer biomarkers (e.g., PSA, HER2, CEA)	[69, 70]
Aptamer	Recognition element that binds to the target	
Transducer	Converts aptamer-target binding to measurable signals	

Table 10.8 Working mechanism of an aptamer-based biosensor

Step	Description	References
Binding	Aptamer binds to its target cancer biomarker	[74–76]
Conformational change	Binding induces a change in the aptamer's shape	
Signal generation	The change is converted into a measurable signal	
Detection	The transducer processes the signal for detection	

This process is summarized in Table 10.8, describing the step-by-step process involved in the creation and detection of signals in a biosensor. The advantage of this mechanism is its high sensitivity and specificity, ensuring that it identifies only the target molecule. This is important for positive cancer diagnosis and proper monitoring [73].

10.4.4 Advantages and Prospects in Aptamer-Based Biosensors

Biosensors based on aptamers benefit from the recent modern diagnostic tools, which appear with several advantages toward applications, including cancer diagnostics and therapy monitoring. Unique benefits over traditional antibody-based sensors apply to these biosensors; however, they raise challenges that must be answered to improve their clinical applicability. Of late, significant improvements in the performance of these biosensors have meant that detecting and visualizing cancer biomarkers has been made much more reliable and efficient [77–79].

10.4.5 Advantages of Aptamer-Based Biosensors

Aptamers possess several critical advantages, summarized in Table 10.9, which makes them ideal candidates for cancer diagnostics. These include high specificity, stability, cost-effectiveness, non-immunogenic properties, and versatility in conjugation with other materials like nanomaterials. These features enhance the overall functionality of biosensors in clinical settings [80, 81].

Table 10.9 Advantages of aptamer-based biosensors

Advantage	Description	References
High specificity	Aptamers exhibit great specificity and excellent binding affinity to the target molecules. This can decrease false positives and ensure more accurate diagnostics, especially in complex biomarker detection	[82]
Stability	Unlike antibodies, aptamers are very stable, i.e., they can maintain their functions under varying environmental conditions. This makes them suitable for long-term usage and transportation without the risk of degradation	[83]
Cost-effectiveness	Aptamer synthesis is a more economical process than antibody production. The cost advantage makes aptamers more accessible for large-scale clinical and diagnostic applications	[84]
Non-immunogenic	Aptamers are synthetic molecules, and as such, they do not trigger immune responses. This ensures their safe use in clinical diagnostics without the complications associated with immunogenicity	[85]
Versatility	Such versatile aptamers can be easily conjugated with other materials, such as nanomaterials, improving the sensitivity and specificity of biosensors in complex biological systems, especially in detecting cancer	[86]

These advantages of aptamers make them promising candidates for cancer diagnostics, contributing to the creation of precise, stable, and cost-effective diagnostic devices [87].

10.4.6 Recent Advances in Aptamer-Based Biosensors

Recent advancements in aptamer-based biosensors also enhanced their efficacy, accuracy, and sensitivity over the current challenges. Among the most critical elements toward achieving the functionality enhancements of aptamer-based biosensors are the incorporation of nanomaterials, the use of signal amplification methods, and aptamer-functionalized nanoprobes for imaging purposes. These have demonstrated a wide enhancement in detecting as well as imaging cancer biomarkers with high sensitivity as well as selectivity [88, 89].

10.4.6.1 Nanomaterial Incorporation

The combination of these nanomaterials with aptamers, namely gold nanoparticles, graphene oxide (GO), and magnetic beads, has drastically changed biosensor performance for the better. The nanomaterial amplifies the signal; the aptamer binds efficiently, with higher sensitivity, and the nanomaterial significantly enhances the overall performance of biosensors. These molecules increase the sensitivity of biosensors to detect cancer biomarkers at lower concentrations, which may be pivotal in the early diagnosis phases [90] (Table 10.10).

These nanomaterial-aptamer combinations enhance detection capabilities, enabling more reliable diagnosis and better treatment outcomes for cancer patients [96].

10.4.6.2 Signal Amplification Strategies

Signal amplification methods, such as RCA and HCR, have been reported to be extremely effective in enhancing aptamer-based biosensor sensitivity. Amplification of the target signal enables the sensing of cancer biomarkers at ultralow concentrations, thereby enhancing early diagnosis opportunities. For example, an aptasensor exploiting the RCA approach has shown the possibility of detecting HER2, which

Table 10.10 Nanomaterial integration in aptamer-based biosensors

Nanomaterial	Application	Advantages	References
Gold nanoparticles	PSA detection	Enhances electrochemical signals, improves biosensor stability, and provides better signal detection	[91, 92]
Graphene oxide	miRNA detection	High surface area increases sensitivity, providing better aptamer binding efficiency	[93, 94]
Magnetic beads	CTC isolation	Facilitates target separation and concentration, improving detection limits and detection precision	[95]

is a breast cancer biomarker, at attomolar concentrations, thus furthering the diagnostic results toward earlier accuracy [97, 98].

10.4.6.3 Aptamer-Functionalized Nanoprobes for Imaging

Aptamer-functionalized nanoprobes have rapidly become an integral part of any cancer-imaging arsenal. These nanoprobes enhance sensitivity and specificity through aptamer conjugation with silica nanoparticles and graphene quantum dots. The probes can be used in sophisticated imaging methods, including fluorescence or magnetic resonance imaging, and are of great importance in the in vivo imaging of cancer tissue [99, 100].

Role of Aptamer-Functionalized Nanoprobes in Cancer Imaging

- *Aptamer Selection and Synthesis*
- Aptamers that are selected are those with a high ability to bind specifically to a cancer biomarker, ensuring high specificity and targeting [101].
- *Conjugation with Nanoprobes*
  Selected aptamers are conjugated using the nanoprobes involved; they are silica nanoparticles or graphene quantum dots. The conjugation process improves the sensitivity and specificity of the aptamers through an enhanced interaction of the nanoprobes with the cancerous tissue [102].
- *Target Binding in Tumor Tissue*
  The aptamer-functionalized nanoprobes will specifically bind the cancer biomarkers on the tumor cells' surfaces. This ensures proper localization as well as minimal off-target binding, which tends to enhance the imaging's accuracy [103].
- *The Generation and Imaging of Signal*

  The aptamer-functionalized nanoprobes, once bound to the tumor tissue, produce detectable signals. These signals work in advanced imaging techniques like fluorescence or MRI to furnish images of the tumor in real time and also in accurate diagnosis and treatment planning [104].

Such improvements in cancer imaging accuracy by the use of aptamer-functionalized nanoprobes have been found to increase the chances for early detection and proper treatment planning.

10.5 Challenges and Limitations of Aptamer-Based Biosensors

Aptamer-based biosensors are a promising frontier in the field of diagnostics and therapeutics, but this field of biosensors suffers from several major challenges and limitations. Overcoming these challenges will be a prerequisite to more general clinical application of such biosensors. In this chapter, the author discusses the biggest challenges and limitations that must be overcome to realize successful applications of aptamer-based biosensors in everyday patient therapy [105–107].

10.5.1 Biological Stability and Degradation

Aptamers are known to be sensitive to degradation in biological environments, primarily by the activity of nucleases. Sensitivity toward enzymatic degradation can compromise the binding efficacy of aptamers and thus nullify the advantages associated with the use of aptamer-based biosensors. Apart from enzymatic degradation, the rapid renal clearance of aptamers also reduces their bioavailability, which may ultimately necessitate frequent administration for therapeutic dosing. All these factors reduce a significant limitation in the use of aptamers for long-term clinical applications [108, 109].

10.5.2 Complex Sample Matrices

One of the main disadvantages of aptamer-based biosensors is their performance within complicated biological matrices, i.e., blood, tissue, and urine. Biological samples contain a wide range of biomolecules, including proteins, cells, and metabolites, which can interfere with the binding of aptamers and their targets. Such interference may reduce the specificity of the biosensor, increase false positives, or reduce its accuracy, making it difficult to detect low-abundance biomarkers reliably. These complexities of sample matrices necessitate further refinement of aptamer-based biosensors toward robust performance across different biological environments [110–112].

10.5.3 Reproducibility and Sensor Integration

The reproducibility of aptamer-based biosensors is another major challenge. Often the synthesis and functionalization of aptamers may cause inconsistent sensor performance. This also involves the challenge of integration into functioning biosensors, with which they can consistently sustain real-world clinical environments, due to instability in the sensor, degradation of the aptamers, and interference from other biomolecules. All these factors ultimately impact the efficiency of the biosensor. To apply these aptamer-based sensors in clinics, integration and reproducibility problems have to be overcome [113, 114].

10.5.4 The Problem of Aptamer Selection

The selection of an aptamer is one of the major concerns in developing biosensors, especially for diagnostics of cancer, among others. The heterogeneous nature of cancer cells, for example, complicates the identification of aptamers that can specifically target cancer biomarkers. It is a challenging task to get highly selective aptamers that function under diverse conditions of physiology, and most aptamers that are identified are not specific enough to make them clinically viable. However, much more sophisticated selection methods and better insight into the character of aptamer-target interactions are going to make a crucial difference for these biosensors [115–117].

10.5.5 In Vivo Performance

Despite the prospective applications of aptamers in diagnostics and therapy, their in vivo performance is far from satisfactory. Aptamers are prone to high enzymatic degradation within the organism. This prevents them from being used for long periods or multiple times. This decreases the half-life and bioavailability, thus limiting the aptamer's application in chronic treatments or serial monitoring. Therefore, stabilization approaches or the creation of more stable aptamers would improve their clinical applications [118, 119].

10.5.6 Aptamer Selection and Specificity Problems

The selection of aptamers is often carried out through the SELEX process, but this procedure may lead to aptamers that have different levels of specificity. Impurities within the target molecules and the existence of several binding sites on the target result in the selection of aptamers with suboptimal affinity or specificity. This variability introduces ambiguities in ensuring the reliability of aptamers for exact biosensing applications. Improving the SELEX process to generate more selective and stable aptamers will be very important for enhancing biosensor performance [120–122].

10.5.7 Aptamer Cross-Reactivity

The general specificity of aptamers may lead to their sometimes unwanted interaction with the unintended target, a phenomenon called cross-reactivity. This might lead to false positives or side effects when the aptamer reacts with nontarget proteins or molecules. In conclusion, cross-reactivity makes using aptamers in clinical diagnostics and therapies difficult, as it can interfere with the biosensor's accuracy. To overcome this problem, researchers have incorporated negative selection steps into the process of SELEX to eliminate the aptamers that might cause cross-reactivity with other biomolecules. This problem still needs more refinement to ensure specificity in aptamers [123].

10.5.8 Limitations of Colorimetric Aptasensors

Colorimetric aptasensors depend on the color change as the signaling for biomarker presence, which is easily interfered with by the color of the sample itself. Biological fluids—such as blood, urine, or tissue samples—may contain interfering substances that alter the color of the sample and thereby mask the diagnostic signal. This can avoid differentiation between several targets or precise determination of the concentration of a given biomarker in the sample. An alternative detection means or approach to minimize sample interference should be developed [124, 125].

10.5.9 Translation to the Clinical Setting Challenges

Despite all the potential advantages of aptamer-based biosensors, the translation into the clinic has been slow. Apart from stability problems, cross-reactivity, degradation, and serious difficulty in achieving high specificity for clinical use, aptamers have additional complications during their transition into therapeutic usage, especially into cancer therapy, due to potential side effects and biocompatibility issues. Overcoming these barriers will require continued research and innovation in improving aptamer stability, specificity, and clinical performance [126–128].

10.6 Prospective Developments and New Trends in Aptamer-Driven Biosensors for Cancer Treatment

The rapid evolution of aptamer-based biosensors has opened new possibilities for targeted cancer therapies and diagnostics. These biosensors, based on the specificity and binding affinity of aptamers, will become a revolutionary technology in oncology. Integration with nanotechnology, artificial intelligence (AI), and electrochemical sensors will enhance the functionality of these biosensors to provide personalized and accurate treatment options for cancer patients. The chapter deals with future directions and emerging trends in aptamer-based biosensors for cancer therapy, with a focus on synergy with novel technologies that can revolutionize cancer treatment and diagnostics [129–132].

10.6.1 Nanotechnology in Aptamer-Based Biosensors

Such potential drivers of innovation exist in aptamer-based biosensors that are driven by nanotechnology. Nanomaterials such as gold nanoparticles (AuNPs), graphene oxide (GO), and quantum dots (QDs) enormously improve the sensitivity, stability, and amplification of the signal from these biosensors [133, 134]. Nanomaterials possess surface properties that give them characteristic optical, electrical, and surface conductivity: this allows for more effective binding of aptamers to their targeted matter, thereby improving the overall performance of biosensors [135, 136].

For example, gold nanoparticles amplify the signal through surface plasmon resonance. They significantly increase the sensitivity of detection, even for low-abundance cancer biomarkers. For instance, high surface-area-to-volume ratios in graphene oxide may enable the binding of more aptamers to increase the sensitivity of a sensor. Fluorescent quantum dots give a robust means of detection that can easily be monitored. These nanomaterials address some of the key limitations in poor sensor stability, low sensitivity, and rapid clearance from the bloodstream, which often makes the practical application of biosensors in clinical settings futile [137–139].

10.6.2 Integration of AI and ML Technologies

Increasingly, artificial intelligence (AI) is being integrated into aptamer-based biosensor systems to enhance the analysis and interpretation of data that might lead to the development of tailored cancer treatment strategies. AI algorithms can help in sensor data analysis to detect subtle patterns that a human clinician could hardly identify. Large amounts of data can be trained in machine learning models to predict the patient outcome based on biomarker profiles, hence tailoring the treatment plan [140–142].

Optimizing the Selection of Aptamers Using AI: Another area where AI can impact the selection of aptamers is in optimizing the selection of aptamers, particularly for identifying individuals with the highest affinity and specificity for cancer biomarkers. The addition of AI to aptamer-based biosensors may see a shift toward more personalized, efficient, and accurate diagnostic and therapeutic cancer solutions in the future. This integration implies the processing of real-time data to ensure timely interventions tailored to each patient's unique molecular profile [143, 144].

10.6.3 Aptamers in Targeted Drug Delivery

Aptamers can bind specifically to cancer biomarkers, which has led them to be utilized in highly targeted delivery systems for drugs. Such specificity limits the off-target actions that are usual with conventional therapies, minimizing the chances for side effects and, in turn, enhancing the overall therapeutic index. By conjugating drug molecules to aptamers, scientists are making new improvements to deliver chemotherapeutic agents to targeted sites on the growth, skipping healthy tissues [130, 145, 146].

The combination of aptamers with nanomaterials, such as liposomes or nanoparticles, further enhances the stability and bioavailability of the drug payloads. Nanomaterials protect the drugs from premature degradation and help overcome challenges related to rapid clearance from the bloodstream. For example, utilization of conjugated nanoparticles with aptamers may increase the circulation time of the therapeutic agents, allowing higher concentrations of the drug to reach the tumor site, thus improving the efficacy of the treatment and decreasing dosage interval [147, 148].

10.6.4 Applications of Immunotherapy

Aptamers are increasingly being explored as part of immunotherapy approaches for cancer treatment. One exciting area is the use of aptamers in immune checkpoint modulation. Immune checkpoints are mechanisms that prevent the immune system from attacking normal cells, but they can also inhibit the immune system from attacking cancer cells. Aptamers that specifically target these checkpoints can block their function, thereby enhancing the body's immune response against tumors [149–151].

Targeting the tumor microenvironment, aptamers could modulate the immune system by enhancing the effectiveness of immune checkpoint inhibitors, such as PD-1 or CTLA-4 inhibitors, which have been so successful in treating some of the worst cancers, such as melanoma and non-small cell lung cancer. Furthermore, aptamers can be used to track immune responses, thereby giving real-time feedback that can allow for tailored immunotherapy approaches. This personalization makes the therapy tailored to the specific needs of the patient, and therefore, it might enhance treatment outcomes [152, 153].

10.6.5 Electrochemical Biosensors in Cancer Detection

Aptamer-based electrochemical biosensors are in focus for their ability to quickly and sensitively identify the presence of cancer biomarkers at a low cost. These biosensors detect cancer biomarkers as a change in electrical signals from binding events between aptamers and their targets, in terms of shifts in voltage and current. The potential of electrochemical sensors to be applied in low-resource settings or point-of-care diagnostics—where quick information can be obtained—is mainly because of their simplicity and affordability [154, 155].

One direction for the future is to integrate electrochemical biosensors with microfluidic systems. Miniaturizing the diagnostic device enables analysis of very small sample volumes, such as a drop of blood that contains enough cancer biomarkers for analysis, possibly leading to portable, real-time diagnostics that could be used in clinical settings or even in patients' own homes—to a whole new level in accessibility and convenience [156, 157].

10.6.6 Point-of-Care Diagnostics

Point-of-care (POC) diagnostics is an intriguing prospect for aptamer-based biosensors. The current classical approach in the detection and diagnosis of cancer in most traditions requires a lot of complex equipment and laboratory settings, which are time-consuming and expensive to implement. POC diagnostics, in contrast, achieve much faster, more cost-effective, and real-time results, usually with portable devices. The interfacing of aptamer-based biosensors into the system has the potential to transform how cancer is detected and monitored [158, 159].

Aptamer-based POC devices are known to enable clinicians to detect biomarkers of cancer in a blood or urine sample taken directly from a patient's bed, which would ultimately lead to earlier diagnosis and better monitoring of disease progression. The real-time capability of diagnostics may allow for quicker decisions about treatment, which improves patient outcomes. Additionally, POC may reduce the need for very expensive laboratory equipment and thereby make it even easier to get cancer detected in underserved or remote areas [160, 161].

10.6.7 Overcoming Challenges for Clinical Integration

Though the potential of aptamer-based biosensors is vast, several challenges need to be overcome before they are adopted extensively in the clinical field. Stability, reproducibility, and integration with sensors are key issues. The requirement here is that aptamers must be stable in a complex biological environment that could be blood or tissue for their use in the clinic. Stepping forward, the incorporation of stabilizing agents or changes in aptamer structures could be done to enhance their durability [161, 162].

Another area of ongoing research is the scalability of aptamer-based biosensors for large-scale clinical applications. Manufacturing processes need to be optimized in terms of batch consistency in quality and performance. Standardized protocols for aptamer selection, sensor calibration, and validation will also be important for these biosensors to meet the severe clinical demands for diagnostics and therapy [163, 164].

10.7 Conclusion

Aptamer-based biosensors represent a new edge in technology related to cancer diagnostics and therapy. This technology involves advantages over traditional antibody-based sensors due to several characteristics, which place them in a high position as powerful tools for sensitive, specific, and noninvasive detection of biomarkers. Integration of aptamers with nanotechnology, signal amplification techniques, or electrochemical sensors has enhanced their performance for increasingly reliable use in clinical applications.

Despite such a wide range of potential, barriers include aptamer selection, sensor integration, stability, reproducibility, and in vivo performance that hinder clinical applications. Recent advances in nanomaterials, aptamer-functionalized nanoprobes, and AI-driven data interpretation are addressing such issues, improving the sensitivity, specificity, and overall reliability of these biosensors.

Aptamer-based biosensors are now changing the landscape of cancer detection, targeted drug delivery, immunotherapy, and personalized medicine. These biosensors will play a vital role in the future of oncology, as they allow for accurate targeting of cancer cells while achieving better therapeutic outcomes. Research and innovation should be continued to overcome all the challenges and unlock the potential of aptamers in cancer care.

With ongoing evolutions, aptamer-based biosensors would revolutionize cancer diagnostics and therapy by offering more efficient, targeted, and accessible treatments. These biosensors, as this area evolves, would become part of personalized cancer care, a platform that opens the door for better patient outcomes and a promising future in cancer management.

References

1. Zakari S, Niels NK, Olagunju GV, Nnaji PC, Ogunniyi O, Tebamifor M, Israel EN, Atawodi SE, Ogunlana OO. Emerging biomarkers for non-invasive diagnosis and treatment of cancer: a systematic review. Front Oncol. 2024;14:1405267.
2. Khazaei M, Hosseini MS, Haghighi AM, Misaghi M. Nanosensors and their applications in early diagnosis of cancer. Sens Bio-Sens Res. 2023;41:100569.
3. Yunussova N, Tilegen M, Pham TT, Kanayeva D. Rapid detection of carcinoembryonic antigen by means of an electrochemical aptasensor. Iscience. 2024;27(5):109637.
4. Mikaeeli Kangarshahi B, Naghib SM, Rabiee N. DNA/RNA-based electrochemical nanobiosensors for early detection of cancers. Crit Rev Clin Lab Sci. 2024;7:1–23.
5. Thevendran R, Citartan M. Assays to estimate the binding affinity of aptamers. Talanta. 2022;1(238):122971.
6. Lin Y, Chen CY, Lin ZQ, Chen BH, Sun YC, Hung KF. A modified SELEX enables the efficient identification of DNA aptamers with potential for specific cancer targeting. Cancer Res. 2024;84(6_Supplement):3761.
7. Shraim AA, Abdel Majeed BA, Al-Binni MA, Hunaiti A. Therapeutic potential of aptamer–protein interactions. ACS Pharmacol Transl Sci. 2022;5(12):1211–27.
8. Zhou H, Li Y, Wu W. Aptamers: promising reagents in biomedicine application. Adv Biol. 2024;8(6):2300584.
9. Chiu ML, Goulet DR, Teplyakov A, Gilliland GL. Antibody structure and function: the basis for engineering therapeutics. Antibodies. 2019;8(4):55.
10. Santarpia G, Carnes E. Therapeutic applications of aptamers. Int J Mol Sci. 2024;25:6742.
11. Kalam SA, Hashmi A, Srivastava P. Aptamers: trending prospective in therapeutics. Int J Res Dev Pharm Life Sci. 2020;8(5):01–9.
12. Pellitero MA, de-los-Santos-Álvarez N, Lobo-Castañón MJ. Aptamer-based electrochemical approaches to meet some of the challenges in the fight against cancer. Curr Opin Electrochem. 2023;39:101286.
13. Tombelli S, Minunni M, Mascini M. Analytical applications of aptamers. Biosens Bioelectron. 2005;20(12):2424–34.
14. Ding Y, Liu J. Quantitative comparison of capture-SELEX, GO-SELEX, and Gold-SELEX for enrichment of aptamers. Anal Chem. 2023;95(39):14651–8.
15. Preeti K, Jain N, Sharma SK. Advances in SELEX methods. In: Aptasensors for food safety. CRC Press; 2024. p. 93–105.
16. Bayat P, Nosrati R, Alibolandi M, Rafatpanah H, Abnous K, Khedri M, Ramezani M. SELEX methods on the road to protein targeting with nucleic acid aptamers. Biochimie. 2018;154:132–55.
17. Gopinath SC. Methods developed for SELEX. Anal Bioanal Chem. 2007;387:171–82.
18. Yang G, Liu W, Zhao Y, Jiang G, Zhu C, Qu F. Induction of binding sites for RecA aptamers by differentiated-competition capillary electrophoresis-SELEX. Talanta. 2024;267:125213.

19. Manea I, Casian M, Hosu-Stancioiu O, de-Los-Santos-Álvarez N, Lobo-Castañón MJ, Cristea C. A review on magnetic beads-based SELEX technologies: applications from small to large target molecules. Anal Chim Acta. 2024;1297:342325.
20. Ştefan G, Hosu O, De Wael K, Lobo-Castañón MJ, Cristea C. Aptamers in biomedicine: selection strategies and recent advances. Electrochim Acta. 2021;20(376):137994.
21. Lim MC, Lim ES, Lim JA, Choi SW, Chang HJ. Efficient screening of pesticide diazinon-binding aptamers using the sol–gel-coated nanoporous membrane-assisted SELEX process and next-generation sequencing. Appl Biochem Biotechnol. 2022 Sep;194(9):3901–13.
22. Guan C, Ma Y, Sun P, Wu Y, Arroyo-Currás N, Chen G, Feng C. Dual-targets binding protection mediated rolling circle transcription with tandem fluorescent RNA aptamers for label-free detection of liver cancer biomarkers. Sensors Actuators B Chem. 2024;408:135521.
23. Ma Y, Shi X, Ding Y, Zhang X, Lu J, Sun D. Aptamer-functionalized quasi-ZIF-67@ methylene blue hybrid nanoprobes for the electrochemical aptasensing of epithelial cancer biomarkers. Chem Eng J. 2024;483:149362.
24. Xu X, Zhang Z, Shen T, Pan H, Chang D. Visual dual-mode aptasensor for non-small cell lung cancer exosome detection via HRP self-coupling enhanced oxidized iridium nanoparticle aggregation. Anal Sci. 2024;40:1459–73.
25. Mohan B, Mehak V, Kumar A, Modi K, Singh G, Garazade IM, Parikh J, Pombeiro AJ, Solovev AA. Detecting cancer biomarkers using electrochemical composite nanomaterials tools. Vietnam J Chem. 2024;63:175.
26. Díaz-Fernández A, Lorenzo-Gómez R, Miranda-Castro R, de-Los-Santos-Álvarez N, Lobo-Castañón MJ. Electrochemical aptasensors for cancer diagnosis in biological fluids–a review. Anal Chim Acta. 2020;1124:1–9.
27. Khanmohammadi A, Aghaie A, Vahedi E, Qazvini A, Ghanei M, Afkhami A, Hajian A, Bagheri H. Electrochemical biosensors for the detection of lung cancer biomarkers: a review. Talanta. 2020;206:120251.
28. Mickert MJ, Farka Z, Kostiv U, Hlaváček A, Horák D, Skládal P, Gorris HH. Measurement of sub-femtomolar concentrations of prostate-specific antigen through single-molecule counting with an upconversion-linked immunosorbent assay. Anal Chem. 2019;91(15):9435–41.
29. Chen S, Svedendahl M, Käll M, Gunnarsson L, Dmitriev A. Ultrahigh sensitivity made simple: nanoplasmonic label-free biosensing with an extremely low limit-of-detection for bacterial and cancer diagnostics. Nanotechnology. 2009;20(43):434015.
30. Chang H, Kang H, Ko E, Jun BH, Lee HY, Lee YS, Jeong DH. PSA detection with femtomolar sensitivity and a broad dynamic range using SERS nanoprobes and an area-scanning method. ACS Sens. 2016;1(6):645–9.
31. Borg KN, Ho YP, Zeng S. Recent developments on optical aptasensors for the detection of pro-inflammatory cytokines with advanced nanostructures. Adv Opt Mater. 2024;12(23):2400608.
32. Naziba AT, Uddin MN. Cancer cell detection biosensor utilizing dual-core PCF-based surface plasmon resonance. In: 2024 third international conference on distributed computing and electrical circuits and electronics (ICDCECE) 2024 Apr 26. IEEE; 2024. p. 1–5.
33. Sohrabi H, Mahmoudi-Maleki R, Majidi MR, Oroojalian F, Mokhtarzadeh AA, de la Guardia M. Recent advances in nanostructure-enhanced optical assays focused on luminescence-based biosensors for cancer biomarkers. TrAC Trends Anal Chem. 2024;176:117753.
34. Eivazzadeh-Keihan R, Pashazadeh-Panahi P, Baradaran B, Maleki A, Hejazi M, Mokhtarzadeh A, de la Guardia M. Recent advances on nanomaterial based electrochemical and optical aptasensors for detection of cancer biomarkers. TrAC Trends Anal Chem. 2018;100:103–15.
35. Davodabadi F, Mirinejad S, Fathi-Karkan S, Majidpour M, Ajalli N, Sheervalilou R, Sargazi S, Rozmus D, Rahdar A, Diez-Pascual AM. Aptamer-functionalized quantum dots as theranostic nanotools against cancer and bacterial infections: a comprehensive overview of recent trends. Biotechnol Prog. 2023;39(5):e3366.
36. Dong JM, Wang RQ, Yuan NN, Guo JH, Yu XY, Peng AH, Cai JY, Xue L, Zhou ZL, Sun YH, Chen YY. Recent advances in optical aptasensors for biomarkers in early diagnosis and prognosis monitoring of hepatocellular carcinoma. Front Cell Dev Biol. 2023;18(11):1160544.

37. Li X, Ma F, Yang M, Zhang J. Nanomaterial based analytical methods for breast cancer biomarker detection. Mater Today Adv. 2022;14:100219.
38. Oladepo SA. Design and characterization of a singly labeled fluorescent smart probe for in vitro detection of miR-21. Appl Spectrosc. 2018 Jan;72(1):79–88.
39. Krishnan T, Odion RA, Wang HN, Vo-Dinh T. Colorimetric detection of microRNA biomarkers using plasmonic nanoplatforms on a smartphone (conference presentation). In: Plasmonics in biology and medicine XX 2023 Mar 16. SPIE; 2023. p. PC123960F.
40. Akim AM, Safdar N, Yasmin A, Sung YY, Muhammad TS. Cancer and disease diagnosis-biosensor as potential diagnostic tool for biomarker detection. J Adv Pharm Technol Res. 2022;13(4):243–7.
41. Kou Q, Yuan H, Zhao G, Li Q, Zhang J, Li M, Li S, Zhao M, Zhang K, Pu G, Li L. Ultrasensitive detection of circulating tumor cells in clinical blood samples by a three-dimensional network nanovehicle-based aptasensor platform. Sensors Actuators B Chem. 2024;404:135172.
42. Wang G, Han D, Zhang Q. Highly sensitive detection of circulating tumour cells based on an ASV/CV dual-signal electrochemical strategy. RSC Adv. 2023;13(47):33038–46.
43. Putri AD, Murti BT, Manga YB, Kanchi S, Huang YJ, Peng CW, Yang PK, Hsieh CM. Whole-cell electrochemical aptasensors for cancer diagnosis: current advances and prospects. Adv Sensor Res. 2024;3(5):2300151.
44. Liu C, Shen X, Yan L, Qu R, Wang Y, He Y, Zhan Z, Chen P, Lin F. Controllable self-assembled DNA nanomachine enable homogeneous rapid electrochemical one-pot assay of lung cancer circulating tumor cells. Biosens Bioelectron. 2024;246:115865.
45. Mao Z, Hu M, Shen Q. Capturing and releasing of hepatocellular carcinoma EpCAM+ and EpCAM-circulating tumor cells based on photosensitive intelligent nanoreactor. Front Bioeng Biotechnol. 2024;12:1443843.
46. Mohammadinejad A, Gaman LE, Aleyaghoob G, Gaceu L, Mohajeri SA, Moga MA, Badea M. Aptamer-based targeting of cancer: a powerful tool for diagnostic and therapeutic aims. Biosensors. 2024;14(2):78.
47. Gilboa-Geffen A, Hamar P, Le MT, Wheeler LA, Trifonova R, Petrocca F, Wittrup A, Lieberman J. Gene knockdown by EpCAM aptamer–siRNA chimeras suppresses epithelial breast cancers and their tumor-initiating cells. Mol Cancer Ther. 2015;14(10):2279–91.
48. Yadav A, Kumar A, Siddiqui MH. Detection of circulating tumour cells in colorectal cancer: emerging techniques and clinical implications. World J Clin Oncol. 2021;12(12):1169.
49. Vidlarova M, Rehulkova A, Stejskal P, Prokopova A, Slavik H, Hajduch M, Srovnal J. Recent advances in methods for circulating tumor cell detection. Int J Mol Sci. 2023;24(4):3902.
50. Wilson RE Jr, O'Connor R, Gallops CE, Kwizera EA, Noroozi B, Morshed BI, Wang Y, Huang X. Immunomagnetic capture and multiplexed surface marker detection of circulating tumor cells with magnetic multicolor surface-enhanced Raman scattering nanotags. ACS Appl Mater Interfaces. 2020;12(42):47220–32.
51. Hashkavayi AB, Cha BS, Hwang SH, Kim J, Park KS. Highly sensitive electrochemical detection of circulating EpCAM-positive tumor cells using a dual signal amplification strategy. Sensors Actuators B Chem. 2021;343:130087.
52. Bhardwaj T, Sharma TK. Various detection techniques for aptasensing. In: Aptasensors for food safety. CRC Press; 2024. p. 155–97.
53. Hachigian TZ. A DNA aptamer transducer designed toward rapid biosensor development: a novel approach to modular biosensing platforms (Doctoral dissertation, Boise State University).
54. Cossettini A, Pasquardini L, Romani A, Feriani A, Pinamonti D, Manzano M. Computational aptamer design for spike glycoprotein (S)(SARS CoV-2) detection with an electrochemical aptasensor. Appl Microbiol Biotechnol. 2024;108(1):259.
55. Malhotra S, Verma A, Tyagi N, Kumar V. Biosensors: principle, types and applications. Int J Adv Res Innov Ideas Educ. 2017;3(2):3639–44.
56. Kaur B, Kumar S, Nedoma J, Martinek R, Marques C. Advancements in optical biosensing techniques: from fundamentals to prospects. APL Photonics. 2024;9(9):100326.

57. Ronkainen NJ, Halsall HB, Heineman WR. Electrochemical biosensors. Chem Soc Rev. 2010;39(5):1747–63.
58. Strianese M, Staiano M, Ruggiero G, Labella T, Pellecchia C, D'Auria S. Fluorescence-based biosensors. In: Spectroscopic methods of analysis: methods and protocols; 2012. p. 193–216.
59. Kaur B, Kumar S, Kaushik BK. Recent advancements in optical biosensors for cancer detection. Biosens Bioelectron. 2022;197:113805.
60. Borisov SM, Wolfbeis OS. Optical biosensors. Chem Rev. 2008;108(2):423–61.
61. Arshad F, Nabi F, Iqbal S, Khan RH. Applications of graphene-based electrochemical and optical biosensors in early detection of cancer biomarkers. Colloids Surf B: Biointerfaces. 2022;212:112356.
62. Wang TT, Huang XF, Huang H, Luo P, Qing LS. Nanomaterial-based optical-and electrochemical-biosensors for urine glucose detection: a comprehensive review. Adv Sens Energy Mater. 2022;1(3):100016.
63. Sarhadi VK, Armengol G. Molecular biomarkers in cancer. Biomolecules. 2022;12(8):1021.
64. de-los-Santos-Álvarez N, Miranda-Ordieres AJ, Tuñón-Blanco P. Aptamers as recognition elements for label-free analytical devices. TrAC Trends Anal Chem. 2008;27(5):437–46.
65. Snook KA, Zhao JZ, Alves CH, Cannata JM, Chen WH, Meyer RJ, Ritter TA, Shung KK. Design, fabrication, and evaluation of high frequency, single-element transducers incorporating different materials. IEEE Trans Ultrason Ferroelectr Freq Control. 2002;49(2):169–76.
66. Negahdary M. Aptamers in nanostructure-based electrochemical biosensors for cardiac biomarkers and cancer biomarkers: a review. Biosens Bioelectron. 2020;152:112018.
67. Cheng AK, Sen D, Yu HZ. Design and testing of aptamer-based electrochemical biosensors for proteins and small molecules. Bioelectrochemistry. 2009;77(1):1–2.
68. Tothill IE. Biosensors for cancer markers diagnosis. In: Seminars in cell & developmental biology 2009 Feb 1, vol. 20(1). Academic. p. 55–62.
69. Zhou J, Battig MR, Wang Y. Aptamer-based molecular recognition for biosensor development. Anal Bioanal Chem. 2010;398:2471–80.
70. Famulok M, Mayer G. Aptamer modules as sensors and detectors. Acc Chem Res. 2011;44(12):1349–58.
71. Hianik T. Aptamer-based biosensors. In: Encyclopedia of interfacial chemistry, vol. 7; 2018. p. 11–9.
72. Kangarshahi BM, Naghib SM. Nanogenosensors based on aptamers and peptides for bioelectrochemical cancer detection: an overview of recent advances in emerging materials and technologies. Discov Appl Sci. 2024;6(2):47.
73. Fitzgerald RC, Antoniou AC, Fruk L, Rosenfeld N. The future of early cancer detection. Nat Med. 2022;28(4):666–77.
74. Qiao Y, Shi Y, Ji M, Wang Z, Bai X, Zhang K, Yin K, Zhang Y, Chen X, Zhang Y, Lu J. Selection and identification of a prohibitin 2-binding DNA aptamer for tumor tissue imaging and targeted chemotherapy. Int J Biol Macromol. 2024;259:129002.
75. Hu X, Zhang D, Zeng Z, Huang L, Lin X, Hong S. Aptamer-based probes for cancer diagnostics and treatment. Life. 2022;12(11):1937.
76. Deng G, Zha H, Luo H, Zhou Y. Aptamer-conjugated gold nanoparticles and their diagnostic and therapeutic roles in cancer. Front Bioeng Biotechnol. 2023;11:1118546.
77. Rusling JF, Forster RJ. Biosensors designed for clinical applications. Biomedicines. 2021;9(7):702.
78. MacKay S, Wishart D, Xing JZ, Chen J. Developing trends in aptamer-based biosensor devices and their applications. IEEE Trans Biomed Circ Syst. 2014;8(1):4–14.
79. Velasco-Garcia M, Missailidis S. New trends in aptamer-based electrochemical biosensors. Gene Ther Mol Biol. 2009;13(1):1.
80. Muhammad M, Huang Q. A review of aptamer-based SERS biosensors: design strategies and applications. Talanta. 2021;227:122188.
81. Xiang W, Lv Q, Shi H, Xie B, Gao L. Aptamer-based biosensor for detecting carcinoembryonic antigen. Talanta. 2020;214:120716.

82. Wu L, Wang Y, Xu X, Liu Y, Lin B, Zhang M, Zhang J, Wan S, Yang C, Tan W. Aptamer-based detection of circulating targets for precision medicine. Chem Rev. 2021;121(19):12035–105.
83. McConnell EM, Nguyen J, Li Y. Aptamer-based biosensors for environmental monitoring. Front Chem. 2020;8:434.
84. Liu S, Xu Y, Jiang X, Tan H, Ying B. Translation of aptamers toward clinical diagnosis and commercialization. Biosens Bioelectron. 2022;208:114168.
85. Kumar Kulabhusan P, Hussain B, Yüce M. Current perspectives on aptamers as diagnostic tools and therapeutic agents. Pharmaceutics. 2020;12(7):646.
86. Yoo H, Jo H, Oh SS. Detection and beyond: challenges and advances in aptamer-based biosensors. Mater Adv. 2020;1(8):2663–87.
87. Malecka K, Mikuła E, Ferapontova EE. Design strategies for electrochemical aptasensors for cancer diagnostic devices. Sensors. 2021;21(3):736.
88. Aslan Y, Atabay M, Chowdhury HK, Göktürk I, Saylan Y, Inci F. Aptamer-based point-of-care devices: emerging technologies and integration of computational methods. Biosensors. 2023;13(5):569.
89. Mu Y, Chen Z, Zhan J, Zhang J. Recent advances in aptamer-based sensors for in vitro detection of small molecules. Anal Sens. 2024;4:e202400027.
90. Sharma R, Ragavan KV, Thakur MS, Raghavarao KS. Recent advances in nanoparticle based aptasensors for food contaminants. Biosens Bioelectron. 2015;74:612–27.
91. Suresh L, Brahman PK, Reddy KR, Bondili JS. Development of an electrochemical immunosensor based on gold nanoparticles incorporated chitosan biopolymer nanocomposite film for the detection of prostate cancer using PSA as biomarker. Enzym Microb Technol. 2018;112:43–51.
92. Pingarrón JM, Yanez-Sedeno P, González-Cortés A. Gold nanoparticle-based electrochemical biosensors. Electrochim Acta. 2008;53(19):5848–66.
93. Zhang C, Miao P, Sun M, Yan M, Liu H. Progress in miRNA detection using graphene material–based biosensors. Small. 2019;15(38):1901867.
94. Kim J, Park SJ, Min DH. Emerging approaches for graphene oxide biosensor. Anal Chem. 2017;89(1):232–48.
95. Li F, Xu H, Zhao Y. Magnetic particles as promising circulating tumor cell catchers assisting liquid biopsy in cancer diagnosis: a review. TrAC Trends Anal Chem. 2021;145:116453.
96. Ren Q, Ga L, Lu Z, Ai J, Wang T. Aptamer-functionalized nanomaterials for biological applications. Mater Chem Front. 2020;4(6):1569–85.
97. Zhang Q, Wang H, Liu Q, Zeng N, Fu G, Qiu Y, Yang Y, Yuan H, Wang W, Li B. Exosomes as powerful biomarkers in cancer: recent advances in isolation and detection techniques. Int J Nanomedicine. 2024;19:1923–49.
98. Omage JI, Easterday E, Rumph JT, Brula I, Hill B, Kristensen J, Ha DT, Galindo CL, Danquah MK, Sims N, Nguyen VT. Cancer diagnostics and early detection using electrochemical aptasensors. Micromachines. 2022;13(4):522.
99. Röthlisberger P, Gasse C, Hollenstein M. Nucleic acid aptamers: emerging applications in medical imaging, nanotechnology, neurosciences, and drug delivery. Int J Mol Sci. 2017;18(11):2430.
100. Dilnawaz F. Multifunctional mesoporous silica nanoparticles for cancer therapy and imaging. Curr Med Chem. 2019;26(31):5745–63.
101. Yüce M, Ullah N, Budak H. Trends in aptamer selection methods and applications. Analyst. 2015;140(16):5379–99.
102. Vandghanooni S, Barar J, Eskandani M, Omidi Y. Aptamer-conjugated mesoporous silica nanoparticles for simultaneous imaging and therapy of cancer. TrAC Trends Anal Chem. 2020;123:115759.
103. Chiu TC, Huang CC. Aptamer-functionalized nano-biosensors. Sensors. 2009;9(12):10356–88.
104. Mahmoudpour M, Ding S, Lyu Z, Ebrahimi G, Du D, Dolatabadi JE, Torbati M, Lin Y. Aptamer functionalized nanomaterials for biomedical applications: recent advances and new horizons. Nano Today. 2021;39:101177.

105. Kudłak B, Wieczerzak M. Aptamer based tools for environmental and therapeutic monitoring: a review of developments, applications, future perspectives. Crit Rev Environ Sci Technol. 2020;50(8):816–67.
106. Han K, Liang Z, Zhou N. Design strategies for aptamer-based biosensors. Sensors. 2010;10(5):4541–57.
107. Li ZH, Ge RT, Zhou J, Zhang YF, Zhang SY. Organocatalytic asymmetric tandem reaction for the enantioselective synthesis of chiral oxindoles to construct CyK dyes. Perspective. 2024;5(2):101188
108. Dunn MR, McCloskey CM, Buckley P, Rhea K, Chaput JC. Generating biologically stable TNA aptamers that function with high affinity and thermal stability. J Am Chem Soc. 2020;142(17):7721–4.
109. Xie S, Wang Z, Fu T, Zheng L, Wu H, He L, Huang H, Yang C, Wang R, Qian X, Qiu L. Engineering aptamers with selectively enhanced biostability in the tumor microenvironment. Angew Chem Int Ed. 2022;61(31):e202201220.
110. Kong D, Thompson IA, Maganzini N, Eisenstein M, Soh HT. Aptamer–antibody chimera sensors for sensitive, rapid, and reversible molecular detection in complex samples. ACS Sensors. 2024;9(3):1168–77.
111. Du S, Ge Y, Lu Z, Du W, Zhang Z, Zhang H. Selection and application of highly specific Salmonella typhimurium aptamers against matrix interference. Biosens Bioelectron. 2024;249:116013.
112. Orlov AV. Real-time detection of molecular markers in complex biological matrices. In: 2022 international conference laser optics (ICLO) 2022 June 20. IEEE; 2022. p. 1.
113. Duan H, Tang SY, Goda K, Li M. Enhancing the sensitivity and stability of electrochemical aptamer-based sensors by AuNPs@ MXene nanocomposite for continuous monitoring of biomarkers. Biosens Bioelectron. 2024;246:115918.
114. Arroyo-Currás N, Dauphin-Ducharme P, Scida K, Chávez JL. From the beaker to the body: translational challenges for electrochemical, aptamer-based sensors. Anal Methods. 2020;12(10):1288–310.
115. Pandey SK, Parul M, Santhanam M. Aptamer-guided selective delivery of therapeutics to breast cancer cells expressing specific biomarkers. Curr Cancer Ther Rev. 2024;20(5):434–60.
116. Paul AR, Falsaperna M, Lavender H, Garrett MD, Serpell CJ. Selection of optimised ligands by fluorescence-activated bead sorting. Chem Sci. 2023;14(35):9517–25.
117. Nordin FJ, Ming LW, Teo MYM, In LLA. Aptamer development for cancer diagnostic. In: Rapid antigen testing. IntechOpen; 2023.
118. Tsai YC, Weng WY, Yeh YT, Chien JC. Dual-aptamer drift canceling techniques to improve long-term stability of real-time structure-switching aptasensors. ACS Sens. 2023;8(9):3380–8.
119. Wu G, Zhang ET, Qiang Y, Esmonde C, Chen X, Wei Z, Song Y, Zhang X, Schneider MJ, Li H, Sun H. Long-term In vivo molecular monitoring using aptamer-graphene microtransistors. bioRxiv. 2023 Oct 20.
120. Fang Z, Feng X, Tang F, Jiang H, Han S, Tao R, Lu C. Aptamer screening: current methods and future trend towards non-SELEX approach. Biosensors. 2024;14(7):350.
121. Le A, Teclemichael E, Krylova S, Krylov S. Quantitative characterization of stringency in SELEX. JACS Au. 2024;4:4910–20.
122. Zhu C, Feng Z, Qin H, Chen L, Yan M, Li L, Qu F. Recent progress of SELEX methods for screening nucleic acid aptamers. Talanta. 2024;266:124998.
123. Alkhamis O, Canoura J, Willis C, Wang L, Perry J, Xiao Y. Comparison of aptamer signaling mechanisms reveals disparities in sensor response and strategies to eliminate false signals. J Am Chem Soc. 2023;145(22):12407–22.
124. Sen A, Poulsen H, Sondhauss S, Hodgkiss JM. How saliva interferes with colorimetric gold nanoparticle aptasensors: understanding and mitigating surface interactions. ACS Sens. 2023;8(4):1841–9.
125. Davydova A, Vorobyeva M. Aptamer-based biosensors for the colorimetric detection of blood biomarkers: paving the way to clinical laboratory testing. Biomedicines. 2022;10(7):1606.

126. Buglak AA, Samokhvalov AV, Zherdev AV, Dzantiev BB. Methods and applications of in silico aptamer design and modeling. Int J Mol Sci. 2020;21(22):8420.
127. Akhlaghi AA, Kaur H, Adhikari BR, Soleymani L. Challenges and opportunities for developing electrochemical biosensors with commercialization potential in the point-of-care diagnostics market. ECS Sens Plus. 2024;3:011601.
128. Zhang Y, Li Y. Clinical translation of Aptamers for COVID-19. J Med Chem. 2023;66(24):16568–78.
129. Mehmood S, Khan AZ, Bilal M, Sohail A, Iqbal HM. Aptamer-based biosensors: a novel toolkit for early diagnosis of cancer. Mater Today Chem. 2019;12:353–60.
130. Huang Z, Wang D, Zhang Q, Zhang Y, Peng R, Tan W. Leveraging aptamer-based DNA nanotechnology for bioanalysis and cancer therapeutics. Acc Mater Res. 2024;5(4):438–52.
131. Shahazi R, Saddam AI, Islam MR, Rahman MM, Paimard G, Kumer A, Alam MM, Mahamud MK. Recent progress in nanomaterial-based biosensors for the detection of cancer biomarkers in human fluids. Nano Carbons. 2024;2(2):1254.
132. Stanciu LA, Wei Q, Barui AK, Mohammad N. Recent advances in aptamer-based biosensors for global health applications. Annu Rev Biomed Eng. 2021;23(1):433–59.
133. Abdel-Karim R. Nanotechnology-enabled biosensors: a review of fundamentals, materials, applications, challenges, and future scope. Biomed Mater Devices. 2024;2(2):759–77.
134. Rahimizadeh K, ul ain Zahra Q, Chen S, Le BT, Ullah I, Veedu RN. Nanoparticles-assisted aptamer biosensing for the detection of environmental pathogens. Environ Res. 2023;238:117123. https://doi.org/10.1016/j.envres.2023.117123.
135. Štukovnik Z, Fuchs-Godec R, Bren U. Nanomaterials and their recent applications in impedimetric biosensing. Biosensors. 2023;13(10):899.
136. Stangherlin S, Liu J. Nanomaterials enabled and enhanced DNA-based biosensors. J Mater Chem B. 2023;11(30):6994–7003.
137. Dkhar DS, Kumari R, Patel V, Srivastava A, Prasad R, Srivastava R, Chandra P. Versatile approaches of quantum dots in biosensing and imaging. Wiley Interdiscip Rev Nanomed Nanobiotechnol. 2024;16(5):e1998.
138. Chiu NF, Tai MJ, Yang HT. Fundamental studies of graphene oxide quantum dots for plasmonic properties and microRNAs in sensing mechanism. In: Biophotonics in point-of-care III 2024 Jun 20, vol. 13008. SPIE; 2024. p. 159–64.
139. Fu L, Lin CT, Karimi-Maleh H, Chen F, Zhao S. Plasmonic nanoparticle-enhanced optical techniques for cancer biomarker sensing. Biosensors. 2023;13(11):977.
140. Bhaiyya M, Panigrahi D, Rewatkar P, Haick H. Role of machine learning assisted biosensors in point-of-care-testing for clinical decisions. ACS Sens. 2024;9(9):4495–519.
141. Chennupati A. Artificial intelligence and machine learning for early cancer prediction and response. World J Adv Eng Technol Sci. 2024;12(1):035–40.
142. Odah M. Artificial Intelligence (AI) and Machine Learning (ML) in diagnosing cancer: current trends.
143. Lee SJ, Cho J, Lee BH, Hwang D, Park JW. Design and prediction of aptamers assisted by in silico methods. Biomedicines. 2023;11(2):356.
144. Perez Tobia J, Huang PJ, Ding Y, Saran Narayan R, Narayan A, Liu J. Machine learning directed aptamer search from conserved primary sequences and secondary structures. ACS Synth Biol. 2023;12(1):186–95.
145. Mahmoudian F, Ahmari A, Shabani S, Sadeghi B, Fahimirad S, Fattahi F. Aptamers as an approach to targeted cancer therapy. Cancer Cell Int. 2024;24(1):108.
146. Manna S, Mahata R, Dey SK, Das Chaudhuri A, Choudhury SM. Multifunctional aptamer grafted targeted nano-drugs execute molecular cross-talks with cancer cells. Appl Res. 2024;3(4):e202300115.
147. Tiwari C, Tomer J, Kumar D. Liposomal drug delivery: progress, clinical outlook, and ongoing challenges. Recent Adv Drug Deliv Formul. 2024;18(3):157–69.
148. Zubair M, Riaz M, Kiani MN, Aslam HM, Fatima AE, Sultan HM, Rehman AU. Application of nanotechnology for targeted drug delivery and nontoxicity. Int J Green Pharm Nanomed. 2024;2(2):57–67.

149. Ayass MA, Tripathi T, Griko N, Okyay T, Ramankutty Nair R, Zhang J, Zhu K, Melendez K, Pashkov V, Abi-Mosleh L. Dual checkpoint aptamer immunotherapy: unveiling tailored cancer treatment targeting CTLA-4 and NKG2A. Cancers. 2024;16(5):1041.
150. Pastor F. Aptamers: a new technological platform in cancer immunotherapy. Pharmaceuticals. 2016;9(4):64.
151. Zhang D, Zheng Y, Lin Z, Liu X, Li J, Yang H, Tan W. Equipping natural killer cells with specific targeting and checkpoint blocking aptamers for enhanced adoptive immunotherapy in solid tumors. Angew Chem. 2020;132(29):12120–6.
152. Xiong H, Liu L, Liu X, Jiang H, Wang X. Aptamer-based immune drug systems (AptIDCs) potentiating cancer immunotherapy. Chemistry. 2023;5(3):1656–80.
153. Ramos C, Ramos C, Senechal V, Ruez R, Delebecq S. Integrative multimodality spatial biomarker analysis for tailoring checkpoint inhibitor therapies in non-small cell lung cancer. J Clin Oncol. 2024;42:e14664.
154. Yao W, Sun W, Fan Y, Xiao J, Wang T, Huang K, Liu L, Wang X, Jiang H. Aptamer-based electrochemical analysis platform for tumor cells and biomarkers detection. J Electroanal Chem. 2024;960:118194.
155. Kiani P, Vatankhahan H, Zare-Hoseinabadi A, Ferdosi F, Ehtiati S, Heidari P, Dorostgou Z, Movahedpour A, Baktash A, Rajabivahid M, Khatami SH. Electrochemical biosensors for early detection of breast cancer. Clin Chim Acta. 2024;564:119923.
156. Ma S, Zhao W, Liu X, Li Y, Ma P, Zhang K, Zhang Q. A novel microfluidic chip integrating with microcolumn array electrodes for rapid and ultrasensitive detection of alpha-fetoprotein. Anal Chim Acta. 2024;1291:342240.
157. Achi F, Attar AM, Lahcen AA. Electrochemical nanobiosensors for the detection of cancer biomarkers in real samples: trends and challenges. TrAC Trends Anal Chem. 2024;170:117423.
158. Futane A, Narayanamurthy V, Jadhav P, Srinivasan A. Aptamer-based rapid diagnosis for point-of-care application. Microfluid Nanofluid. 2023;27(2):15.
159. Ponnada S, Yadav S, Gorle DB, Devi M, Palariya A, Bose RS, Sharma RK. Challenges and advances in aptamer-based biosensing approaches. In: Aptasensors for point-of-care diagnostics. p. 248–70.
160. Tabar FS, Yazdian F, Rashedi H, Rahdar A, Fathi-karkan S, Ferreira LF. Ultrasensitive aptamer-based electrochemical nanobiosensor in diagnosis of prostate cancer using 2D: 2D reduced graphene oxide/graphitic carbon nitride decorated with Au nanoparticles. Eur J Med Chem Rep. 2024;12:100192.
161. Chen L, Yang G, Qu F. Aptamer-based sensors for fluid biopsies of protein disease markers. Talanta. 2024;276:126246.
162. Hemdan M, Ali MA, Doghish AS, Mageed SS, Elazab IM, Khalil MM, Mabrouk M, Das DB, Amin AS. Innovations in biosensor technologies for healthcare diagnostics and therapeutic drug monitoring: applications, recent progress, and future research challenges. Sensors (Basel, Switzerland). 2024;24(16):5143.
163. Olejnik B, Kozioł A, Brzozowska E, Ferens-Sieczkowska M. Application of selected biosensor techniques in clinical diagnostics. Expert Rev Mol Diagn. 2021;21(9):925–37.
164. Lafi Z, Gharaibeh L, Nsairat H, Asha N, Alshaer W. Aptasensors: employing molecular probes for precise medical diagnostics and drug monitoring. Bioanalysis. 2023;15(23):1439–60.

Aptamer-Based Biosensors for Cancer Therapy Monitoring

11

Ashok Thulluru, Sarad Pawar Naik Bukke,
Bala Sai Soujith Nidamanuri, and Nawaz Mohammed

11.1 Introduction

Cancer represents the leading cause of global mortality while also acting as the main disease factor, yet it requires never-ending improvements regarding diagnostic and therapeutic strategies. Patient results improve, and side effects decrease whenever medical assessments evaluate cancer treatments through drug measurement and personalized patient response evaluation [1]. Cancer monitoring techniques through imaging and biomarker methods currently fail to achieve real-time diagnoses because they do not include efficient response speed and sensitive measurement features with specific identification capabilities. Aptamers apply solutions to the current healthcare system issues [2]. The selectivity of aptamer function in biosensing relies on the single-stranded nucleic acid's ability to achieve high specificity in binding. According to research data, single-stranded nucleic acid aptamers offer superior performance to antibodies by maintaining stability at affordable production prices for cancer surveillance biosensors [3]. Real-time cancer management systems can achieve their objectives with biosensors that perform therapeutic drug

A. Thulluru (✉)
Department of Pharmaceutics, Sandip University School of Pharmaceutical Sciences, Nashik, Maharashtra, India

S. P. N. Bukke
Department of Pharmaceutics, School of Pharmacy, Kampala International University, Western Campus, Ishaka, Uganda

B. S. S. Nidamanuri
Department of Health Informatics, Governor's State University, Chicago, IL, USA

N. Mohammed
Department of Pharmaceutics, Raghavendra Institute of Pharmaceutical Education and Research (Autonomous), Anantapur, Andhra Pradesh, India

S. Srivastava et al. (eds.), *Biosensors and Aptamers*,
https://doi.org/10.1007/978-981-96-8387-1_11

observation, cancer biomarker identification, and molecular treatment assessment procedures [4]. Aptamer sensors benefit from precise setting methods to achieve rapid, noninvasive medical tests for individualized treatments that do not need biopsy specimens for patient examination [5]. Biosensor principles built on aptamers are explored through studies focusing on both development methods while analyzing their rising importance for enhancing monitoring systems used in cancer treatment [6].

11.1.1 Overview of Cancer Therapy Monitoring

Oncology depends heavily on cancer therapy analysis to determine outcomes with reduced adverse effects during real-time evaluations. Biopsies combined with blood tests and imaging test monitoring methods display insufficient sensitivities, which limit their ability to detect in real time. Traditional monitoring techniques are inadequate for detecting rapid changes between drug performance levels and drug treatment effectiveness and changing drug amounts. The increase in market demand in recent years has led to the parallel development of sophisticated monitoring solutions. The scientific community has verified that aptamer-based biosensors are potential tools for ongoing cancer therapy observation. The fast, Highly sensitive, and noninvasive properties of these sensors achieve better measurement outcomes when compared to typical detection platforms for cancer biomarkers and drug tracking operations. Accurate monitoring is vital to healthcare providers since future cancer treatment depends on exact measurement protocols. Medical professionals can modify treatment plans by studying live monitoring data, which presents information about tumor markers and drug concentrations to help identify drug-resistant diseases soon after their emergence. This method enables practitioners to develop improved drug therapy techniques and dosage adjustment capabilities that aid in forecasting adverse drug responses to achieve superior results [7]. Through aptamer-based biosensors, medical practice gains better patient monitoring capabilities by evaluating disease development alongside drug responsiveness. New technologies grant patients better comfort and financial advantages through the ability to minimize invasive patient treatment requirements [8–10].

11.1.2 Importance of Biosensors in Cancer Management

Biosensors have become essential tools for modern cancer patient management since their devices help quickly identify sensitive biomarkers to assess cancer development and therapeutic results. The medical procedure based on imaging tests along with biopsies proves inadequate for therapy monitoring because it requires extensive time and invasive methods that prevent early relapse detection. Implementing biosensors with aptamers enables medical cancer treatment to function more efficiently without causing serious invasive complications. Biosensors enable fast marker detection of biomolecular and cancer-specific elements, enabling physicians to reorganize therapy approaches and create tailored treatment plans to improve patient care [11, 12]. Incorporating biosensors in cancer therapy monitoring facilitates ongoing, real-time evaluation of drug concentrations, treatment effectiveness, and the development of therapeutic resistance. Through biosensing systems, aptamers enable the detection of very small biomarker concentration changes to observe cancer treatment responses at every developmental stage. The healthcare provider uses distinct patient responses to adapt medication dosages when offering personalized cancer patient care [13]. The microfluidic systems with lab-on-a-chip (LoC) networks include biosensors as their main components, which perform simultaneous multiple biomarker detection functions [14]. Biosensor technology enables nonsurgical diagnostic procedures with precise results alongside unaltered accuracy levels. Healthcare facilities benefit from archives through two primary functions: satisfactory patient care and economical medical service delivery. Nanomaterial-enhanced sensors utilizing signal amplification methods became better through research development for standard clinical cancer management applications [15, 16].

11.1.3 Aptamers: A Concise Overview and Their Function in Biosensing

DNA or RNA nucleic acid sequences form short single-stranded sequences that evolve through the Systematic Evolution of Ligands by Exponential Enrichment (SELEX) selection process. The target detection capability of aptamers extends to proteins, small compounds, and whole cells using this method. Through their synthetic origin, aptamers achieve higher performance characteristics than biological receptors, especially antibodies. The synthesis process for aptamers remains easy to execute, while their environmental stability covers a broad spectrum, and their application options can be tailored to diverse purposes [17]. Aptamers offer powerful binding specificities and exceptional affinity properties, which qualify them as advanced biosensing compounds for biomarker analytical work in cancer therapy oversight [18]. These properties in aptamers enable their effective use within multiple biosensing applications. Highly specific detection of low-abundance targets can be achieved using biosensors that link aptamers with transducers. The detection portion of biosensing platforms depends on optical sensors, electrochemical sensors, and mass-based sensors. Information from these platforms becomes measurement-ready because of how aptamers interact with their targets [19]. Medical professionals gain accurate biomarker detection capacities for fluid diagnoses alongside treatment assessment frameworks through aptamer-based biosensors used in cancer therapy. The detection system integrates sensors that enable biomarker analysis while monitoring the behavior changes that cancer responds to treatment [20]. Aptamers are fundamental medical technology because healthcare experts use them to develop personalized medicine strategies. The diverse applications of aptamers make them critical assets for biosensors, and their capacity to measure treatment effects precisely enables better cancer monitoring tools for oncology diagnostics and treatment strategy improvement [21].

11.2 Fundamentals of Aptamer-Enhanced Biosensors

The binding affinity between aptamers and their specific target molecules, which often include cancer indicators, enables the operation of these biosensors. Numerous transduction methods enable the signal detection resulting from the target molecule binding with its aptamer counterpart. Due to their strong target selectivity, aptamers are suitable tools for accurate cancer screening procedures and medical therapy assessments [22–24]. Oncological treatment yields substantial potential from aptamers that include DNA and RNA sequences, peptides, and small molecules as well as cellular structures. These specific aptamers bind to cancer-relevant sites to be used for accurate diagnostic tests, delivery systems, and therapeutic approaches that enable gene suppression, early-stage cancer recognition, and customized therapeutic plans [25].

DNA Aptamers DNA aptamers have gained scientists' attention in cancer treatment because they provide excellent specificity, high-affinity properties, and easy adaptability. Single-stranded DNA oligonucleotide molecules have unique binding characteristics to seek out cancer cell receptors and proteins, allowing for exact treatment of specific cancers. Research shows that DNA aptamers create a successful method to guide cancer cell targeting while delivering medicine to specific cells through immunological response control systems. The research community assessed the capability of DNA aptamers to target epidermal growth factor receptor (EGFR) for cancer treatment to provide specific therapeutic drug delivery or immune response strengthening against tumor cells. DNA aptamers present a practical solution for resolving the medical problems faced by traditional medicines, including adverse effects and systemic toxicity. Xenoparticle-aptamer complexes developed recently enable directed chemotherapy delivery to cancer cells, thus creating more effective treatment outcomes accompanied by fewer side effects [26, 27]. Medical diagnosis platforms gain improved capabilities in detecting unique biomarkers of malignant tissue through the integration of aptamers. DNA aptamers hold promising clinical utility for cancer immunotherapy according to bioengineering research, and these aptamers work better with immune checkpoint inhibitors to enhance treatment effects [28, 29].

RNA Aptamers RNA aptamers serve as modern therapeutic instruments in cancer treatment due to their enhanced capability to bind to specific locations. The delivery of cancer-related medications uses aptamers as diagnostic instruments, therapeutic agents, and target-specific tools. Molecular compounds maintain a high level of adaptability in the detection of cancer-related proteins and their interactions with cell receptors and nucleic acids [30–33]. The delivery system created by chemotherapies and radiolabeled substances bound to aptamers improves therapeutic results while minimizing adverse drug reactions. Because of their binding properties, RNA aptamers find applications in cancer immunotherapy by promoting immune checkpoint inhibitor effects and helping T cell activation despite cancer cell immune escape mechanisms [34, 35]. Researchers have conducted studies during the past years to evaluate RNA aptamers as potential therapeutic weapons against cancer stem cells (CSCs) because of these cells' immune resistance properties. Aptamers function as marker detectors on cancer stem cells (CSCs) through their specific recognition ability to develop therapeutic drug guides that shrink tumors and reduce recurrence threats. Metastasis develops incidentally when scientists create aptamers that limit cancer cell signaling to stop locomotion and invasion processes [36]. Research teams seeking clinical applications of RNA aptamers for cancer treatment dedicate efforts to create stability boosters and immunologic protections as well as to develop delivery frameworks [37]. Precision oncology medical care needs aptamer medical applications combined with nanotechnology and gene editing platforms to create better-advanced treatment options.

Peptide Aptamers The modern field of cancer treatment research involves developing short synthetic peptides that bind exclusively to their target locations. Research verifies that these substances present opportunities to function as next-generation molecular devices that selectively attack cancer cells and retard tumor development. Aptamers function as cancer biomarker-specific adhesives to produce platforms for drug delivery systems and diagnostic equipment delivery platforms. The specific treatment method removes unwanted side effects commonly found in chemotherapy to yield improved therapeutic gains for patients. Targeted medication delivery serves as a significant application where peptide aptamers act as cancer treatment guides to isolate therapy delivery exclusively to cancer cells. Modern research shows that aptamers improve nanoparticle drug delivery systems through nanomedicine by specifically directing cancer cells for treatment with reduced injury to healthy tissue [38]. Scientific researchers study aptamers as potential therapeutic immunology agents during their investigations. The immune response performs better with aptamers targeting immunological checkpoints or regulating immune system activities [39]. Scientific investigation demonstrates how peptide aptamers can detect cancer at early stages by recognizing cancer-associated antigens for proper medical interventions [40]. Recent developments have not eliminated the stability-related issues and expense concerns scientists must handle. Research groups dedicate themselves to finding solutions for the limitations of creating peptide aptamers suitable for cancer therapy.

Small-Molecule Aptamers Medical molecules are powerful therapeutic instruments in cancer treatments because they feature biomarker binding attributes, specific target attachment features, and species selection. Scientific engineering produces short molecules, creating RNA or DNA structures that focus exclusively on cancer cell biomolecules and proteins or lipids. Aptamer size has medical value in cancer therapy by cutting expenses while removing unintentional antigen-based binding effects [41]. Small-molecule aptamers demonstrate confirmed therapeutic potential as specific therapeutic agents based on results obtained from multiple scientific investigations. The epidermal growth factor receptor (EGFR) binds aptamers to stop cancer progression and metastasis in lung cancer patients with EGFR overexpression as well as those with breast cancer. Scientists created additional aptamers that specifically targeted PD-L1, which allowed successful treatment of tumor immune evasion through combination use with immune checkpoint inhibitors, according to [4]. Biomedical research demonstrates that aptamers achieve higher therapeutic potential when medical personnel combine them with transportation agents, including chemotherapeutic agents and siRNA and nanoparticles, to improve delivery effectiveness while minimizing side effects. Drug delivery systems that involve aptamers have demonstrated their therapeutic ability to overcome standard cancer therapy barriers [42].

Cell-Based Aptamers The production of these compounds occurs through engineering processes to detect surface proteins that exist exclusively on cancer cells. Scientific research confirms that aptamers function effectively together with therapeutic agents containing cytotoxic drugs, siRNA, and nanoparticles to improve their delivery parameters for cancer cells. The epidermal growth factor receptor (EGFR) is the target for aptamers discovered in research experiments that show strong suppression of breast cancer cell growth in model experiments [43]. The association between aptamers and immunotherapy in cancer treatment research aims to identify novel approaches against cancer cell immune evasion mechanics. Scientists optimize the target affinity of aptamers and their stability level to enhance drug effectiveness in therapeutic treatment [44]. The potential for future application of aptamers faces technical difficulties in biological environment stability and delivery system creation alongside immunological reaction control systems. Recovery processes that combine nanoparticles with stable aptamers now create improved solutions for therapeutic outcomes [1]. Table 11.1 displays different operative mechanisms of aptamer-based biosensors used for cancer therapy while illustrating their current medical applications.

11.2.1 Mechanisms of Aptamer-Target Interactions

Aptamers employ their distinctive binding selectivity to detect various targets, including proteins, nucleic acids, molecules, and additional target classes. Nucleic acids called aptamers fold into distinct shapes that allow their binding to target molecules through noncovalent molecular bonds. Among noncovalent forces aptamers use to bond with their targets are strong hydrogen bonds, van der Waals interactions, and electrostatic forces as well as base stack interactions. Aptamer structures make possible the identification of various targets, including cancer biomarkers consisting

Table 11.1 Categories of aptamer-based biosensors for cancer therapy classified by their operational principles and applications

Type	Principle	Applications	Ref.
DNA aptamers	DNA aptamers are synthetic oligonucleotides that bind specifically to target molecules through hydrogen bonding and base pairing	Used for targeted cancer therapy, cancer biomarker detection, and diagnostic purposes	[45]
RNA aptamers	RNA aptamers are single-stranded RNA molecules that bind to targets via specific sequences and secondary structures	Applied in drug delivery, tumor imaging, and targeted cancer therapies	[46]
Peptide aptamers	Peptide aptamers are short peptides that fold into specific structures to bind their targets with high specificity	Used in targeting cancer cell receptors and as inhibitors of cancer-related pathways	[47]
Small-molecule aptamers	Small-molecule aptamers bind to low molecular weight compounds, allowing detection or inhibition of specific molecules	Applied in drug development, biomarker detection, and diagnosis of cancer	[48]
Cell-based aptamers	Cell-based aptamers target specific surface proteins or receptors on cancer cells, facilitating targeted drug delivery	Used for targeted delivery of therapeutic agents to cancer cells and immune modulation	[49]

of tumor-specific antigens together with extracellular matrix proteins as well as circulating tumor DNA. The biomarker detection features of aptamers yield high precision to identify minimal levels of molecular indicators that reside in malignant cells. Aptamers enable outstanding cancer disease monitoring because they permit treatment outcome assessment while forecasting therapeutic resistance development throughout cancer treatment duration. The target recognition mechanism of aptamers operates by induced-fit binding, which causes aptamers to structurally reform through binding interactions. Aptamer-target binding strength increases because of their ability to rearrange their structure. The capability helps researchers find particular biomarkers for therapy monitoring that provide essential tumor activity data in specified treatment periods.

The binding performance of biosensors depends directly on both aptamer interaction mechanisms and their affinity for binding targets. A biosensor's sensitivity results from two factors: the aptamer used to recognize its target and its release following recognition. High binding strength and quick dissociation kinetics are essential for aptamers that perform effective cancer therapy monitoring because they eliminate measurement interruptions from interference.

11.2.2 Types of Aptamer-Based Biosensors

Inside biosensors, the exact interactions between aptamers and their targets become measurable as they generate tools with multiple detection capabilities. The sensors' classification depends on transduction methods because these methods convert aptamer-target binding into detectable signals. The employed transduction methods serve as classifiers for aptamer-based biosensors. Assessments of cancer therapy by aptamer-based biosensors primarily rely on optical detection systems and electrochemical systems as well as mass-based detection systems.

(a) ***Optical Aptamer-Based Biosensors:*** The optical biosensing system operates largely for biosensing evaluations by producing real-time high-resolution information from operations that do not need labeled samples or complicated processing protocols. The detection methods in optical sensor systems measure bindings between aptamers and targets through light parameter changes in absorbance and fluorescence and surface plasmon resonance (SPR). Aptamers operate as fluorescent components to identify particular cancer biomarkers in patient serum when bound to fluorescent molecules in a biosensor system. Biomarker concentration evaluation for drug therapy monitoring or tumor marker detection happens when target substances link to sensor devices, which causes fluorescence light signals to change [50].
(b) ***Electrochemical Aptamer-Based Biosensors:*** Electrochemical aptamer-based biosensors utilize aptamers as biorecognition elements for specific target detection. These sensors convert biomolecular interactions into measurable electrical signals, offering high sensitivity, selectivity, and real-time analysis. Their compact design and low cost make them ideal for clinical diagnostics, environmental monitoring, and point-of-care applications. [51].
(c) ***Mass-Based Aptamer-Driven Biosensors:*** Mass variations can be detected at biosensor surfaces by mass-sensitive instruments, specifically surface plasmon resonance (SPR) and quartz crystal microbalance (QCM) sensors. These sensors show better sensitivity because they detect low cancer indicator amounts instantaneously. Changes in the sensor surface refractive index detected by SPR technology indicate aptamer binding to targets for the purpose of label-free and real-time cancer biomarker assessment. The sensors are indispensable for measuring present-day cancer treatments' success rate [52]. A pictorial representation of aptamer-based biosensors for cancer therapy according to their transduction methods appears in Table 11.2. Fig. 11.1 shows the methods used to detect aptamers in cancer therapy using transduction techniques.

11.2.3 Advantages of Aptamers over Traditional Bioreceptors

Aptamers demonstrate essential traits that surpass traditional bioreceptor antibodies, which makes them an excellent choice for cancer therapy monitoring. Biosensing applications exploit aptamer properties, including high stability, adaptable specificity, and easy manufacturing methodology. Aptamers become more affordable to produce and easier to synthesize due to their synthetic origins compared to antibodies. The production of conventional antibodies requires multiple animal-based operations throughout manufacturing, yet developers must implement extensive tests to

Table 11.2 Categorization of aptamer-based biosensors for cancer therapy according to their transduction mechanisms

Transduction mechanism	Principle	Ref.
Optical sensors	Detect changes in light absorption or fluorescence when aptamer binds to target	[50]
Electrochemical sensors	Measure changes in the electrical properties of a sensor surface upon aptamer binding	[51]
Mass-sensitive sensors	Detect shifts in mass as aptamers interact with target molecules [e.g., surface plasmon resonance (SPR) or quartz crystal microbalance (QCM)]	[52]

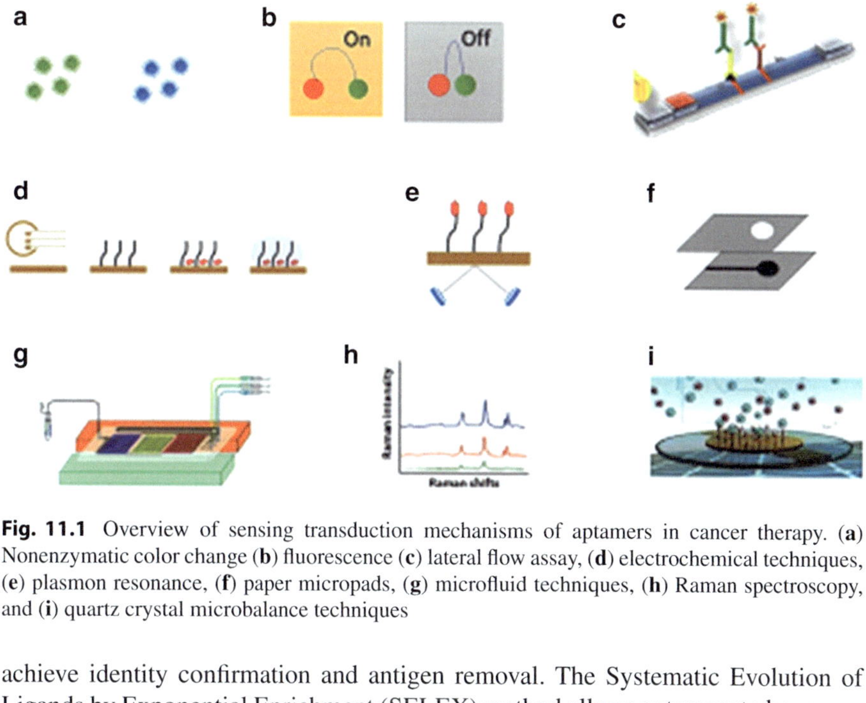

Fig. 11.1 Overview of sensing transduction mechanisms of aptamers in cancer therapy. (**a**) Nonenzymatic color change (**b**) fluorescence (**c**) lateral flow assay, (**d**) electrochemical techniques, (**e**) plasmon resonance, (**f**) paper micropads, (**g**) microfluid techniques, (**h**) Raman spectroscopy, and (**i**) quartz crystal microbalance techniques

achieve identity confirmation and antigen removal. The Systematic Evolution of Ligands by Exponential Enrichment (SELEX) method allows aptamers to be manufactured through laboratory processes, yielding quick production capacities while eliminating animal usage [53]. Enhancements in aptamer stability occur from various situations within laboratory settings. Aptamers possess structural features that maintain their binding capacity under various temperature conditions pH levels and storage conditions as well as resist multiple environmental factors. Such environmental elements cause decreased stability in antibodies compared to aptamers. Biosensors require dependable operation for cancer monitoring because patients face unpredictable and unfavorable health conditions. The chemical modification process enables aptamers to withstand enzyme degradation and grow their operational durability over time. The ability of aptamers to make flexible adjustments in specificity represents their major distinct feature. Aptamer specificity outperforms antibodies because their development process allows for one-target recognition combined with unwanted interaction blocking, but antibodies yield both false-positive and false-negative results due to their cross-reactivity. Measurement values for cancer treatment from the biosensor become more accurate because its exact biomarker detection capability blocks interference from background molecules [5]. Marine aptamers enable multiple biomarker detection on biosensors since they can simultaneously hold numerous aptamer molecules. Such real-time biomarker surveillance provides significant value to overall cancer therapy observation by measuring relevant treatment effects or evasion indicators. The primary advantages of aptamers compared to conventional receptors, which are essential for effective cancer therapy control, are:

Signal Amplification Methods The addition of nanoparticles is an effective technique for improving aptamer-based sensor sensitivity. The detection method delivers optimal recognition of scarce biomarkers that maintain essential status for cancer treatment evaluation [54, 55].

Aptamers Can Be Designed for Enhanced Stability These sensing systems offer superior performance when used in volatile cancer therapy monitoring environments because of their excellent stability. This stability facilitates continuous monitoring even in adverse physiological conditions [3, 56].

11.3 Design and Fabrication of Aptamer-Based Biosensors

To produce aptamer-based biosensors for cancer therapy monitoring, researchers must execute necessary procedures, starting with aptamer selection and optimization of surface immobilization techniques and signal amplification strategies. A biosensor system contains these fundamental components that produce sensitive and specific detection methods to identify rare cancer biomarkers in complicated biological test samples. The production method showing aptamer-based biosensor fabrication for cancer therapy monitoring is shown in Table 11.3.

Table 11.3 Development and construction of aptamer-based biosensors for monitoring cancer therapy

Parameter	Key points	Ref. no.
11.3.1. Aptamer selection and optimization	Aptamers are selected using SELEX to target cancer biomarkers They bind to molecules like circulating tumor DNA, cancer antigens, or drugs Optimized for better binding, stability, and resistance to degradation	[57]
11.3.2. Immobilization techniques for aptamers on sensor surfaces	Aptamers are immobilized using covalent bonding, physisorption, or affinity interactions Example: Aptamers bind to gold electrodes using thiol groups in electrochemical sensors In optical sensors, aptamers attach via flexible linkers to reduce binding interference	[16]
11.3.3. Signal amplification strategies for enhanced sensitivity	Nanomaterials (gold nanoparticles, carbon nanotubes, graphene) amplify signals by increasing surface area Enzyme labels and quantum dots enhance sensitivity to detect low biomarker levels	[58, 59]

11.4 Aptamer-Based Biosensors in Cancer Therapy Monitoring

The real-time analysis of cancer development, drug-resistant biomarkers, and treatment effectiveness represents a significant strength of aptamer-based biosensors used for cancer therapy monitoring. Short synthetic oligonucleotides known as aptamers bind precisely to target molecules that possess therapeutic medications, cancer biomarkers, and biological tumor proliferation contents. Exact binding capabilities, affordable nature, and adjustable properties help aptamer technology deliver the required sensitive biosensors for cancer treatment monitoring. Various biosensors that incorporate aptamers serve as machinery for cancer therapeutic monitoring, and Table 11.4 includes the complete list. The illustrations depicting aptamer use in cancer detection and treatment applications can be found in Fig. 11.2.

Table 11.4 Utilization of aptamer-based biosensors in monitoring cancer therapy

Application	Key points	Ref. no.
11.4.1. Detection of cancer biomarkers during treatment	Aptamers detect cancer biomarkers like ctDNA, proteins, and exosomes to assess therapeutic response and early relapse Helps identify minimal residual disease (MRD) and drug resistance Example: In breast cancer, aptamers bind to HER2 for monitoring targeted therapies	[57]
11.4.2. Monitoring therapeutic drug levels	Aptamers monitor drug levels in real time Helps adjust dosages for optimal efficacy and minimal toxicity Crucial for drugs with narrow therapeutic windows	[16]
11.4.3. Multiplexed detection for comprehensive monitoring	Multiplexed biosensors detect multiple biomarkers simultaneously for a comprehensive treatment overview Tracks DNA mutations, protein expression, and circulating tumor cells Helps predict relapse and resistance	[58]
11.4.4. Real-time tracking of treatment efficacy	Aptamers track treatment efficacy by monitoring biomarkers in real time Allows oncologists to adjust treatments based on patient response Example: Monitoring VEGF levels to assess antiangiogenic therapy effectiveness	[59]

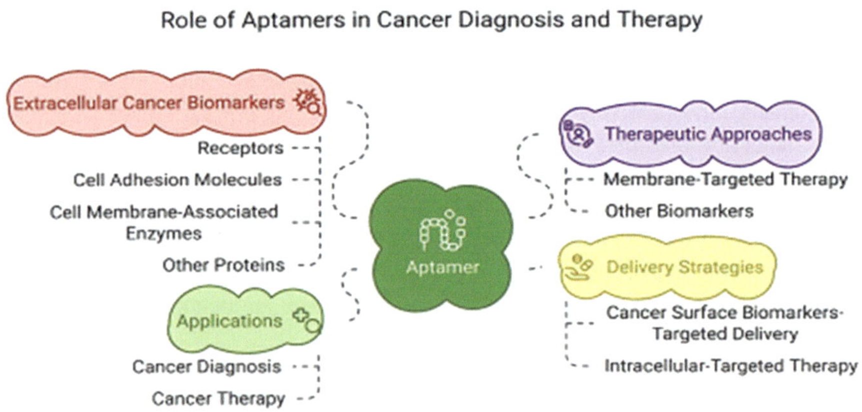

Fig. 11.2 Role of aptamers in cancer diagnosis and therapy

11.5 Advances in Aptamer-Based Biosensing Technologies

Through enhanced aptamer development and biosensing methods, doctors can perform precise treatment evaluations for cancer patient follow-up. Aptamer-based sensors show rapid development because they combine more accurate and sensitive

Table 11.5 Progress in aptamer-enhanced biosensing technologies for cancer therapy monitoring

Advancement	Key points	Ref. no.
11.5.1. Integration with microfluidics and lab-on-a-chip systems	Combines aptamers with microfluidics for fast, portable biomarker detection Enables detection from small samples, ideal for point of care (POC) Supports simultaneous biomarker detection for comprehensive tumor profiling	[16, 57]
11.5.2. Role of nanomaterials in enhancing sensor performance	Nanomaterials (e.g., gold nanoparticles, CNTs, graphene) boost sensor sensitivity Gold nanoparticles allow for precise detection through light scattering CNTs/graphene enhance electrochemical sensors for quicker, more accurate results	[58, 59]
11.5.3. Development of multiplex biosensors for comprehensive monitoring	Multiplex biosensors detect multiple biomarkers at once Provides a full picture of tumor progression and treatment response Nanomaterials enhance signal strength and data accuracy	[60, 61]

operations with the flexibility achieved through microfluidic systems combined with nanomaterials and multiplexed detection methods. Scientific innovations of today allow for real-time tumor tracking to develop aptamer-based monitoring systems that guide personal cancer treatment development. The investigation summarizes findings about aptamer-based biosensing method utilization for cancer therapy monitoring (Table 11.5).

11.6 Challenges and Limitations

The potential use of aptamer-based biosensors for cancer therapy monitoring has emerged. However, they face various obstacles in addition to their superior sensitivity, selectivity, and adjustment capabilities. Many hurdles and bounds prevent the widespread adoption of these sensors in clinical settings despite their favorable features. Conversion to clinical cancer therapy monitoring remains challenging since the sensors require improvements toward increased sensitivity, better stability, reduced cost, and enhanced repeatability. The current research summarizes (Table 11.6) to summarize the obstacles and boundaries that aptamer-based biosensors face when used to monitor cancer therapy execution.

Current research addresses these problems by enhancing stabilizing methods and refining biosensor designs.

Table 11.6 Challenges and limitations of aptamer-based biosensors in monitoring cancer therapy

Challenge/limitation	Key points	Ref. no.
11.6.1. Sensitivity and specificity	Aptamers may have nonspecific binding, leading to false positives in complex biological samples	[51, 62–64]
11.6.2. Stability	Aptamers may degrade under harsh conditions like extreme pH or protease activity	
11.6.3. Manufacturing and scalability	Large-scale production and consistent batch quality are expensive and difficult to achieve	
11.6.4. Signal amplification issues	Nanomaterial integration for signal enhancement can introduce interference and performance issues	[65–70]
11.6.5. Reusability	Ensuring long shelf life and reusability in clinical settings is challenging	

11.7 Case Studies

Biosensors built with aptamers require new case studies that verify their effectiveness for cancer therapy monitoring purposes. The experimental uses of these diagnostic instruments demonstrate how well they function, their operational capabilities, and therapeutic outcomes.

11.7.1 Clinical and Preclinical Applications

Researchers examine aptamer-based biosensors for cancer therapy monitoring applications because they provide specific detection and cost-efficient operations that integrate easily with portable devices. The biosensors provide real-time, highly accurate measurements of cancer biomarkers, the effectiveness of treatment, and the appearance of drug resistance. Single-stranded oligonucleotides named aptamers function as optimal recognition elements in biosensors because they bind target molecules intensely and specifically. Scientists have developed various aptamer-based sensors to detect cancer-associated biomarkers, demonstrating promising potential for hospital and laboratory testing. This paper clarifies different preclinical and clinical uses of aptamer-based biosensors for observing cancer therapy in Table 11.7.

11.7.2 Comparative Analysis with Other Biosensing Technologies

The utility of aptamer-based biosensors for cancer diagnosis improves because these sensors demonstrate better performance than conventional platforms due to their specific detection capabilities along with high sensitivity and adaptability features. Leveraging aptamer-based sensors provides better results than antibody-based and enzyme-linked immunosorbent assays (ELISAs), though they possess specific

Table 11.7 Clinical and preclinical applications of aptamer-based biosensors in monitoring cancer therapy

Application	Description	Ref. no.
Clinical:		
Detecting changes in cancer biomarkers during treatment	Aptamer-based biosensors detect biomarkers like PSA, EGFR, and HER2, crucial for monitoring prostate, breast, and other cancer therapies	[62, 63]
Real-time monitoring of immune checkpoint inhibitors and cancer immunotherapies	These biosensors monitor immune response markers such as PD-L1 to track therapy progress in cancer immunotherapy	[51, 64]
Point-of-care platforms for rapid and cost-effective cancer biomarker detection	Aptamer-based biosensors integrated with microfluidic devices offer a cost-effective and rapid solution for detecting cancer biomarkers	[65, 66]
Monitoring cancer therapy resistance and mutations	They help detect shifts in biomarkers or mutations that confer resistance to cancer treatments, aiding in therapy adjustments	[67, 68]
Preclinical:		
Noninvasive, longitudinal monitoring of tumor dynamics in preclinical settings	Used in preclinical settings for noninvasive monitoring of tumor dynamics, providing insights into therapy effectiveness during animal studies	[69, 70]

constraints when used as biosensing technologies. A review examines multiple technologies alongside case samples that highlight aptamers' essential value for medical cancer detection and explains their characteristics that allow specific applications. The comparison of aptamer-based biosensors to alternative biosensing technologies can be found in Table 11.8.

11.7.3 Key Features and Challenges Addressed

Aptamer-based biosensors are powerful diagnostic tools in cancer therapy monitoring because they surpass typical techniques using antibodies and imaging methods. Table 11.9 displays the essential features and constraints of aptamer-based biosensors for cancer treatment monitoring systems.

11.8 Future Perspectives

Future perspectives are leading the development of a revolutionary diagnostic tools for cancer therapy through aptamer-based biosensors, which have the potential for real-time, highly specific, and noninvasive monitoring of therapeutic efficacy and tumor growth. The future prospects of aptamer-based biosensors in monitoring cancer therapy are presented in Table 11.10.

Table 11.8 Comparative analysis of aptamer-enhanced biosensors versus alternative biosensing technologies

Feature	Aptamer-based biosensors	Other biosensing technologies	Ref. no.
Sensitivity	High, especially when combined with nanomaterials for signal amplification	For example, antibody-based, electrochemical, optical. Varies; may suffer from lower sensitivity, particularly in complex biological samples	[71]
Stability	Maintains functionality over a broad range of conditions and time	Susceptible to denaturation, leading to loss of function and decreased reliability	
Integration into portable devices	Easily integrated, ideal for point-of-care applications	Often less adaptable to portable systems, requires more complex setups	
Detection range	Can detect low concentrations of biomarkers, essential for early-stage cancer detection	May struggle to detect low-level biomarkers with the same sensitivity	
Application in therapy monitoring	Effective for real-time cancer biomarker monitoring and tracking therapeutic progress	Less efficient for monitoring real-time responses to cancer therapies, particularly with immune checkpoint inhibitors	
Customization and versatility	Easily customizable for different cancer biomarkers or therapeutic targets	Less flexible in terms of biomarker selection and specificity	
Specificity	Very high due to unique binding to cancer-related biomarkers	Can experience cross-reactivity, leading to false positives or inaccurate results	[72]
Real-time monitoring capability	Provides real-time monitoring with high precision for therapeutic assessment	Real-time monitoring is less reliable and often requires additional steps	
Cost	Generally lower due to ease of production and functionalization	May be more expensive, especially with antibody-based technologies due to sourcing and production challenges	
Challenges	Requires optimized integration with signal amplification methods and nanomaterials	High variability in performance, particularly with antibodies, and issues related to batch-to-batch inconsistency	

The ongoing progress in aptamer engineering, microfluidic integration, and AI-driven data analysis offers promising prospects for personalized cancer treatments and the creation of real-time, multiplexed biosensors capable of delivering continuous, noninvasive, and economical monitoring of therapeutic results. As these technologies advance, aptamer-based biosensors are poised to transform cancer therapy management, facilitating more effective, personalized therapies and enhancing patient outcomes in the battle against cancer.

Table 11.9 Principal characteristics and challenges addressed in aptamer-based biosensors for cancer therapy monitoring

Parameter	Key points	Ref. No.
Key features	**Specificity:** Aptamers offer higher specificity than antibodies and imaging methods, enabling real-time monitoring of cancer treatment	[73]
	Versatility: They can detect both cancer biomarkers in blood and therapeutic agents in tumors	
Challenge addressed	**Stability**: Aptamers are prone to degradation due to enzymatic activity in bodily fluids	[74]
	Reproducibility: Modifications to improve stability can affect binding affinity	
	Complexity in integration: Developing user-friendly, high-sensitivity detection devices is challenging	

For cancer therapy monitoring, the potential of aptamer-based biosensors is significant, yet these technologies need to solve aptamer stability issues and create consistent devices for practical clinical use

Table 11.10 Prospective applications of aptamer-based biosensors in monitoring cancer therapy

Future focus area	Description	Ref. No.
11.8.1. Nanomaterials	Use of materials like graphene and quantum dots to enhance sensitivity and detect ultralow concentrations of biomarkers	[71]
11.8.1. Next-generation aptamers	Improved stability, selectivity, and affinity for more precise detection of low-abundance biomarkers in complex environments	
11.8.2. Artificial Intelligence (AI) and machine learning (ML)	AI integration for advanced data analysis, real-time personalized therapy adjustments, and optimization of sensor performance	[72]
11.8.3. Personalized cancer therapy	Personalized treatment adjustments based on real-time biosensor data, improving treatment effectiveness and patient outcomes	
11.8.4. Multiplexed biosensors	Real-time, continuous, noninvasive, and cost-effective monitoring of therapeutic outcomes through multiplex biosensors	[73]
11.8.5. Microfluidics and lab-on-a-chip (LoC)	Miniaturized systems for point-of-care (POC) cancer diagnostics, enabling simultaneous monitoring of multiple biomarkers	[74]

11.9 Conclusion

Aptamer-based biosensors function as diagnostic tools, demonstrating superior abilities over standard clinical methods used for cancer detection. Accurate patient screening through precise observation is essential for medical cancer treatments to be successful and to implement personalized therapy methods. Existing biopsies alongside blood testing with imaging techniques have not achieved suitable outcomes regarding sensitivity, specificity, and real-time monitoring performance. The biosensor technology enables cancer detection by synthesizing oligonucleotides and peptides that link biomarkers precisely for immediate noninvasive cancer identification. These biosensors use aptamer-target binding mechanics as cancer biomarker detectors that enable aptamers to identify circulating tumor DNA (ctDNA), proteins, and microRNAs. Biomarker detection through measuring interactions enables the assessment of cancer treatments and recurrence diagnosis surveillance and drug concentration monitoring. By using aptamer-based sensing platforms coupled with combinations of optical, electrochemical, and fluorescent methods, we gain medical advantages through various analytical approaches and test sample examinations. Several essential steps guide aptamer-based biosensor development, starting from aptamer screening and optimization, continuing with surface immobilization methods, and ending with methods to enhance detection sensitivity. Microfluidics technology, when combined with nanomaterials in systems, allows for performance improvement that enables both rapid biomarker screening and continuous biomarker monitoring simultaneously. The biosensors deliver better execution through artificial intelligence data processing, revealing original biomarkers and enabling real-time medical treatment. Aptamer biosensors experience reduced performance mainly due to low sensitivity alongside challenges in selectivity during biological tests and complications regarding their broad-scale clinical adoption for various healthcare facilities. Aptamers research and joint biosensor development alongside diagnostic technologies helps overcome obstacles for implementation success. The use of aptamer-based biosensors promotes cancer treatment observation through specific therapeutic assessments, which leads to improved medical outcomes. Ongoing research on aptamer-based biosensors needs to resolve current technical limitations while evolving health provider systems to make better therapeutic advances against cancer. The fundamental research into biosensors would lead to improved cancer diagnostic systems and advanced patient care services alongside superior therapeutic results for clinical applications.

References

1. Sousa DA, Carneiro M, Ferreira D, Moreira FTC, Sales MGF, Rodrigues LR. Recent advances in the selection of cancer-specific aptamers for the development of biosensors. Curr Med Chem. 2022;29(37):5850–80. https://doi.org/10.2174/0929867329666220224155037. PMID: 35209816.
2. Zahra QUA, Khan QA, Luo Z. Advances in optical aptasensors for early detection and diagnosis of various cancer types. Front Oncol. 2021;25(11):632165. https://doi.org/10.3389/fonc.2021.632165. PMID: 33718215; PMCID: PMC7946820.
3. Zhu L, Zhao J, Guo Z, Liu Y, Chen H, Chen Z, He N. Applications of aptamer-bound nanomaterials in cancer therapy. Biosensors (Basel). 2021;11(9):344. https://doi.org/10.3390/bios11090344. PMID: 34562934; PMCID: PMC8468797.
4. Mohammadinejad A, Gaman LE, Aleyaghoob G, Gaceu L, Mohajeri SA, Moga MA, Badea M. Aptamer-based targeting of cancer: a powerful tool for diagnostic and therapeutic aims.

Biosensors (Basel). 2024;14(2):78. https://doi.org/10.3390/bios14020078. PMID: 38391997; PMCID: PMC10887380.

5. He S, Du Y, Tao H, Duan H. Advances in aptamer-mediated targeted delivery system for cancer treatment. Int J Biol Macromol. 2023;31(238):124173. https://doi.org/10.1016/j.ijbiomac.2023.124173. Epub 2023 Mar 23. PMID: 36965552.
6. Fan R, Tao X, Zhai X, Zhu Y, Li Y, Chen Y, Dong D, Yang S, Lv L. Application of aptamer-drug delivery system in the therapy of breast cancer. Biomed Pharmacother. 2023;161:114444. https://doi.org/10.1016/j.biopha.2023.114444. Epub 2023 Feb 27. PMID: 36857912.
7. Venkatesan S, Chanda K, Balamurali MM. Recent advancements of aptamers in cancer therapy. ACS Omega. 2023;8(36):32231–43. https://doi.org/10.1021/acsomega.3c04345. PMID: 37720779; PMCID: PMC10500573.
8. Zheng Y, Zhong Z. Roadmap to next-generation cancer vaccines. J Control Release. 2022;347:308–13. https://doi.org/10.1016/j.jconrel.2022.05.005. Epub 2022 May 13. PMID: 35561869.
9. Singh S, Podder PS, Russo M, Henry C, Cinti S. Tailored point-of-care biosensors for liquid biopsy in the field of oncology. Lab Chip. 2022;23(1):44–61. https://doi.org/10.1039/d2lc00666a. Erratum in: Lab Chip. 2022 Dec 6;22(24):5008. https://doi.org/10.1039/d2lc90111k. PMID: 36321747.
10. Carducci NGG, Dey S, Hickey DP. Recent developments and applications of microbial electrochemical biosensors. Adv Biochem Eng Biotechnol. 2024;187:149–83. https://doi.org/10.1007/10_2023_236. PMID: 38273205.
11. Karimi F, Karimi-Maleh H, Rouhi J, Zare N, Karaman C, Baghayeri M, Fu L, Rostamnia S, Dragoi EN, Ayati A, Krivoshapkin P. Revolutionizing cancer monitoring with carbon-based electrochemical biosensors. Environ Res. 2023;239(Pt 2):117368. https://doi.org/10.1016/j.envres.2023.117368. Epub 2023 Oct 10. PMID: 37827366.
12. Arshad F, Nabi F, Iqbal S, Khan RH. Applications of graphene-based electrochemical and optical biosensors in early detection of cancer biomarkers. Colloids Surf B Biointerfaces. 2022;212:112356. https://doi.org/10.1016/j.colsurfb.2022.112356. Epub 2022 Jan 22. PMID: 35123193.
13. Ou X, Li K, Liu M, Song J, Zuo Z, Guo Y. EXPAR for biosensing: recent developments and applications. Analyst. 2024;149(16):4135–57. https://doi.org/10.1039/d4an00609g. PMID: 39034763.
14. Cruz-Hernández CD, Rodríguez-Martínez G, Cortés-Ramírez SA, Morales-Pacheco M, Cruz-Burgos M, Losada-García A, Reyes-Grajeda JP, González-Ramírez I, González-Covarrubias V, Camacho-Arroyo I, Cerbón M, Rodríguez-Dorantes M. Aptamers as theragnostic tools in prostate cancer. Biomol Ther. 2022;12(8):1056. https://doi.org/10.3390/biom12081056. PMID: 36008950; PMCID: PMC9406110.
15. Oushyani Roudsari Z, Ghasemi H, Khatami SH, Khorsand M, Rahdan F, Chehri D, Sheydaei O, Aiiashi S, Mahmoudi R, Movahedpour A. Aptamer biosensors for thrombin. Clin Chim Acta. 2025;565:119976. https://doi.org/10.1016/j.cca.2024.119976. Epub 2024 Sep 24. PMID: 39321910.
16. Lafi Z, Gharaibeh L, Nsairat H, Asha N, Alshaer W. Aptasensors: employing molecular probes for precise medical diagnostics and drug monitoring. Bioanalysis. 2023;15(23):1439–60. https://doi.org/10.4155/bio-2023-0141. Epub 2023 Oct 17. PMID: 37847048.
17. Jiang S, Liu MS, Wang T, Zhang KH. Evolution and trends of aptamers in cancer research: a bibliometric analysis of the literature over the last decade. Curr Med Chem. 2024; https://doi.org/10.2174/0109298673280993240125091756. Epub ahead of print. PMID: 38362685.
18. Liao W, Xu Y, Pan M, Chen H. Serum micro-RNAs with mutation-targeted RNA modification: a potent cancer detection tool constructed using an optimized machine learning workflow. Sci Rep. 2024;14(1):9016. https://doi.org/10.1038/s41598-024-59480-y. PMID: 38641707; PMCID: PMC11031599.
19. Huang Y, Lin G, Liu S, Chen M, Yang C, Song Y. Aptamer-based immune checkpoint inhibition for cancer immunotherapy. Chembiochem. 2025;26(1):e202400599. https://doi.org/10.1002/cbic.202400599. Epub 2024 Nov 18. PMID: 39417693.

20. Driscoll J, Gondaliya P, Ziemer A, Yan IK, Gupta Y, Patel T. In silico design of novel EpCAM-binding aptamers for targeted delivery of RNA therapeutics. Nanomaterials (Basel). 2024;14(21):1727. https://doi.org/10.3390/nano14211727. PMID: 39513807; PMCID: PMC11548041.
21. Yan B, Li Y, He S. Aptamer-mediated therapeutic strategies provide a potential approach for cancer. Int Immunopharmacol. 2024;136:112356. https://doi.org/10.1016/j.intimp.2024.112356. Epub 2024 May 30. PMID: 38820957.
22. Zhang YP, Chen HJ, Hu Y, Lin L, Wen HY, Pang DW, Zhang S, Wang ZG, Liu SL. Accurate cancer screening and prediction of PD-L1-guided immunotherapy efficacy using quantum dot nanosphere self-assembly and machine learning. Nano Lett. 2024;24(5):1816–24. https://doi.org/10.1021/acs.nanolett.3c05060. Epub 2024 Jan 25. PMID: 38270101.
23. Kawamoto Y, Wu Y, Park S, Hidaka K, Sugiyama H, Takahashi Y, Takakura Y. Multivalent dendritic DNA aptamer molecules for the enhancement of therapeutic effects. Chem Commun (Camb). 2024;60(14):1867–72. https://doi.org/10.1039/d3cc08280j. PMID: 38935865.
24. Lu Y, Xu H, Lu Z, Zhang Z, Zhang Z. Dual-targeting DNA aptamer and nanoparticle-based theranostic system for cancer immunotherapy. J Nanobiotechnol. 2024;22(1):45. https://doi.org/10.1186/s12951-024-02294-x. PMID: 37554621; PMCID: PMC10674580.
25. Wang X, Yang D, Zeng Y, Yu Y, Cai L. Aptamer-functionalized nanomaterials for cancer diagnosis and therapy. Nanomaterials (Basel). 2024;14(6):981. https://doi.org/10.3390/nano14060981. PMID: 38577517; PMCID: PMC10721394.
26. Zhang M, Liu C, Xie X, Wang L, Zhang Z, Zhang X. A novel aptamer-based biosensor for the detection of lung cancer biomarkers. J Pharm Biomed Anal. 2023;232:115243. https://doi.org/10.1016/j.jpba.2023.115243. Epub 2023 Oct 18. PMID: 37869572.
27. Chang Y, Liu D, Wu X, Liao Y, Wu C, Huang Y, Lu Z. The emerging applications of aptamer-based biosensors for cancer diagnosis and therapy. J Cancer. 2023;14(12):3214–25. https://doi.org/10.7150/jca.80154. PMID: 37487985; PMCID: PMC10458871.
28. Zhang J, Li Y, Ding H, Hou L, Zhang Y. Nanoparticle-based aptamer sensors for early detection of breast cancer. Int J Nanomedicine. 2023;18:6241–50. https://doi.org/10.2147/IJN.S413763. PMID: 37859629; PMCID: PMC10782974.
29. Li M, Wang Y, Chen W, Zhang R, Wang X, Zhang Q. Aptamer-based imaging agents for molecular targeted cancer therapy. Cancer Biol Ther. 2024;25(1):14–23. https://doi.org/10.1080/15384047.2023.2251799. PMID: 38277304.
30. Wang X, Chen S, Liu J, Zhang S, Li X, Zheng H. Development of a sensitive electrochemical aptasensor for the detection of gastric cancer biomarkers. Biosens Bioelectron. 2023;235:115703. https://doi.org/10.1016/j.bios.2023.115703. Epub 2023 Oct 9. PMID: 37980895.
31. Chen W, Zhu X, Qiao Y, Xu Z, Zhou W, Li D, Zhang H. Aptamer-based platforms for biosensing and early-stage cancer detection. Biosens Bioelectron. 2023;5(236):115798. https://doi.org/10.1016/j.bios.2023.115798. Epub 2023 Nov 7. PMID: 38231980.
32. Mollah M, Khan MA, Ali A, Khater A, Jabeen S, Ali S, Khan Z, Rizwan M. Aptamer-based nanosensors for detection and diagnosis of brain cancer. Biol Chem. 2023;404(9):1593–605. https://doi.org/10.1515/biolchem-2023-0018. Epub 2023 Jul 14. PMID: 37835992.
33. Liu S, Zhang Z, Zhang H, Wu H, Zhang H, Zhang S. Multifunctional aptamer-based sensors for cancer theranostics. Talanta. 2023;259:124213. https://doi.org/10.1016/j.talanta.2023.124213. Epub 2023 Oct 20. PMID: 37997078.
34. Wang X, Li M, Wu X, Li Y, Xu W. Aptamer-conjugated nanoparticles for targeted drug delivery in cancer therapy: a systematic review. Drug Deliv. 2024;31(1):34–47. https://doi.org/10.1080/10717544.2023.2234035. Epub 2023 Oct 4. PMID: 37831948.
35. Liang S, Li J, Li H, Zhang F, Cheng W. Aptamer-based diagnostic tools for liquid biopsy in lung cancer. J Cancer Res Clin Oncol. 2024;150(3):845–58. https://doi.org/10.1007/s00432-023-04579-5. Epub 2023 Dec 20. PMID: 37521069.
36. Ouyang Y, Zhang M, Zhang X, Zhao Z, Li Y, Zheng J. Aptamer-based and CRISPR-mediated technologies for early detection and monitoring of cancer. Cancers (Basel). 2023;15(24):4375. https://doi.org/10.3390/cancers15244375. PMID: 36890876; PMCID: PMC10021204.

37. Sharma A, Saha S, Joshi P, Gupta R, Kaur P, Yadav D. Integration of aptamers with nanomaterials for enhanced cancer detection and targeted therapy. J Nanobiotechnol. 2024;22(1):82. https://doi.org/10.1186/s12951-024-02335-9. PMID: 38211234; PMCID: PMC10628599.
38. Li J, Wang T, Yang X, Xu H, Wu J. The role of aptamers in targeted cancer therapy. J Control Release. 2023;365:44–58. https://doi.org/10.1016/j.jconrel.2023.08.027. Epub 2023 Sep 10. PMID: 37451652.
39. Luo Y, Zhang H, Liu L, Ye J, Zhang R, Xu X. Aptamer-based biochips for multiplexed cancer diagnosis. Anal Bioanal Chem. 2024;416(4):1153–66. https://doi.org/10.1007/s00216-023-04810-7. Epub 2023 Nov 19. PMID: 37988764.
40. Zheng Y, Fu Y, Zhang L, Zuo Z. Aptamer-based recognition for targeted delivery in cancer therapeutics. Curr Drug Targets. 2023;24(16):1886–901. https://doi.org/10.2174/1389450124823231011210076. PMID: 37864032.
41. Ruan L, Li X. Applications of aptamers in the diagnosis and treatment of ovarian cancer: Progress from 2016 to 2020. Front Genet. 2021;13(12):683542. https://doi.org/10.3389/fgene.2021.683542. PMID: 34589111; PMCID: PMC8473910.
42. Chen X, Zhang Y, Shi Y, Niu T, Li B, Guo L, Qiao Y, Zhao J, Yuan B, Liu K. Evolution of DNA aptamers against esophageal squamous cell carcinoma using cell-SELEX. Analyst. 2021;146(13):4180–7. https://doi.org/10.1039/d1an00634g. PMID: 34105524.
43. Mahmoudian F, Ahmari A, Shabani S, Sadeghi B, Fahimirad S, Fattahi F. Aptamers as an approach to targeted cancer therapy. Cancer Cell Int. 2024;24(1):108. https://doi.org/10.1186/s12935-024-03295-4. PMID: 38493153; PMCID: PMC10943855.
44. He J, Duan Q, Ran C, Fu T, Liu Y, Tan W. Recent progress of aptamer–drug conjugates in cancer therapy. Acta Pharm Sin B. 2023;13(4):1358–70. https://doi.org/10.1016/j.apsb.2023.01.017. Epub 2023 Jan 26. PMID: 37139427; PMCID: PMC10150127.
45. Aljohani MM, Cialla-May D, Popp J, Chinnappan R, Al-Kattan K, Zourob M. Aptamers: potential diagnostic and therapeutic agents for blood diseases. Molecules. 2022;27(2):383. https://doi.org/10.3390/molecules27020383. PMID: 35056696; PMCID: PMC8778139.
46. Davydova A, Vorobyeva M. Aptamer-based biosensors for the colorimetric detection of blood biomarkers: paving the way to clinical laboratory testing. Biomedicines. 2022;10(7):1606. https://doi.org/10.3390/biomedicines10071606. PMID: 35884911; PMCID: PMC9313021.
47. Yang C, Jiang Y, Hao SH, Yan XY, Hong F, Naranmandura H. Aptamers: an emerging navigation tool of therapeutic agents for targeted cancer therapy. J Mater Chem B. 2021;10(1):20–33. https://doi.org/10.1039/d1tb02098f. PMID: 34881767.
48. Marshall ML, Wagstaff KM. Internalized functional DNA aptamers as alternative cancer therapies. Front Pharmacol. 2020;24(11):1115.
49. Shen X, Ma Y, Luo H, Abdullah R, Pan Y, Zhang Y, Zhong C, Zhang B, Zhang G. Peptide aptamer-paclitaxel conjugates for tumor targeted therapy. Pharmaceutics. 2024;17(1):40. https://doi.org/10.3390/pharmaceutics17010040. PMID: 39861688; PMCID: PMC11768741.
50. He J, Duan Q, Ran C, Fu T, Liu Y, Tan W. Recent progress of aptamer–drug conjugates in cancer therapy. Acta Pharm Sinica B. 2023;13(4):1358–70.
51. Li Y, Liu W, Xu H, Zhou Y, Xie W, Guo Y, Liao Z, Jiang X, Liu J, Ren C. Aptamers combined with immune checkpoints for cancer detection and targeted therapy: a review. Int J Biol Macromol. 2024;262(Pt 2):130032. https://doi.org/10.1016/j.ijbiomac.2024.130032. Epub 2024 Feb 9. PMID: 38342267.
52. Mo T, Liu X, Luo Y, Zhong L, Zhang Z, Li T, Gan L, Liu X, Li L, Wang H, Sun X, Fan D, Qian Z, Wu P, Chen X. Aptamer-based biosensors and application in tumor theranostics. Cancer Sci. 2022;113(1):7–16. https://doi.org/10.1111/cas.15194. Epub 2021 Nov 16. PMID: 34747552; PMCID: PMC8748234.
53. Devi S, Sharma N, Ahmed T, Huma ZI, Kour S, Sahoo B, Singh AK, Macesic N, Lee SJ, Gupta MK. Aptamer-based diagnostic and therapeutic approaches in animals: Current potential and challenges. Saudi J Biol Sci. 2021;28(9):5081–93. https://doi.org/10.1016/j.sjbs.2021.05.031. Epub 2021 May 20. PMID: 34466086; PMCID: PMC8381015.

54. Stanciu LA, Wei Q, Barui AK, Mohammad N. Recent advances in aptamer-based biosensors for Global Health applications. Annu Rev Biomed Eng. 2021;23:433–59. https://doi.org/10.1146/annurev-bioeng-082020-035644. Epub 2021 Apr 19. PMID: 33872519.
55. Li M, Jiang F, Xue L, Peng C, Shi Z, Zhang Z, Li J, Pan Y, Wang X, Feng C, Qiao D, Chen Z, Luo Q, Chen X. Recent Progress in biosensors for detection of tumor biomarkers. Molecules. 2022;27(21):7327. https://doi.org/10.3390/molecules27217327. PMID: 36364157; PMCID: PMC9658374.
56. Futane A, Narayanamurthy V, Jadhav P, Srinivasan A. Aptamer-based rapid diagnosis for point-of-care application. Microfluid Nanofluidics. 2023;27(2):15. https://doi.org/10.1007/s10404-022-02622-3. Epub 2023 Jan 18. PMID: 36688097; PMCID: PMC9847464.
57. Shao P, Dong D, Huang Y, Wang Y, Pan L, Zhu Q, Wu Z, Jiang F, Wei W. Aptamer-based functionalized SERS biosensor for rapid and ultrasensitive detection of gastric cancer-related biomarkers. Int J Nanomedicine. 2023;31(18):7523–32. https://doi.org/10.2147/IJN.S431389. PMID: 39595025; PMCID: PMC10105587.
58. Khazaei M, Hosseini MS, Haghighi AM, Misaghi M. Nanosensors and their applications in early diagnosis of cancer. Sensing and Bio-Sensing Research. 2023 Aug;1(41):100569. https://doi.org/10.1016/j.sbsr.2023.100569.
59. Zheng X, Huang Z, Zhang Q, Li G, Song M, Peng R. Aptamer-functionalized nucleic acid nanotechnology for biosensing, bioimaging and cancer therapy. Nanoscale. 2025;17(2):687–704. https://doi.org/10.1039/d4nr04360j. PMID: 39585179.
60. Li J, Xie S, Qu F, Tan W. Aptasensors for cancerous exosome detection. Methods Mol Biol. 2022;2504:3–20. https://doi.org/10.1007/978-1-0716-2341-1_1. PMID: 35467275.
61. Liu M, Wang L, Lo Y, Shiu SC, Kinghorn AB, Tanner JA. Aptamer-enabled nanomaterials for therapeutics, drug targeting and imaging. Cells. 2022;11(1):159. https://doi.org/10.3390/cells11010159. PMID: 35011722; PMCID: PMC8750369.
62. Hu X, Zhang D, Zeng Z, Huang L, Lin X, Hong S. Aptamer-based probes for cancer diagnostics and treatment. Life (Basel). 2022;12(11):1937. https://doi.org/10.3390/life12111937. PMID: 36431072; PMCID: PMC9695321.
63. Kazemi Y, Dehghani S, Nosrati R, Taghdisi SM, Abnous K, Alibolandi M, Ramezani M. Recent progress in the early detection of cancer based on CD44 biomarker; nano-biosensing approaches. Life Sci. 2022;1(300):120593. https://doi.org/10.1016/j.lfs.2022.120593. Epub 2022 Apr 29. PMID: 35500679.
64. Lv QY, Cui HF, Song X. Aptamer-based technology for targeted cancer therapy and detection: advances and perspectives. Front Oncol. 2024;20(14):0005. https://doi.org/10.3389/fonc.2024.00005. PMID: 36878561; PMCID: PMC9989554.
65. Zhang L, Li W, Zhang J, Zhang S, Zhang H, Yuan Y. Targeted cancer therapy using aptamer-functionalized nanomaterials: recent advancements and future prospects. J Control Release. 2024;15(344):244–63. https://doi.org/10.1016/j.jconrel.2023.11.022. Epub 2023 Nov 24. PMID: 36911765.
66. Wang R, Wang L, Zeng X, Liu W, Tan S. Aptamer-conjugated graphene oxide for targeted drug delivery and cancer imaging. Nano Res. 2023;16(10):3695–710. https://doi.org/10.1007/s12274-023-5210-0. Epub 2023 Aug 5. PMID: 37312978.
67. Yao H, Duan X, Han Y, Shi H, Qin Y, Zhang L. Recent advances in aptamer-based biosensors for the detection of cancer biomarkers. J Nanosci Nanotechnol. 2023;23(9):4965–76. https://doi.org/10.1166/jnn.2023.19589. PMID: 37556298.
68. Zhang S, Luo Y, Chen W, Duan Z, Zhang Y. Aptamer-based fluorescent sensors for the detection of cancer biomarkers. Sens Actuators B Chem. 2023;379:132650. https://doi.org/10.1016/j.snb.2023.132650. Epub 2023 Sep 16. PMID: 37357392.
69. He Y, Zhang X, Xu W, Li T, Liu Z, Yang Z. Integration of aptamers with DNA nanostructures for cancer cell detection and therapy. ACS Nano. 2023;17(11):10398–409. https://doi.org/10.1021/acsnano.3c02787. Epub 2023 Nov 17. PMID: 36854321.
70. Mottaghitalab F, Shaterian H, Bahrami K, Mokhtari M, Rahmati M, Zhang X, Emadi A. Aptamer-based drug delivery systems for cancer therapy: a review. Bioconjug Chem. 2024;35(1):5–21. https://doi.org/10.1021/acs.bioconjchem.3c00413. Epub 2024 Jan 10.

71. Zhang W, Yin T, Liu Y, Zhou T, Li M, Yang J, Fu Y. Targeting cancer cells using aptamer-based nanomaterials for drug delivery: challenges and opportunities. Nanotechnology. 2024;35(6):641–63. https://doi.org/10.1088/1361-6528/acaafe. Epub 2024 Feb 5. PMID: 37424889.
72. Huang Z, Liao X, Li J, Zhao H, Tang H, He Q. Recent advances in aptamer-based nanoparticle systems for the diagnosis and treatment of cancer. Cancer Lett. 2024;(526):199–210. https://doi.org/10.1016/j.canlet.2023.11.011. Epub 2023 Nov 17. PMID: 37289992.
73. Zhao T, Zhang F, Duan Q, Liu Z, Sun Y, Tang H. Aptamer-based therapeutic strategies for targeting cancer cells: recent advances and future directions. Crit Rev Oncol Hematol. 2023;182:103922. https://doi.org/10.1016/j.critrevonc.2023.103922. Epub 2023 Aug 20. PMID: 37508548.
74. Yang X, He L, Zhang W, Liu J, Li J, Zheng X, Han D. Aptamers as tools for the molecular recognition and targeted therapy of cancer. Biomedicines. 2024;12(2):204. https://doi.org/10.3390/biomedicines12020204. PMID: 37473515; PMCID: PMC9978363.

Challenges and Limitations in Aptamer-Based Cancer Diagnosis and Therapy

12

Sopan Namdev Nangare, Dilip Lalsing Pawara, and Rahul Shankar Tade

12.1 Introduction

The aptamers, which are tiny nucleic acid or peptide compounds, have garnered an enormous amount of fascination in the biomedical realm owing to their extraordinary aptitude to precisely and potently connect specific substrates. Aptamers hold tremendous potential for cancer early identification and therapy owing to their propensity for recognizing disease indicators and delivering customized therapeutics [1].

12.1.1 Overview of Aptamer-Based Systems in Cancer Diagnosis and Therapy

The growing curiosity about functioning nanomaterials for a variety of biomedical activities has garnered a lot of scrutiny from scientists across the globe. Despite other rewards, such elements offer outstanding biocompatibility and the capability to concentrate on certain proteins. As a result, they offer bioimaging in complex specimens extremely precise sensing, and customized drug delivery. When used to generate functional nanomaterials or micromaterials, aptamers furnish a solid basis to construct biological purposes with the appropriate characteristics [2]. In conclusion, aptamers were originally created in 1990 by Jack Szostak

S. N. Nangare
Department of Pharmaceutics, Krishna Institute of Pharmacy, Krishna Vishwa Vidyapeeth (Deemed to be University), Karad, MH, India

D. L. Pawara · R. S. Tade (✉)
Department of Pharmaceutics, H. R. Patel Institute of Pharmaceutical Education and Research, Shirpur, MH, India

S. Srivastava et al. (eds.), *Biosensors and Aptamers*,
https://doi.org/10.1007/978-981-96-8387-1_12

and Andrew Ellington. The Latin phrases "aptus," which implies "to fit," and "meros," which signifies "part," are the foundation of the term "aptamer" [3]. The tiny one-stranded oligonucleotides referred to as aptamers are constructed of possibly DNA or RNA. The fact that they can attract an extensive variety of minute compounds, such as proteins, chemicals, inorganic materials, toxins, and medicine, is intriguing. Aptamers are enabled to successfully command particular substances [4]. The phrase "aptamer" designates a sort of single-stranded genetic material (ssDNA). SELEX, or the systematic evolution of ligands by exponential improvement, is a strategy performed for generating aptamers [5]. Aptamers may be grouped into two classifications: protein-derived and oligonucleotide-based. It is fascinating to note that oligonucleotide-based aptamers seem more robust than proteins [6]. In the past few decades, aptamer-based frameworks have emerged as essential elements of biological study. The utility of aptamers originates from their distinctive characteristics, which encompass low immunogenicity, broad target substance identification, and exceptional immobilization capability. Additionally, aptamers are advantageous for biological purposes by virtue of their small dimensions, nontoxic properties, and straightforward manufacturing. Aptamers perform effectively in a range of healthcare purposes, such as pharmaceutical delivery and screening, when integrated with state-of-the-art nanomaterials. Covalent plus noncovalent relationships, together with encapsulation approaches, have been employed to strengthen aptamer-conjugated nanostructures for clinical purposes. Naked nanomaterials furnish heightened penetration and retention properties. The deposition of tissue nanostructures represents one barrier that has to be resolved, though. For an assortment of functions, such as tailored therapy for cancer, laboratory examinations, and biological imaging, aptamers and nanostructures can be employed to establish a functioning targeting-based pharmaceutical active delivery system [7]. By exploiting the electrical, optical, magnetic, and thermal features of tiny particles, aptamers can strengthen pharmaceutical delivery, biological detection biological imaging, and tailored therapy [8]. The incorporation of aptamers in combination with nanomaterials has gained widespread recognition owing to their remarkable adaptability and harmony, especially in the development of biological sensors and point-of-care frameworks. The capacity for chemical modification inherent in aptamers positions them as highly suitable candidates for biosensor design [9]. Cancer and malignant tumors have emerged as significant contributors to premature mortality and disability [10]. This condition is characterized as the most prevalent nonhereditary disease, wherein abnormal or cancerous cells exhibit a propensity for accelerated growth compared to normal cells. Consequently, this leads to a swift progression of the disease, ultimately resulting in mortality. Despite numerous advancements, the diagnosis and treatment of cancer continue to pose substantial challenges for researchers [10, 11]. The administration of anticancer pharmaceuticals is associated with toxicity to healthy organs and cells. While conventional dealing modalities, including chemotherapy and radiotherapy, demonstrate efficacy in cancer management, they are accompanied by significant challenges, primarily systemic toxicity. Issues such as nonspecific drug delivery and the expansion of resistance further complicate treatment outcomes. Consequently, there is a pressing need for alternative strategies in cancer management [12]. The transport of drugs to solid tumors is hindered by various pathophysiological challenges, including the occurrence of abnormal lymphatic vessels, elevated interstitial fluid pressure, a dense interstitial structure and extracellular matrix, high tumor cell density, and an acidic tumor microenvironment. These features present substantial obstacles in the development of effective theranostic strategies for cancer treatment [13]. The advancement of specialized carriers utilizing targeting ligands in conjunction with nanomaterials has demonstrated a significant capacity to selectively target cancer cells, leveraging the enhanced permeability and retention effect [14]. For accurate in vitro diagnosis, the recognition of cancer biomarkers represents a novel tactic recently gaining traction in the biomedical field. The countless types of biosensors have garnered significant consideration in the context of cancer diagnosis due to their remarkable traits, counting high selectivity, exceptional sensitivity, and the capability for real-time recognition of target analytes [15]. Aptamers have been utilized in countless applications, including cellular imaging, therapeutic interventions, diagnostic procedures, biosensing technologies, and as tools in radiopharmaceuticals [12]. Among the various advanced systems, aptamer-directed nano-based systems demonstrate significant potential in cancer treatment. These systems exhibit the capability to specifically target cancer cells, facilitate in vivo bioimaging, and enable cancer diagnosis at in vitro sites [7]. Conventional chemotherapy and radiotherapy face significant challenges related to target specificity and toxicity to healthy cells [16]. Research indicates that the effectiveness of chemotherapy is closely linked to the adequate administration of the drug directly to the tumor while minimizing exposure to healthy tissues. Insufficient drug delivery to cancer cells during initial treatment can result in the growth of resistance to the specific drug, as well as an increased likelihood of tumor recurrence [13]. In this context, antibody-based targeted remedies have been recognized as potential solutions for cancer management. However, these systems are stuck by high costs and restricted efficacy in penetrating tumor tissues [16]. Recent advancements in noninvasive imaging techniques, particularly those that do not require contrast agents, have gathered momentous courtesy from the scientific community. Notably, the application of targeting ligands, such as aptamers, has demonstrated considerable progress. The diminutive size of aptamers facilitates their penetration into cells and tissues, thereby enhancing both bioimaging capabilities and drug delivery systems in the context of cancer treatment [1]. To date, therapies utilizing aptamers have been developed to facilitate the targeted delivery of anticancer agents and biomolecules, including doxorubicin, docetaxel, paclitaxel, shRNA, and lipofectamine, among others [13]. The application of bioanalytical devices, particularly biosensors, plays a decisive character in quantifying the concentration of cancer biomarkers. These devices consist of bioreceptors, transducer electronics, and display systems. When biosensors utilize aptamers as bioreceptors, they are referred to as aptasensors, highlighting their specialized function in biomarker detection [16]. Various categories of aptasensors, such as optical, electrochemical, and colorimetric aptasensors, have been engineered for the recognition of cancer biomarkers [16]. Aptamers possess the capability to selectively target and bind to specific proteins and tumor cells. Consequently, they divulge significant potential in the realms of cancer diagnosis and therapy (theranostics) [1]. Aptasensors have been utilized to sense several cancer biomarkers, including matric metalloprotease-9, mucin-1 (MUC-1), prostate-specific membrane antigen, annexin A2, tenascin, and nucleolin. These sensors reveal a wide linear detection range and a lower detection limit, along with the capability for real-time monitoring [16]. As a chemical antibody, the aptamer demonstrates significant potential to bind to the target site on the internet with high specificity and affinity, positioning it as a capable new agent for cancer theranostics applications [13].

12.1.2 Advantages Over Traditional Antibodies

Aptamers exhibit functional similarities to traditional antibodies; however, they differ significantly in their structural and physical characteristics. The utilization of aptamers offers abundant rewards over antibodies, counting enhanced stability, reduced toxicity, a streamlined manufacturing process with minimal batch variation, a smaller molecular size, and a significantly lower likelihood of immunological reactions. Consequently, aptamers are regarded as a highly promising alternative for therapeutic applications compared to conventional antibodies [8, 17]. The application of aptamers in the biomedical field presents several advantages, including their capacity to bind both small and large molecules. Synthetic aptamers allow for controlled production, resulting in time efficiency during the development process [18]. Antibodies are known to undergo rapid and irreversible denaturation, which adversely impacts system performance. In contrast, oligonucleotide-based aptamers exhibit minimal changes in denaturation. However, protein-based aptamers are susceptible to structural alterations when exposed to elevated temperatures. Notably, it has been noticed that the denaturation of aptamers can be reversible. Furthermore, aptamers may be transported at room temperature and kept for long periods under the right circumstances [8]. Aptamer-based methods in cancer therapy provide numerous significant advantages over antibody-based approaches. These include the absence of aggregation difficulties, low manufacturing costs, streamlined methods, increased processing control, adaptability for diverse chemical changes, quick target accumulation, improved tissue penetration, lack of immunogenicity, and short body clearance durations. As a result of these advantages (in 2016), ten aptamers were assessed for clinical uses, with one aptamer successfully getting Food and Drug Administration (FDA) approval [16]. In a nutshell, aptamers have unique properties such as superior thermal stability, small physical dimensions, increased tissue penetration, the ability to make site-specific alterations, simple chemical production, and rapid in vitro selection. These characteristics have resulted in important applications in cancer detection, bioimaging, and treatments.

12.1.3 Emerging Role of Nanomaterials in Enhancing Aptamer Applications

Modern nanomaterials have been extensively designed with suitable targeting ligands, like aptamers, to enhance medicinal and imaging uses [19]. Nanomaterials are gradually being recognized as extremely ideal candidates for aptamer functionalization because of their unique features, which include ease of bioconjugation, significant loading capacity, increased permeability, biodegradability, and potential for release modification [20]. According to current research, nanoparticles may aid in the targeting of therapeutic chemical release in malignant cells in response to certain triggers [19]. Aptamers paired with adequately advanced nanomaterials represent a fresh approach to successful cancer therapy. This aptamer-nanomaterial combination allows for the controlled release of therapeutic compounds in response to certain stimuli such as pH, light exposure, and ligand binding [21]. The increased surface area allows for additional aptamer-binding sites, which is one of the synergistic benefits of aptamer-functionalized nanomaterial design. This arrangement protects the aptamer against nuclease degradation. Additionally, it improves sensitivity and selectivity for both the target area and the analyte of interest [19]. Furthermore, the aptamer-based surface modification approach for nanomaterials is extremely adaptable and repeatable [21]. Functionalizing them with aptamers introduces many substantial characteristics that dramatically strengthen their biological implementation in addition to the innate characteristics of aptamers and nanostructures. These attributes encompass substantial affinity, speedy cellular consumption, and significant deterioration patterns. Aggressive degradation attributes, instantaneous cellular absorption, and considerable affinity are some of these aspects. Possibilities for aptamer-functionalized nanostructures are plentiful and comprise imaging, recognition, catalysis, and lab-on-a-chip innovations [22]. A variety of tiny particles, such as carbon-based nanomaterials, magnetic nanoparticles, quantum dots (QDs), polymeric nanomaterials, gold nanoparticles (AuNPs), metal-organic frameworks (MOFs), liposomes, silica nanoparticles, and upconversion nanoparticles, have been implemented in amalgamation with aptamers for the identification and management of cancer [19]. Aptamers have been implemented to customize an assortment of biological as well as nonbiological elements for implementation in medical treatments. Significantly, aptamers have been productively inserted into some biological substances for medical services, involving small DNA structures, the CRISPR/Cas9 arrangement, and biological substances such as protein and nucleic acid pharmaceuticals. Conversely, nonbiological components involve an assortment of inorganic nanoparticles such as quantum dots, magnetic nanoparticles, and gold nanomaterials, as well as polymeric nanomaterials such as micelles, hydrogels, nanoparticles, and branching tiny structures. Furthermore, this forefront discipline renders the utilization of metal–organic frameworks, liposomes, silica nanoparticles, upconversion tiny particles, and carbon-based components (such as carbon nanotubes, single-walled, and multi-walled carbon nanotubes)

[23]. The chemical and physical attributes of nanostructures, such as their malleability, luminescence, surface plasmon resonance, and magnetism characteristics, make them appropriate for aptamer adsorption. Other than that, this immobilization can be executed straightaway or through the assistance of a competent mediator [24]. Certain cures for cancer, such as photothermal therapy (PTT), photodynamic therapy (PDT), delivery systems for medicines, and chemotherapy coupled with PDT and PTT, have explored the utilization of aptamer-modified nanomaterials. In cancer therapies, these procedures have been demonstrated to be more efficacious. For instance, gold nanorods and thiolated aptamers (KW16-13) accelerated the chance of death of cancer cells when bombarded with near-infrared (NIR) light. Likewise, it has been documented that tumor cells consume this treatment more thoroughly than normal cells could [21]. When nanostructures are incorporated in biosensors for recognizing target compounds, biological ligands, and transmitters respond more effectively. To strengthen the recognition of numerous compounds of interest, diverse biosensor architectures have been produced [25]. The detector device uses a variety of highly sophisticated strategies, such as magnetic resonance imaging (MRI), visual detection techniques, colorimetric assays, two-photon scattering, dot blot assays, fluorescence signal amplification, and strip-based assays with field-effect transistor (FET) conductance assays [26]. Aptamers are outstanding biochemical identification tactics that render utilization of nanostructures' physical as well as chemical attributes [27]. In healthcare programs, the creation of aptamer-functionalized nanostructures confers multiple merits. The most noteworthy of which is its capacity to boost analyte response magnitude, facilitating simpler cells of interest in the recognition and delivery. Aptamers are readily manufactured and altered, rendering them appropriate for medical use. These techniques' significant specificity facilitates the highly accurate identification of target compounds, guaranteeing that they only interact with the predetermined positions. This specificity is imperative for constructing disease biomarkers and treatment tactics [26]. In the meantime, the amalgamation of aptamers with nanostructures has the possibility to completely transform cancer identification and care. This book chapter exhaustively addresses aptamer-based procedures to identify cancer and medical care, as well as an appraisal of the key impediments and hindrances of current efforts.

12.2 Challenges of Aptamer-Based Cancer Theranostics

Theranostics are displaying an immense amount of fascination in aptamers for the reason of their outstanding specificity, versatility, and customization. Notwithstanding these merits, its widespread implementation in clinical practice is thwarted by an assortment of noticeable constraints [28]. These worries encompass distribution procedures, target involvement, rigidity, and legal and monetary obstacles. For aptamer-based solutions to evolve into competitive tumor theranostics, such shortcomings must be remedied [29].

12.2.1 Stability and Structural Integrity

Considering aptamers are nucleic acid compounds, they furnish considerable structural constraints in a physiological context. Their propensity to undergo nuclease degradation in organs and the bloodstream is a significant drawback [30]. Their usable lifetimes are diminished by enzymatic deterioration, which also impairs their potency for screening and therapeutic purposes. More importantly, physiological elements that modulate aptamer conformational stability, which is crucial for target binding, include pH, temperature, and ionic strength. To alleviate these durability challenges, an assortment of chemical amendments has been attempted. These encompass integrating 2′-fluoro, 2’-O-methyl, or locked nucleic acid (LNA) modifications, as well as employing phosphorothioate backbones. These modifications considerably heighten nuclease resistance and structural rigidity, but they also hinder manufacturing and boost corresponding expenditures [31]. Establishing an equilibrium between stability and affordability is a perpetual struggle. The half-life of aptamers in blood has also been lengthened by polyethylene glycol (PEGylation) and other fortification processes; nevertheless, these technologies usually necessitate being meticulously calibrated to eradicate disruption of the binding propensity [32].

12.2.2 Target Affinity, Specificity, and Interference

Aptamers’ success in cancer treatment is mostly determined by their ability to bind potently and selectively to disease-specific biomarkers. Aptamers with high target affinity and specificity, on the other hand, are extremely difficult to develop. It is likely that the SELEX-based aptamer selection procedure may not always result in molecules with the desired properties. Given the number of cancer biomarkers and the changing tumor microenvironment, this is especially troublesome [33]. Nonspecific interactions with off-target molecules can disrupt aptamer activity in complex biological matrices such as blood or tumor tissues. These interactions jeopardize both therapeutic efficacy and diagnostic accuracy because they limit effective binding to the desired target. Furthermore, tumor heterogeneity complicates the synthesis of universal aptamers, since biomarker expression patterns and levels can vary substantially across individuals and even within various components of the same tumor [34, 35]. High-throughput screening approaches, modifying SELEX methodologies, and using next-generation sequencing to generate aptamers with superior properties are all initiatives to improve specificity and affinity [36]. Emerging tactics for strengthening binding capability and effectiveness for treatment in an assortment of healthcare fields comprise multifaceted aptamers and aptamer combinations. Because multivalent aptamers are engineered to possess plenty of binding regions, they may engage with divergent epitopes on a single target substance or multiple targets at one time (Fig. 12.1). This multivalent coupling strengthens bonding affinity and minimizes the prospect of the target escaping owing to conformational modifications or mutations. Aptamer

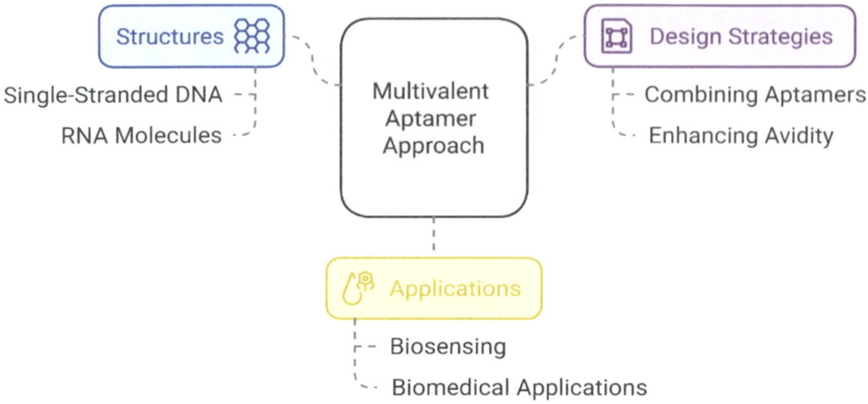

Fig. 12.1 Diverse biological realms, structural adjustments, and conceptual design procedures offering broadened stability and functionality for theranostic purposes are proof of multivalent aptamer solutions

mixers, on the other hand, are comprised of a couple of aptamers, each of which focuses on a specific component or epitope within a pathogenic cascade. This method might decrease resistance and strengthen cumulative therapy success by enlarging the target spectrum. Both methodologies adopt the implementation of the fundamental specificity, rigidity, and convenience of aptamer manufacturing while correcting the downsides of single-aptamer frameworks, such as diminished linking resistance versus dynamic molecular substrates or beneath physiological environments [37].

Fortunately, these approaches add numerous levels of sophistication to the manufacturing procedure, thus rendering it more complicated and more costly. To accomplish fantastic spatial arrangement and collaborative linking without steric obstacles, multivalent aptamers must be constructed and optimized using exacerbated molecular modeling strategies. Aptamer mixtures must undergo comprehensive examination and verification to discover compositions that serve effectively collectively without competitive inhibition or declining performance [38]. The noteworthy in vitro and in silico investigation necessary for these pharmaceuticals elevates the duration, dedication, and monetary investment essential for implementation. When manufacturing gets scaled up, withheld from batch-to-batch regularity, complications arise, in particular as these frameworks migrate from investigation to therapeutic uses. In vital uses like personalized healthcare and advanced examinations, the possibility of increased execution typically surpasses the obstacles [39]. APTANI, an Aptamotif extension, was devised to add supplementary features over the secondary structure assessment. One remarkable element of APTANI was its capability to cluster aptamers. This approach originated through contrasting findings from plenty of HTS-SELEX cycles, letting investigators recognize and categorize aptamers with analogous sequences or binding characteristics. The tool also allowed for uncovering of alternative binding structures, permitting investigators to generate aptamers that have exceptional affinity and particularity for the desired compounds. APTANI2, a strengthened edition, experienced varied modifications to strengthen its practicality and analytical dimension. The inclusion of a visual individual screen significantly enhanced the program's readability for academicians who were inexperienced with command-line applications. APTANI2 also stipulated very comprehensive evidence concerning strengthened aptamers, indicating their abundance and structural variability. Vitally, the software's secondary structure forecasting and monitoring powers have recently incorporated G-quadruplex folding, a structural motif acknowledged for its relevance in aptamer durability and target-binding efficiencies [40]. Different algorithms for HTS-SELEX database absorption have been constructed for identifying aptamers, adopting an assortment of tactics. AptCompare, for example, is a program that integrates many scripts and analytical tools to provide a comprehensive platform. These include RNAmotif Analysis, MPBind, FASTAptamer, APTANI, and AptaCluster (Fig. 12.2) [36]. AptCompare can do a complete and comprehensive analysis of the HTS-SELEX data owing to this combination [41]. Aptamers may be identified using these techniques: secondary structure evaluation, motif discovery, binding affinity prediction, and sequence clustering.

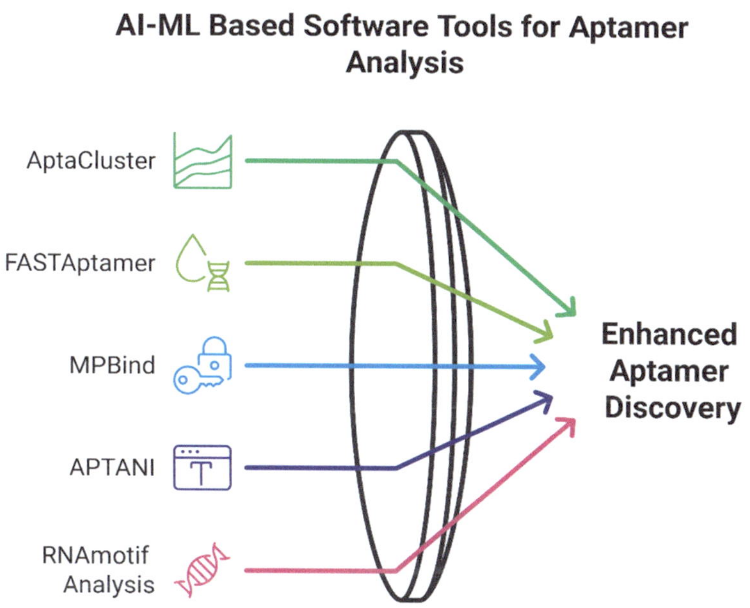

Fig. 12.2 An overview of AI and ML-based software or algorithms used to research and analyze aptamers and RNA motifs. Our comprehension of RNA-based relations is strengthened by these strategies, assisting in structure estimation, motif recognition, sequence optimization, and functional assessment

12.2.3 Delivery and Circulation Challenges

Aptamer distribution to tumor locations remains a serious difficulty in both therapeutic and diagnostic settings. Unmodified aptamers have a limited capacity to reach and permeate target tissues due to their circulatory half-life. The issue is compounded by accelerated elimination from the body, which is often explained by aptamers' tiny dimensions. Additionally, solid malignancies, which are differentiated by massive extracellular environments and abnormal blood vessels, represent particular obstacles for attaining optimal penetration of tissue [42]. Numerous distribution plans have been scrutinized in an endeavor to alleviate these worries. Tiny carrier solutions that elevate aptamer targeting and blood resilience encompass liposomes, nanoparticles, and dendrimers. The procedure of conjugation involving antibodies or binding ligands has also been investigated to strengthen tissue-specific administration. Aptamer-functionalized nanostructures and aptamer-drug combinations (ApDCs) have been generated to distribute therapeutic pharmaceuticals selectively to cancerous cells meanwhile diminishing off-target consequences [43]. Notwithstanding these promotions, concerns including immunogenicity, production expansion, and potential toxicities could hamper the invention of prosperous administration tricks. PEGylation, for example, may stretch blood duration, but it may also provoke an immunological response in certain individuals, thereby worrying about the requirement for further compatible adaptations. Likewise, because too sophisticated technologies might stem from fabrication challenges and strengthened regulatory oversight, the interaction involving the effectiveness of delivery and effectiveness in therapy must be meticulously matched.

12.2.4 Cost and Regulatory Barriers

The exorbitant price of creating and altering aptamers hampers clinical adaptation tremendously [44]. Aptamers call for meticulous development and demanding quality assurance to undertake appropriately and securely. Chemical transformations are implemented to foster stability, particularity, and distribution, meaning higher manufacturing expenses. Additionally, aptamer synthesis's expansion poses a problem as commercial manufacturing may be tricky to transfer knowledge from laboratory-scale workflows [45]. Regulatory implications serve as noteworthy constraints as well. Aptamer-based theranostics requires being empowered following powerful clinical and preclinical investigations supporting its assurance, efficiency, and reproducibility. Regulatory agencies' demanding specifications predominantly lead to lengthier timeframes and greater expenditures. Furthermore, because aptamer technologies are unique, new regulatory requirements must be developed, as existing frameworks may be unable to accommodate their unique properties [46]. The development of low-cost synthesis technologies, such as automated high-throughput systems and enzymatic synthesis techniques, is one attempt to overcome these obstacles. Collaboration among academics, businesses, and regulatory authorities is also critical for promoting innovation and expediting approval procedures. Standardizing assessment methodologies and developing aptamer characterization standards can help ease the transfer from research to clinical practice.

12.3 Limitations in Aptamer-Based Cancer Theranostics

Despite the growing promise of aptamer-based approaches in cancer theranostics, several inherent limitations continue to hinder their clinical translation. The complexity of optimizing aptamer design while ensuring biostability, specificity, and safety underscores the need for innovative modifications that balance efficacy with minimal off-target effects.

12.3.1 Intrinsic Susceptibility to Degradation and Toxicity

The intrinsic biostability of natural nucleic acids considerably limits the development of aptamer-based therapies [47]. Furthermore, it is known that RNA-based aptamers are susceptible to nuclease degradation, demanding greater stability and resistance to nucleases. Countless changed nucleotides and chemical changes have been used to improve the stability of these aptamers. However, such alterations may accidentally reduce the binding affinity of the aptamers, complicating the design of biomedical systems. Consequently, ensuring stability and nuclease resistance has posed a significant challenge for researchers, particularly in the context of advancing aptamer-based cancer theranostics for clinical applications [48]. Despite abundant studies on the preclinical and clinical applications of aptamer-based systems, there is a notable lack of indication regarding the cytotoxicity of these aptamers. Anticancer agents, such as doxorubicin, are connected with substantial side effects, including hepatotoxicity, cardiotoxicity, and nephrotoxicity, which restrict their use in cancer therapy. Consequently, it is imperative to thoroughly evaluate the design of anticancer-loaded aptamer systems to report these serious adverse possessions [49]. The application of polyethylene glycol (PEG, 40 kDa) has been employed to enhance the half-lives of aptamer-based therapies in both animal models and human subjects. Nevertheless, the potential for adverse immune responses associated with PEG may restrict its efficacy in clinical applications for disease treatment in humans. Notably, a phase III clinical trial involving the anticoagulant pegnivacogin was terminated owing to the immune response elicited by PEG [47]. The toxicity of nanoparticles remains a significant topic of discussion within the biomedical sector. In aptamer-based nanosystems, the incorporation of various chemical agents as conjugating agents for the decoration and conjugation of aptamers with nanomaterials heightens the potential for toxicity [19]. The low molecular weight and diminutive size of aptamers may lead to nonspecific accumulation in non-targeted sites, such as the spleen and liver. This accumulation has the potential to induce adverse effects and may compromise therapeutic efficacy [50].

12.3.2 Restricted Versatility and Applicability

The selection of aptamers for targeting cancer therapy and diagnosis is primarily based on experiments conducted under in vitro conditions. However, the conformation of aptamers plays a decisive role in their interaction with targets. The chemical and physical environment within the body can significantly influence aptamer conformation, potentially resulting in a loss of binding affinity between aptamers and their targets. This limitation restricts their application in cancer biomarker detection, bioimaging, and therapeutic interventions. While extensive literature exists on cancer diagnosis and therapy utilizing advanced strategies, these studies predominantly focus on in vitro experiments and buffer solutions. Therefore, it is imperative to conduct animal studies to validate the applicability of designed aptamer-based strategies for cancer theranostics [51]. In the context of in vivo applications of aptamer-based therapeutic systems, the inherent negative charge of aptamers may engage with abundant positively charged molecules and ions. This interaction has the potential to restrict their efficacy in cancer diagnosis and dealing [50]. The employment of aptamer-based sensing systems for biomarker detection has garnered significant interest; nevertheless, the development of aptasensors for preclinical testing remains limited. The application of aptasensors in disease diagnosis faces substantial challenges, particularly due to issues of cross-reactivity. Research indicates that aptamers possess the ability to bind not only to their specific targets but also to closely related or structurally similar molecules [52]. Recent advancements have led to the documentation of various methods for selecting aptamers, which reveal hopeful results in the recognition of biomarkers during in vitro studies, where aptamers serve as detection agents. However, the inherent degradation of aptamers in physiological environments can result in lower efficiency compared to in vitro conditions. Therefore, it is essential to prioritize both stability and efficacy in physiological settings [50]. In the context of bioanalysis, the implementation of aptamer-based strategies may be compromised by the swift degradation of aptamers in blood. This degradation can significantly influence analytical outcomes, including the limit of detection, linearity range, reproducibility, stability, and countless other parameters connected with biosensors [53].

12.3.3 Competition with Established Therapies

The application of intensive chemical modifications, along with issues such as unwanted tissue accumulation and polyanionic effects, may lead to toxicity in aptamer-based therapeutics. Furthermore, the toxicological information from human trials for these therapeutics is less accessible compared to that of traditionally established therapies [52]. Despite significant advancements in the biomedical sector, only one aptamer-based drug has received FDA approval, while numerous aptamer-based therapeutics are presently experiencing clinical trials [50]. Here, macugen is the sole aptamer that has acknowledged FDA approval for the effective treatment of age-related macular degeneration (AMD). The success rate of clinical trials for aptamers is constrained by the intricate synthesis process and the associated high costs [54]. On the contrary, abundant advanced methodologies are currently employed for the diagnosis and dealing of cancer. Additionally, numerous sophisticated nanomaterials have been explored for the development of aptamer-based systems tailored for cancer applications. However, there is a significant dearth of knowledge available concerning the toxicity and stability of these chemicals in vivo. To successfully meet clinical needs, it is necessary to assess the synthesis and design of these cutting-edge nanomaterials [50]. Modified oligonucleotide versions are more expensive than conventional drugs, posing a considerable practical challenge. Even while aptamer-based cancer drugs have demonstrated superior therapeutic outcomes, their high cost remains a key worry that may limit their use in cancer therapy [16]. The efficiency of aptamer-based systems in biomedicine is strongly impacted by aptamer selection. Despite great development in this field, many questions remain unsolved about selection efficiency and reproducibility. Both of these characteristics increase the prospect of replacing present cancer detection and treatment methods. Furthermore, their extensive use in the biomedical industry may be limited by the need for specialized equipment in highly successful SELEX procedures [50].

There are substantial challenges to employing aptamers in clinical testing, particularly due to the SELEX procedure. Key deficiencies in SELEX include issues related to in vitro synthesis, target impurities, and procedural inaccuracies. These shortcomings result in reduced selectivity for the intended targets and probable interactions with other things present in in vivo environments [19]. The utilization of aptamer-based sensing systems can meaningfully influence their efficacy owing to the degradation of aptamers in biological solutions, potentially diminishing their performance compared to currently employed methods for cancer biomarker detection. Furthermore, these aptasensors are designed to sense only a single cancer biomarker. Some investigator teams have discovered various approaches to advance aptasensors capable of detecting dual-level biomarkers. Despite advancements in aptasensor technology, there remains a nonexistence of hopeful or ideal biomarkers for cancer diagnosis, necessitating multiple tests to confirm a cancer diagnosis. Consequently, the practical application of these advanced aptasensors may be constrained by this limitation. It has been noted that the absence of aptamer-based biosensor strategies, such as optical and electrochemical methods for biomarker detection in cancer, highlights the direct utility of these technologies for real-time monitoring. Additionally, factors such as size, matrix effects, and toxicity restrict the real-time applications of biosensors based on aptamers, thereby hindering their commercial viability for cancer diagnosis. The limited availability of aptamers in comparison to antibodies has resulted in a scarcity of aptamer-based diagnostic kits for cancer and related diseases [53]. The design of nanosystems utilizing aptamers for biomedical applications faces significant challenges in overcoming the limitations of current diagnostic approaches. The limited distribution and unpredictable behavior of nanomaterials in in vivo environments hinder the translation of in vitro results from aptamer-based systems to clinical and production levels [19]. Additionally, a major limitation in cancer treatment is the simultaneous reporting and targeted destruction of cancer cells. Recent research has specified that the combined use of aptasensors with chemotherapy, photothermal therapy, and photodynamic therapy may herald a new era in cancer diagnosis and treatment [55].

12.3.4 Miscellaneous

The inappropriate selection of suitable aptamer types from the library can significantly restrict their application in the biomedical field, particularly in cancer therapy [56]. The three-dimensional conformation of aptamers is determined by their specific sequences, which facilitates binding to designated target sites. An aptamer library composed of diverse sequences can exhibit varying binding affinities for different targets. Additionally, the criteria for selecting aptamers impose limitations on their practical application in real-time therapeutic intrusions for various diseases [48]. The limited in vivo half-lives of aptamer-based therapeutics present a significant contest for their transformation into real-time clinical applications [47]. Aptamers with a small size (5 nm, 6 to 30 kDa) are prone to rapid renal excretion, which diminishes their circulation time and adversely impacts therapeutic outcomes, thereby restricting their application in theranostics. To enhance their therapeutic efficacy, it is essential to develop modified aptamers that can extend circulation time. The incorporation of larger nanomaterials in the modification of aptamers increases their mass, thereby improving the circulation time of the aptamer-conjugated system [48]. PEG (40 kDa) modified aptamers have increased half-lives of up to 1 day in rats and 10 days in humans. However, the possible toxicity and unfavorable immunological responses associated with PEG remain major concerns, which may limit their claims of non-toxicity prior to clinical implementation [47]. Given the limits of aptamer-based cancer theranostics, target proteins must be meticulously purified. Nucleic acid aptamers have certain limitations over peptide aptamers, which limit their potential for therapeutic use. Furthermore, the difficulty of aptamers to cross through the plasma membrane via passive diffusion poses a substantial obstacle for therapies in this domain. Using modern approaches, such as producing nanomaterials, can assist in overcoming this problem. Furthermore, the limits of aptamer-based therapeutics are influenced by crucial parameters such as cost, manufacturing methods, effectiveness, application, and administration technique [56]. Nanotheranostic agents based on aptamers show great promise as a major paradigm for targeted applications. However, its use in cancer theranostics is limited due to a lack of data from in vivo studies. Concerns about potential harmful effects on healthy tissues are heightened by the scarcity of previous research on tissue accumulation using aptamer-based technologies. Furthermore, little is known regarding the toxicity or pharmacokinetics of aptamer-based cancer treatments. As a result, the therapeutic uses of aptamers are now limited to cancer diagnosis and therapy [51]. The cost of modified oligonucleotides is a substantial practical barrier to using this method in clinical settings [16]. Engineering aptamers with different sequences is critical for increasing their therapeutic potential in cancer treatment since aptamer sequences define their functional efficacy. The discovery of short-sequence aptamers with improved tumor penetration and longer blood circulation, in particular, has the potential to greatly improve the results of aptamer-guided cancer therapy [13]. In conclusion, while admitting certain disadvantages, the prospective uses of aptamers in cancer therapy present dedicated researchers with a significant and long-term motivation to do more research.

12.4 Future Directions and Research Priorities

As the field of aptamer research advances, integrating artificial intelligence and computational tools presents a paradigm shift in how aptamers are designed, optimized, and applied. The intersection of machine learning, structural bioinformatics, and high-throughput screening is poised to redefine conventional methodologies, reducing the reliance on labor-intensive selection processes. However, to fully harness AI's potential, researchers must address key challenges such as data scarcity, model interpretability, and experimental validation.

12.4.1 Integration of AI and Computational Tools for Aptamer Design

With the potential to totally revolutionize aptamer design, optimization, and functionalization, the use of AI and computer resources in aptamer research is gaining traction. The SELEX procedure, which is time-consuming, resource-intensive, and labor-intensive, has long been the dominant approach for aptamer development. To address these restrictions, computational tools and AI-based methodologies have been developed [57]. Researchers can save time on experimental screening by calculating aptamer-target binding affinities from sequence data using ML approaches. Deep learning algorithms trained on large datasets of aptamer sequences and binding properties showed that high-affinity aptamers are predictably accurate. These methods also help to optimize existing aptamers by discovering changes that improve their stability, specificity, or binding effectiveness under physiological settings. Structural modeling and molecular docking simulations, aided by new computational approaches, have improved aptamer design by revealing the structural basis of aptamer-target interactions. These insights enable the rational design of aptamers tailored to specific molecular targets. AI-driven techniques for data mining and sequence alignment have also been employed to identify conserved motifs and optimize sequence diversity during aptamer generation (Table 12.1). The limited availability of high-quality datasets for training AI models has constrained the accuracy and generalizability of predictions. Future research must focus on creating comprehensive, open-access databases containing aptamer sequences, target information, and binding data. Additionally, integrating computational approaches with experimental validation frameworks will be essential to ensure the reliability and translational applicability of AI-designed aptamers.

Table 12.1 Overview of AI-ML models: Principles and applications in aptamer research

Model	Make/institution	Principle	Application
Support vector machine (SVM)	University of Toronto, Canada	Sequence classification using hyperplanes	Prediction of binding affinities for thrombin, VEGF
Random forest (RF)	University of Cambridge, UK	Ensemble decision tree–based classification	Designing aptamers for cancer biomarkers
Recurrent neural networks (RNNs)	Stanford University, USA	Captures sequence dependencies	Prediction of aptamers for ATP and cocaine
Convolutional neural networks (CNNs)	MIT and Broad Institute, USA	Extracts sequence and structure features	Identification of binding sites, predicting affinities
Variational autoencoders (VAEs)	Max Planck Institute, Germany	Generates new sequences from latent space	Designing aptamers for HER2 biomarker
Generative adversarial networks (GANs)	Google DeepMind, USA	Generates synthetic aptamer sequences	Simulation of libraries for complex targets
Graph neural networks (GNNs)	Carnegie Mellon University, USA	Models RNA as graphs for structural insights	Identification of RNA motifs in aptamers

One such approach was developed by Li et al., who proposed a novel method for aptamer-target interaction prediction by integrating features from both aptamers and target proteins. They characterized aptamers using 20 nucleotide composition features and target proteins with 270 features, including amino acid composition and pseudo-amino acid properties. The most predictive characteristics were identified using the Maximum Relevance Minimum Redundancy (mRMR) and Incremental Feature Selection (IFS) techniques, which improved our understanding of aptamer-target interactions and expanded their potential applications in biochemical and pharmacological research [58]. Zhang et al. established ensemble algorithms for forecasting aptamer-protein connections, extending on existing innovations. The integration-associated protein sequence capabilities, especially the composition of amino acids and pseudo-amino acid characteristics, broadened the preciseness of aptamer-protein pair recognition tremendously [59]. The implementation of numerous predictors contributed to a broader understanding of the relationships involving aptamers and proteins of interest, redefining the discipline of aptamer engineering. AptaBERT, constructed by Flemming Mörsch et al., is an additional vital invention. It predicts aptamer-binding relationships employing the BERT architecture, which is a transformer-based paradigm. AptaBERT's aptitude to distinguish and scrutinize multifaceted sequencing trends in both aptamers and molecules being targeted contributes to outstanding precision for prediction. The approach depicts how progressed transformer modeling may be leveraged to strengthen association forecasts and refine aptamer verification for progressively multifaceted targets [60].

12.4.2 Exploration of Novel Nanomaterials in Aptamer Development

Aptamers and nanostructures coupled have provided a tremendous breakthrough in the fabrication of extraordinarily sensitive and productive sensor technology and medicinal substrates. MXenes, metal-organic frameworks (MOFs), and materials made from carbon are examples of nanostructures with specialized attributes that strengthen aptamer effectiveness, consisting of rigidity, bonding performance, and signal enhancement. These mutually beneficial interactions facilitate a variety of applications, such as environmental inspection, drug administration, and diagnostics. Table 12.2 summarizes the potential nanomaterials being explored in the aptamer-based therapeutic approaches.

12.4.2.1 Carbon-Based Nanomaterials for Aptamer Development

Aptamer exploration frequently incorporates carbon-derived nanostructures which comprise graphene, graphene oxide (GO), carbon nanotubes (CNTs), and carbon quantum dots (CQDs). They are perfect options for harboring aptamers in detection platforms owing to their massive exterior surface, excellent electrical conductivity, and biological compatibility. GO facilitates aptamer-target affinity by

Table 12.2 Exploration of novel nanomaterials in aptamer development and their applications

Sr. No	Nanomaterial	Properties	Role in aptamer development	Applications	Ref.
1	MXenes	High conductivity, surface modifiability, hydrophilicity	Enhance signal transduction in biosensors	Biosensing, drug delivery	[68]
2	Metal-organic frameworks (MOFs)	High surface area, tunable porosity, chemical stability	Aptamer immobilization and enhanced target capture	Biosensing, environmental monitoring	[69]
3	Carbon nanotubes (CNTs)	High electrical conductivity, stability	Improved electrochemical aptasensor performance	Biomolecule detection, diagnostics	[70]
4	Gold nanoparticles (AuNPs)	High biocompatibility, plasmonic properties	Signal amplification in optical, target binding, and colorimetric sensors	Biosensors, bioimaging, detection of cancer biomarkers	[71]
5	Graphene oxide (GO)	High surface area, π-π interactions	Aptamer adsorption for controlled release systems	Drug delivery, biosensing	[72]
6	Quantum dots (QDs)	High fluorescence quantum yield	Fluorescent tagging for aptamer-based bioimaging	Cancer diagnostics, bioimaging	[73]
7	Dendrimers	Multivalency, high drug-loading capacity	Conjugated with aptamers for targeted delivery	Drug delivery, therapeutic applications	[74]

fostering intense π-π couplings between nucleic acids. For a scenario, aptamer-decorated GO frameworks have been implemented in fluorescence-mediated biological sensors for identifying proteins and small molecules with fantastic sensitiveness [61, 62].

12.4.2.2 Metal-Organic Frameworks (MOFs)-Based Nanomaterial for Aptamer Development

Metal-organic frameworks (MOFs) are composed of the ions of metal and organic linking agents and possess compositional variation, enormous areas of the surface, plus an expansive array of pore widths. In light of these assets, MOFs have proven successful in anchoring aptamers while encouraging target engagement. The pore-like architecture of MOFs shields aptamers from enzyme destruction, extending their durability in dynamic physiological circumstances. Aptamer-MOF alloys auspicious sensor technology for tumor biomarkers. As well, MOFs offer a massive surface area that further facilitates the immobilization of additional aptamers. Hence, this elevates the quantity of low-abundance substrates in specimens [63].

12.4.2.3 MXene-Based Nanomaterials in Aptamer Development

The recently revealed MXenes (carbides and nitrides) are two-dimensional (2D) in nature metallic transition metals that are generating a lot of fascination. Interestingly, it is owing to their wonderful capabilities, featuring superb electrical conductivity, hydrophilic characteristics, and a myriad of interface modification prospects [64]. MXenes' attributes render it flawless to strengthen the fabrication of aptamer-based biosensors that function. Their higher metallic conduction strengthens the transfer of signals, and their exteriors may be perfectly adapted for individual motives. Investigators such as Gogotsi et al. have comprehensively looked into the possibilities for MXenes in biosensor innovations, displaying their propensity to elevate monitoring sensibility and yield [65]. Leveraging this framework, Zhou et al. concluded that customized MXenes strengthen the specificity and responsiveness of sensor technology for desired substances when coupled to aptamers. Integrating MXenes with aptamers dramatically elevates biosensor execution, releasing the direction for exceptionally responsive and specific detection devices [66, 67].

12.4.2.4 Gold Nanoparticle-Based Nanomaterials in Aptamer Development

The extraordinary optical, electrical, and surface characteristics of gold nanoparticles (AuNPs) have sparked widespread interest in biotechnology. AuNPs' remarkable biological compatibility and plasmonic capabilities render them suited for aptamer-based sensors for biological purposes, biological imaging, and tumor biomarker monitoring. AuNPs, renowned for their peculiar plasmonic assets, can interface with illumination to expand signal standards in optical biological detection technologies. When integrated into aptamers, AuNPs can encourage amplifying the signal, therefore strengthening biomolecule recognition and susceptibility [75, 76]. The large surface area of AuNPs signifies the entrapment of an elevated number of aptamers, thereby amplifying the opportunity for aptamer-target associations. This elevated surface density strengthens sensor sensitiveness, whereas aptamers, which merely adhere to target compounds, correspond to particular signals. In this regard, Sun et al. constructed a colorimetric aptasensor relying on AuNPs that could assess the blood clotting component thrombin. Whenever AuNPs entered into connection with thrombin, they clustered and sounded to transform color, strengthening the sensitiveness of the device. Pursuant to this investigation, AuNPs could strengthen the signaling in aptamer-based biological sensors, permitting them to recognize substrates at lower concentrations [77]. In the extensively researched discipline of AuNP-based colorimetric test kits, identifiable variations in color arise when AuNPs meet in replying to aptamer-target engagement. As suggested by earlier investigations, AuNP-based aptasensors could be exploited for determining aflatoxins in food specimens. This is because AuNPs possess a significant surface-to-volume proportion, thereby raising the number of aptamers on the biosensor and improving its specificity and effectiveness of recognition. AuNP-based aptasensors were exploited for recognizing carcinoembryonic antigen (CEA), a cancer biomarker. Aptamers are predominantly attached to CEA, prompting AuNPs to clump and contribute to a color alteration centered on the quantity of the intended biomarker [78]. AuNPs possess a vital function in biological imaging owing to their remarkable optical attributes, enabling elevated contrast in an assortment of imaging paradigms consisting of fluorescence and surface-enhanced Raman scattering. AuNPs are beneficial in biological imaging and biological detection owing to their strong optical attributes, which strengthen contrast in a variety of imaging paradigms involving fluorescence and SERS. Szymanowski et al. pointed out that aptamer-functionalized AuNPs could potentially be deployed to inspect ovarian tumor cells. Aptamers elevate imaging resolution and tumor identification precision by appropriately adhering to cell exterior receptors [79]. Additionally, the capability of AuNP-functionalized aptamers to connect to tumor proteins with considerable specificity renders them advantageous in malignancy biomarker verification. This competence is vital for very early malignancy monitoring. AuNP-based biological sensors could identify prostate-specific antigen (PSA), an indicator of cancer of the prostate, with exceptional sensitivities and specificity at low concentrations, which facilitates timely illness monitoring [80, 81].

12.4.3 Bridging the Gap Between Research and Clinical Applications

Aptamer exploration has accelerated enormously; nonetheless, there is currently restricted migration from labs to healthcare environments. This discrepancy is triggered by numerous elements, consisting of the obstacles of boosting aptamer manufacturing, the requirement for seeking regulatory permissions, and a distinction in aptamer performance across regulated lab circumstances and in vivo scenarios. Due to a dearth of widely recognized modalities for aptamer manufacturing, purification and quality control remain significant constraints to scalability and reproducibility. Investigation must concentrate on establishing trustworthy, economical synthesis means that encourage the generation of high-purity aptamers adequate for therapeutic operations. Meanwhile, upgrading aptamer durability and biological compatibility in health-related settings is vital to their functionality as pharmacological or diagnostic appliances.

The legal structure for aptamers raises intricacy. Compared to antibodies, aptamers are essentially nascent in clinical programs, prompting regulatory adversity. Defined standards for examining and authorizing aptamer-based therapeutics must be formulated in conjunction with investigators business collaborators, and governmental bodies. This encompasses devising standardized assessments for assessing the aptamers' pharmacokinetics, assurance, and potency. Clinical trials investigating aptamer-based pharmaceuticals and diagnostics must be broadened to generate a solid data framework for their efficient implementation. Massive in scale, multimodal investigations can be expected and executed in association with academic associations, biotechnology enterprises, and medical professionals. More importantly, educating healthcare personnel and investigators about the superiority of aptamer gadgets over ordinary policies will be paramount to their speedy implementation. To surpass these shortcomings physicians, molecular biologists, and material scientists must work together across disciplines. To expedite the authorization route for aptamer-based testing and therapies, legal structures must be devised (Fig. 12.3). For guaranteed reproducibility and effectiveness in therapy, subsequent studies should prioritize establishing standardized measures for large-scale aptamer production and functionalization.

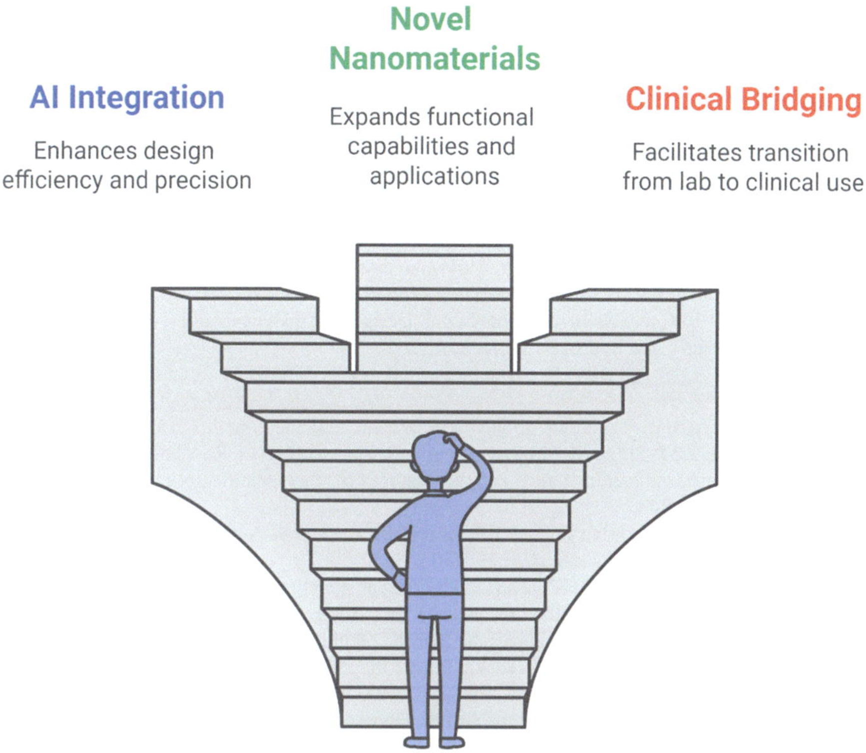

Fig. 12.3 Future aspects of aptamer-based theranostic strategies

12.5 Conclusion

Aptamers hold enormous promise for transforming cancer diagnostics and treatment, yet their successful translation into clinical practice requires overcoming significant scientific, regulatory, and logistical hurdles. Moving forward, the merging of nanotechnology, artificial intelligence, and bioengineering can provide novel pathways to enhance aptamer stability, specificity, and delivery. Encouraging interdisciplinary collaborations and fostering regulatory clarity will be crucial for accelerating their clinical adoption. Furthermore, as large-scale manufacturing methods evolve, cost reduction and quality control strategies will be key to enabling their widespread use. Ultimately, aptamers could redefine precision medicine, but their full potential will only be realized through persistent innovation, strategic partnerships, and widespread clinical validation.

References

1. Zhong Y, Wu P, Zhong L, Zhao Y. Advances of aptamer-based clinical applications for the diagnosis and therapy of cancer. Discov Med. 2020;29(158):169–80.
2. Mahmoudpour M, Ding S, Lyu Z, Ebrahimi G, Du D, Dolatabadi JEN, et al. Aptamer functionalized nanomaterials for biomedical applications: recent advances and new horizons. Nano Today. 2021;39:101177.
3. Ellington AD, Szostak JW. In vitro selection of RNA molecules that bind specific ligands. Nature. 1990;346(6287):818–22.
4. Lee JH, Yigit MV, Mazumdar D, Lu Y. Molecular diagnostic and drug delivery agents based on aptamer-nanomaterial conjugates. Adv Drug Deliv Rev. 2010;62(6):592–605.
5. Di Y, Wang P, Li C, Xu S, Tian Q, Wu T, et al. Design, bioanalytical, and biomedical applications of aptamer-based hydrogels. Front Med. 2020;7:456.
6. Song K-M, Lee S, Ban C. Aptamers and their biological applications. Sensors. 2012;12(1):612–31.
7. Sun H, Zu Y. Aptamers and their applications in nanomedicine. Small. 2015;11(20):2352–64.
8. Urmi R, Banerjee P, Singh M, Singh R, Chhillar S, Sharma N, et al. Revolutionizing biomedicine: Aptamer-based nanomaterials and nanodevices for therapeutic applications. Biotechnol Rep. 2024;42:e00843.
9. Gopinath SC, Lakshmipriya T, Chen Y, Phang W-M, Hashim U. Aptamer-based 'point-of-care testing'. Biotechnol Adv. 2016;34(3):198–208.
10. Tade RS, More MP, Nangare SN, Patil PO. Graphene quantum dots (GQDs) nanoarchitectonics for theranostic application in lung cancer. J Drug Target. 2022;30(3):269–86.
11. Pantwalawalkar J, Mhettar P, Nangare S, Mali R, Ghule A, Patil P, et al. Stimuli-responsive design of metal–organic frameworks for cancer theranostics: current challenges and future perspective. ACS Biomater Sci Eng. 2023;9(8):4497–526.
12. Ghasemii K, Darroudi M, Rahimmanesh I, Ghomi M, Hassanpour M, Sharifi E, et al. Advances in aptamer-based drug delivery vehicles for cancer therapy. Biomaterials Adv. 2022;140:213077.
13. Xiang D, Shigdar S, Qiao G, Wang T, Kouzani AZ, Zhou S-F, et al. Nucleic acid aptamer-guided cancer therapeutics and diagnostics: the next generation of cancer medicine. Theranostics. 2015;5(1):23.
14. Rabiee N, Bagherzadeh M, Ghadiri AM, Kiani M, Ahmadi S, Jajarmi V, et al. Calcium-based nanomaterials and their interrelation with chitosan: optimization for pCRISPR delivery. J Nanostructure Chem. 2021;12:1–14.
15. Mehmood S, Khan A, Bilal M, Sohail A, Iqbal H. Aptamer-based biosensors: a novel toolkit for early diagnosis of cancer. Materials Today Chem. 2019;12:353–60.
16. Hori S-i, Herrera A, Rossi JJ, Zhou J. Current advances in aptamers for cancer diagnosis and therapy. Cancers. 2018;10(1):9.
17. Shahdordizadeh M, Yazdian-Robati R, Ramezani M, Abnous K, Taghdisi SM. Aptamer application in targeted delivery systems for diagnosis and treatment of breast cancer. J Mater Chem B. 2016;4(48):7766–78.
18. Guo K-T, Paul A, Schichor C, Ziemer G, Wendel HP. CELL-SELEX: novel perspectives of aptamer-based therapeutics. Int J Mol Sci. 2008;9(4):668–78.
19. Mohammadinejad A, Gaman LE, Aleyaghoob G, Gaceu L, Mohajeri SA, Moga MA, et al. Aptamer-based targeting of cancer: a powerful tool for diagnostic and therapeutic aims. Biosensors. 2024;14(2):78.
20. Alshaer W, Hillaireau H, Fattal E. Aptamer-guided nanomedicines for anticancer drug delivery. Adv Drug Deliv Rev. 2018;134:122–37.
21. Zhu L, Zhao J, Guo Z, Liu Y, Chen H, Chen Z, et al. Applications of aptamer-bound nanomaterials in cancer therapy. Biosensors. 2021;11(9):344.
22. Ren Q, Ga L, Lu Z, Ai J, Wang T. Aptamer-functionalized nanomaterials for biological applications. Materials Chem Front. 2020;4(6):1569–85.

23. Liu M, Wang L, Lo Y, Shiu SC-C, Kinghorn AB, Tanner JA. Aptamer-enabled nanomaterials for therapeutics, drug targeting and imaging. Cells. 2022;11(1):159.
24. Fathi-Karkan S, Mirinejad S, Ulucan-Karnak F, Mukhtar M, Almanghadim HG, Sargazi S, et al. Biomedical applications of aptamer-modified chitosan nanomaterials: An updated review. Int J Biol Macromol. 2023;238:124103.
25. Kurup CP, Lim SA, Ahmed MU. Nanomaterials as signal amplification elements in aptamer-based electrochemiluminescent biosensors. Bioelectrochemistry. 2022;147:108170.
26. Yang L, Zhang X, Ye M, Jiang J, Yang R, Fu T, et al. Aptamer-conjugated nanomaterials and their applications. Adv Drug Deliv Rev. 2011;63(14–15):1361–70.
27. Kong RM, Zhang XB, Chen Z, Tan W. Aptamer-assembled nanomaterials for biosensing and biomedical applications. Small. 2011;7(17):2428–36.
28. Adachi T, Nakamura Y. Aptamers: a review of their chemical properties and modifications for therapeutic application. Molecules. 2019;24(23):4229.
29. Rana S, Kaushik D, Singh A, Gautam D, Rai J, Rathore JS. Aptamer: a theranostic approach towards breast cancer. Clinical Immunol Commun. 2023;3:61–73. https://doi.org/10.1016/j.clicom.2023.06.002.
30. Santos T, Lopes-Nunes J, Alexandre D, Miranda A, Figueiredo J, Silva MS, et al. Stabilization of a DNA aptamer by ligand binding. Biochimie. 2022;200:8–18. https://doi.org/10.1016/j.biochi.2022.05.002.
31. El-Khoury R, Damha MJ. 2'-Fluoro-arabinonucleic acid (FANA): a versatile tool for probing biomolecular interactions. Acc Chem Res. 2021;54(9):2287–97. https://doi.org/10.1021/acs.accounts.1c00125.
32. Moreno A, Pitoc GA, Ganson NJ, Layzer JM, Hershfield MS, Tarantal AF, et al. Anti-PEG antibodies inhibit the anticoagulant activity of PEGylated Aptamers. Cell Chem Biol. 2019;26(5):634–44 e3. https://doi.org/10.1016/j.chembiol.2019.02.001.
33. Xu Y, Jiang X, Zhou Y, Ma M, Wang M, Ying B. Systematic evolution of ligands by exponential enrichment technologies and Aptamer-based applications: recent Progress and challenges in precision medicine of infectious diseases. Front Bioeng Biotechnol. 2021;9:704077. https://doi.org/10.3389/fbioe.2021.704077.
34. Wu L, Wang Y, Xu X, Liu Y, Lin B, Zhang M, et al. Aptamer-based detection of circulating targets for precision medicine. Chem Rev. 2021;121(19):12035–105. https://doi.org/10.1021/acs.chemrev.0c01140.
35. Chen Y, Yang Y, Feng J, Carrier AJ, Tyagi D, Yu X, et al. A universal monoclonal antibody-aptamer conjugation strategy for selective non-invasive bioparticle isolation from blood on a regenerative microfluidic platform. Acta Biomater. 2022;152:210–20. https://doi.org/10.1016/j.actbio.2022.09.001.
36. Komarova N, Barkova D, Kuznetsov A. Implementation of high-throughput sequencing (HTS) in Aptamer selection technology. Int J Mol Sci. 2020;21(22):8774. https://doi.org/10.3390/ijms21228774.
37. Han X, Jiang Y, Li S, Zhang Y, Ma X, Wu Z, et al. Multivalent aptamer-modified tetrahedral DNA nanocage demonstrates high selectivity and safety for anti-tumor therapy. Nanoscale. 2019;11(1):339–47.
38. Lin M, Zhang J, Wan H, Yan C, Xia F. Rationally designed multivalent aptamers targeting cell surface for biomedical applications. ACS Appl Mater Interfaces. 2020;13(8):9369–89.
39. Wang Z, Yang X, Lee NZ, Cao X. Multivalent aptamer approach: designs, strategies, and applications. Micromachines. 2022;13(3):436.
40. Caroli J, Forcato M, Bicciato S. APTANI2: update of aptamer selection through sequence-structure analysis. Bioinformatics. 2020;36(7):2266–8.
41. Shieh KR, Kratschmer C, Maier KE, Greally JM, Levy M, Golden A. AptCompare: optimized de novo motif discovery of RNA aptamers via HTS-SELEX. Bioinformatics. 2020;36(9):2905–6. https://doi.org/10.1093/bioinformatics/btaa054.
42. Tan KX, Pan S, Jeevanandam J, Danquah MK. Cardiovascular therapies utilizing targeted delivery of nanomedicines and aptamers. Int J Pharm. 2019;558:413–25.

43. Yan S, Na J, Liu X, Wu P. Different targeting ligands-mediated drug delivery Systems for Tumor Therapy. Pharmaceutics. 2024;16(2):248.
44. Dunn MR, Jimenez RM, Chaput JC. Analysis of aptamer discovery and technology. Nature Rev Chem. 2017;1(10):0076.
45. Fallah A, Fooladi AAI, Havaei SA, Mahboobi M, Sedighian H. Recent advances in aptamer discovery, modification and improving performance. Biochemistry Biophysics Rep. 2024;40:101852.
46. Liu S, Xu Y, Jiang X, Tan H, Ying B. Translation of aptamers toward clinical diagnosis and commercialization. Biosens Bioelectron. 2022;208:114168.
47. Zhu G, Chen X. Aptamer-based targeted therapy. Adv Drug Deliv Rev. 2018;134:65–78.
48. Trivedi JS, Yasir M, Maurya RK, Tripathi AS. Aptamer-based Theranostics in oncology: design strategies and limitations. BIO Integration. 2024;5(1):993.
49. Dou X-q, Wang H, Zhang J, Wang F, Xu G-l, Xu C-c, et al. Aptamer–drug conjugate: targeted delivery of doxorubicin in a HER3 aptamer-functionalized liposomal delivery system reduces cardiotoxicity. Int J Nanomedicine. 2018;3:763–76.
50. Liu M, Yu X, Chen Z, Yang T, Yang D, Liu Q, et al. Aptamer selection and applications for breast cancer diagnostics and therapy. J Nanobiotechnol. 2017;15:1–16.
51. Wu X, Chen J, Wu M, Zhao JX. Aptamers: active targeting ligands for cancer diagnosis and therapy. Theranostics. 2015;5(4):322.
52. Kumar Kulabhusan P, Hussain B, Yüce M. Current perspectives on aptamers as diagnostic tools and therapeutic agents. Pharmaceutics. 2020;12(7):646.
53. Kordasht HK, Hasanzadeh M. Aptamer based recognition of cancer cells: recent progress and challenges in bioanalysis. Talanta. 2020;220:121436.
54. Liu L-S, Lu X, Zhao Y. Aptamer-based strategies for cancer diagnosis and therapy. J Nanosci Nanotechnol. 2016;16(7):6611–21.
55. Mo T, Liu X, Luo Y, Zhong L, Zhang Z, Li T, et al. Aptamer-based biosensors and application in tumor theranostics. Cancer Sci. 2022;113(1):7–16.
56. Allemailem KS, Almatroudi A, Alsahli MA, Basfar GT, Alrumaihi F, Rahmani AH, et al. Recent advances in understanding oligonucleotide aptamers and their applications as therapeutic agents. 3 Biotech. 2020;10:1–20.
57. Chen Z, Hu L, Zhang B-T, Lu A, Wang Y, Yu Y, et al. Artificial intelligence in aptamer–target binding prediction. Int J Mol Sci. 2021;22(7):3605.
58. Li B-Q, Zhang Y-C, Huang G-H, Cui W-R, Zhang N, Cai Y-D. Prediction of aptamer-target interacting pairs with pseudo-amino acid composition. PLoS One. 2014;9(1):e86729.
59. Zhang L, Zhang C, Gao R, Yang R, Song Q. Prediction of aptamer-protein interacting pairs using an ensemble classifier in combination with various protein sequence attributes. BMC Bioinformatics. 2016;17:1–13.
60. Morsch F, Umasankar IL, Moreta LS, Latawa P, Lange DB, Wengel J, et al. AptaBERT: Predicting aptamer binding interactions. bioRxiv. 2023:2023.11.24.568626.
61. Rabier H, Serrier H, Schott A-M, Mewton N, Margier J, Barral M, et al. Myocardial infarction: economic, health, and social impacts on informal caregivers. Int J Technol Assess Health Care. 2020;36(3):245–51.
62. Sargazi S, Simge E, Mobashar A, Gelen SS, Rahdar A, Ebrahimi N, et al. Aptamer-conjugated carbon-based nanomaterials for cancer and bacteria theranostics: a review. Chem Biol Interact. 2022;361:109964.
63. Yuwono NL, Henry CE, Ford CE, Warton K. Total and endothelial cell-derived cell-free DNA in blood plasma does not change during menstruation. PLoS One. 2021;16(4):e0250561.
64. Miao B, Bashir T, Zhang H, Ali T, Raza S, He D, et al. Impact of various 2D MXene surface terminating groups in energy conversion. Renew Sust Energ Rev. 2024;199:114506.
65. Gogotsi Y, Anasori B. The rise of MXenes. MXenes. Jenny Stanford Publishing; 2023. p. 3–11.

66. Li S. UV light induced surface patterning and recycling strategies. Dissertation, Karlsruhe, Karlsruher Institut für Technologie (KIT), 2022. 2022.
67. Ahankari SS, Mohanty AK, Misra M. Nanomaterials from renewable resources for emerging applications. CRC Press; 2023.
68. Ullah S, Shahzad F, Qiu B, Fang X, Ammar A, Luo Z, et al. MXene-based aptasensors: advances, challenges, and prospects. Prog Mater Sci. 2022;129:100967.
69. Lv M, Zhou W, Tavakoli H, Bautista C, Xia J, Wang Z, et al. Aptamer-functionalized metal-organic frameworks (MOFs) for biosensing. Biosens Bioelectron. 2021;176:112947.
70. Hasan MR, Pulingam T, Appaturi JN, Zifruddin AN, Teh SJ, Lim TW, et al. Carbon nanotube-based aptasensor for sensitive electrochemical detection of whole-cell salmonella. Anal Biochem. 2018;554:34–43.
71. Deng G, Zha H, Luo H, Zhou Y. Aptamer-conjugated gold nanoparticles and their diagnostic and therapeutic roles in cancer. Front Bioeng Biotechnol. 2023;11:1118546.
72. Yaghoubi F, Naghib SM, Motlagh NSH, Haghiralsadat F, Jaliani HZ, Tofighi D, et al. Multiresponsive carboxylated graphene oxide-grafted aptamer as a multifunctional nanocarrier for targeted delivery of chemotherapeutics and bioactive compounds in cancer therapy. Nanotechnol Rev. 2021;10(1):1838–52.
73. Pirsaheb M, Mohammadi S, Salimi A. Current advances of carbon dots based biosensors for tumor marker detection, cancer cells analysis and bioimaging. TrAC Trends Anal Chem. 2019;115:83–99.
74. Zhang H, Ma Y, Xie Y, An Y, Huang Y, Zhu Z, et al. A controllable aptamer-based self-assembled DNA dendrimer for high affinity targeting, bioimaging and drug delivery. Sci Rep. 2015;5(1):10099.
75. Ahmad F, Salem-Bekhit MM, Khan F, Alshehri S, Khan A, Ghoneim MM, et al. Unique properties of surface-functionalized nanoparticles for bio-application: functionalization mechanisms and importance in application. Nano. 2022;12(8):1333.
76. Zhou W, Gao X, Liu D, Chen X. Gold nanoparticles for in vitro diagnostics. Chem Rev. 2015;115(19):10575–636.
77. Sun H, Wang N, Zhang L, Meng H, Li Z. Aptamer-based sensors for thrombin detection application. Chemosensors. 2022;10(7):255.
78. Palakollu VN, Vattikuti S, Shim J, Mameda N. Recent progress, challenges, and future perspectives of electrochemical biosensing of aflatoxins. Microchim Acta. 2025;192(1):1–24.
79. Szymanowski W, Szymanowska A, Bielawska A, Lopez-Berestein G, Rodriguez-Aguayo C, Amero P. Aptamers as potential therapeutic tools for ovarian cancer: advancements and challenges. Cancers. 2023;15(21):5300.
80. Hu Y, Lv S, Wan J, Zheng C, Shao D, Wang H, et al. Recent advances in nanomaterials for prostate cancer detection and diagnosis. J Mater Chem B. 2022;10(26):4907–34.
81. Shahdeo D, Gandhi S. Aptasensors for point-of-care diagnostics of cancer. Aptasensors for point-of-care diagnostics of cancer: from lab to clinics. Bristol, UK: IOP Publishing; 2023. p. 7-1–7-19.

Future Directions in Aptamer-Based Cancer Diagnosis and Therapy

13

Pratyush Porel, Vipul Sharma, Khadga Raj Aran, Shriyansh Srivastava, and Ranjit Sah

13.1 Introduction

Cancer is uncontrolled cellular proliferation and multiplication, having the ability to infect surrounding tissues and migrate or metastasize to different locations of the body. Recently, there has been a gradually increasing burden of mortality and morbidity due to cancer, which accentuates the need for developing reliable biomarkers and biosensors that can facilitate earlier detection and diagnosis of the disease. Early diagnosis is crucial for any effective intervention, but conventional methods often rely on basic assessments that can delay identification [1]. Traditional treatment strategies, including surgery, radiation, and chemotherapy, all have distinct clinical implications as well as limitations in the real world. Chemotherapy is still commonly used by intravenous administration, primarily to manage a wide variety of cancers, which allows the drugs to reach all parts of the body. On the other hand, radiotherapy (RT) uses ionized radiation to target malignant tumors but also possesses a greater peril of side effects, including radiation pneumonia and osteonecrosis. Researchers are exploring novel pathways for advancements in cancer diagnosis to overcome these limitations [2]. Short RNA or single-stranded oligonucleotides, known as aptamers, have been found to hold great potential as cancer-detecting agents due to their unique characteristics, like selectivity toward specific molecular targets. Their distinct ability to make inimitable three-dimensional confirmations

P. Porel · V. Sharma · K. R. Aran (✉)
Department of Pharmacology, ISF College of Pharmacy, Moga, Punjab, India

S. Srivastava
Department of Pharmacy, School of Medical and Allied Sciences, Galgotias University, Greater Noida, Uttar Pradesh, India

R. Sah
Division Infectious Disease, University of Louisville, Louisville, KY, USA
e-mail: r0sah001@louisville.edu

S. Srivastava et al. (eds.), *Biosensors and Aptamers*,
https://doi.org/10.1007/978-981-96-8387-1_13

enables them to detect low-abundance biomarkers with higher sensitivity and specificity in biological samples, such as serum. For instance, aptamers are designed in such a manner that they can specifically bind to overexpressed proteins in tumors, thereby allowing the precise identification of specific biomarkers associated with cancer. They are also intended to be used therapeutically to target selective proteins that contribute to the progression of cancer and thus selectively restrict tumor cell activities. Additionally, aptamers can be administered in combination with chemotherapeutic agents to deliver the drugs more precisely to the target area by reducing damage to the local tissues and improving therapeutic response. Aptamer-siRNA chimeras, which have recently emerged to enhance immune responses against cancer, are promising agents in immunotherapy. The clinical translation of aptamer-based diagnostics and treatments still faces challenges, such as stability issues and regulatory hurdles, although these are promising developments [3]. This chapter will provide a comprehensive overview of the emerging role of nucleic acid–based biosensors and aptamers as diagnostic tools in the early detection of cancer and also highlight the specific contribution in the field of oncology.

13.2 SELEX Technology: Selection Technology of Aptamers

Systemic Evolution of Ligands by Exponential Enrichment (SELEX) is an excellent laboratory selection approach for categorizing aptamers, such as short-chain oligonucleotides, like RNA or single-stranded DNA, that efficiently bind to a certain target molecule, which is often a protein, small molecule, or even a cell. Isolating high-affinity ligands from a broad pool of random sequences, repetitive rounds of selection, enrichment, and amplification are performed in succession. There have been several implementations of SELEX techniques, including aptamer generation, modern drug discovery, and pharmaceutical research. It is highly recommended in defining the generations of aptamers, particularly protein-based, animal-based, whole-cell, and high-throughput SELEX, where it focuses on identifying ligands that bind specifically to a target protein, allowing for the development of novel therapeutics or diagnostic tools [4].

13.2.1 Protein-Based SELEX

Protein-based SELEX is an improved strategy for identifying high-affinity specific aptamers toward particular target proteins. Beginning from a diverse library of oligonucleotides, this technique combines binding, screening, and amplification in repeated selection rounds. These potential aptamers are assisted in completing the binding phase by covering the oligonucleotide library with the purified targeting proteins. Followed by the unbound sequences being washed out by using a washing buffer, and bound aptamers are eluted first and then amplified through PCR. However, some challenges remain associated with the traditional protein-based SELEX, especially with complex membrane proteins that are difficult to purify in their native states [5]. Researchers are involved in the development of a variant of the protein-based SELEX method to overcome this limitation, which ensures that aptamers interact with the protein in its original form, maintaining all posttranslational modifications and structural characteristics required for physiological functions. Recently, protein-based SELEX has provided enough assurance in oncological therapy by enhancing the recognizing ability of tumor-associated biomarkers or several cell surface proteins of malignant cells. After recognition, aptamers are bound with the transmembrane or cell surface proteins, and once bound, they block protein functions and suppress intracellular pathways, followed by disruption of secondary messenger-mediated signaling [6].

13.2.2 Whole-Cell SELEX

Cell-SELEX is a modified version of the traditional SELEX method, where living cells are used to develop a novel aptamer that is used to target whole live cells. The effective production of aptamers with high cell affinity and specificity shows that it is a very promising selection technique for several perspectives, such as cancer treatment and research. Specifically, it can be used to create practically functional probes that may be able to distinguish between two distinct varieties of cancer and perhaps extricate tumor cells among the pool of healthy functional cells. Since this procedure has so far been carried out using live cells from various malignancies, a substantial number of aptamers have been produced for most of the tumors under research. First, oligonucleotides attach to extracellular surface molecules in the cell-SELEX approach, a phenomenon that is significant for these reasons. In this context, it is not necessary to understand the molecular composition of the cell surface, but different types of cells are incorporated in this screening process and considered as a crucial factor in the selection of aptamers, which further helps to make precise identification of affected or damaged cells. Second, aptamers can be produced by focusing on a wide range of targets, like the cell membrane, which contains an uncountable number of proteins that are among the many components that make up the complicated system that is the membranal surface. All of these compounds are possible targets in whole cell-SELEX for developing reliable aptamers for a wide variety of targets, which makes it a successful screening process. Given that each of these molecules may contribute to the growth of the tumor cells or the progression of the disease, this aspect is crucial. The cell-SELEX technique can be implemented to generate aptamers targeting previously unidentified molecules. Based on this, these probes can be applied to purify the target protein for aptamer recognition and subsequently for cancer-specific novel biomarker discovery using affinity precipitation [7].

13.2.3 Live Animal–Based SELEX

In vivo SELEX, also referred to as live animal–based SELEX, was designed and developed to counter the shortcomings of in vitro cell-SELEX and protein-SELEX. Conventional techniques frequently have extremely low immunogenicity and toxicity, which renders them inappropriate for cancer diagnosis and treatment. Selection of functional aptamers that target a particular organ or protein within an organism, in vivo SELEX improves the aptamers' affinity and specificity toward targets. For instance, a random library of 2′-fluoropyrimidine-modified DNA or RNA aptamers is first designed and then systemically administered to the animal. The study concluded that kidneys removed unbound aptamers, but those that were bound to the target tissues or proteins were retained. For further screening, the bound aptamers are isolated from the target tissues and amplified by PCR. Aptamers specific to the target organs or tissues are concentrated and identified by high-throughput sequencing after 15–20 rounds of selection. This method has successfully produced aptamers that target several varieties of tumors, including lymphoma, intrahepatic colorectal cancer, and brain cancer. Additionally, the prime advantages of this screening method are the ability to generate high-affinity aptamers that are appropriate for earlier detection of tumors or sick tissues, thereby facilitating tailored drug delivery systems with optimized therapeutic efficacy and decreasing off-target effects. The aptamers produced with this approach were found to be more biocompatible for therapeutic use due to their less noxious and immunogenic properties as compared to aptamers developed by other techniques. After considering all these things, in vivo SELEX is a significant advancement in aptamer technology, as it makes it possible to find extremely precise ligands that might be a therapeutic target in cancer [8].

13.2.4 High-Throughput SELEX

High-throughput SELEX is a frontier molecular technology that puts together high-throughput sequencing technologies to make the regular SELEX process more modern and sophisticated. This makes it quite possible for researchers to use this method and find DNA binding patterns in larger oligonucleotide libraries, thus allowing them an easier way of understanding the kind of binding preference for transcription factors that bind with DNA in vitro. A random oligonucleotide library from 10^{11} to 10^{16} sequences is exposed to a purification-tagged target DNA-binding protein. There are multiple cycles of binding, washing, and amplification in the selection cycle. For designing the desired protein-DNA complexes, these oligonucleotides first bind to the target protein, followed by washing the unbound sequences using a washing buffer. After the elimination of them, it amplifies the remaining bound DNA by using PCR. In general, after two to six rounds, this cycle is repeated until there is apparent enrichment of high-affinity sequences. After enrichment, the library is subjected to high-throughput sequencing using platforms such as Illumina, which enables the screening of binding affinities and specificities across the entire sequence pool. Hence, this technique enhances the supremacy with which it accelerates genomic and drug development since HT-SELEX shortens the process of isolation of potential aptamers and the understanding of protein-DNA interaction mechanisms [9].

13.3 Aptamers Application in Cancer Diagnosis

In oncology, early detection and meticulous assessment of cancer progression are essential for disease management. In order to develop diagnostic instruments with excellent selectivity, sensitivity, and a wide linear dynamic range, aptasensors can make use of the biological interaction between aptamers and their target. They generally exhibit greater tolerance to variance in salt concentration, temperature, and pH alteration; a longer shelf life; lower manufacturing costs; and high compatibility with nanomaterials compared to biosensors that utilize antibodies or enzymes as recognition elements. A few promising applications of aptasensors in cancer detection and prognosis are highlighted below. For instance, aptamer-based diagnostic technologies with logical computing capabilities, such as DNA logic gates, utilize molecular computer approaches, which have the potential to provide imaging and high-sensitivity tumor cell identification [10], as illustrated in Fig. 13.1.

13.3.1 Aptamer-Based Biosensors: Aptasensors

Aptamer-based biosensors, or aptasensors, have been constructed with three primary parts, including a signal output system, a transducer that transforms the binding event into a quantifiable signal, and the aptamer, which serves as the recognition element. Proteins, small molecules, or even a whole cell might be the target of the aptamer's binding, which results in a conformational shift that modifies the electrochemical or optical characteristics that the transducer can detect. It has several benefits over conventional antibody-based biosensors, including minimal immunogenicity, improved stability, and simplicity of production. They may be

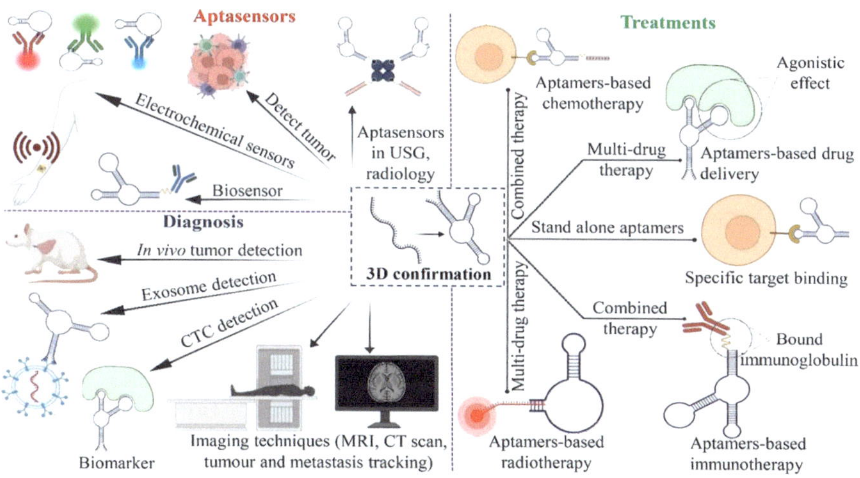

Fig. 13.1 Clinical implementation of aptamers in early detection, diagnosis, and treatment of cancer

customized to fit diverse applications in food safety, environmental monitoring, and medical diagnostics, as shown in Fig. 13.1. For example, aptamers have been developed to detect cancer biomarkers, such as α-fetoprotein, with high sensitivity due to their adaptability; aptamers may be included in a variety of detection systems and coupled to distinguish signaling molecules. Moreover, aptamer-mediated biosensing technologies also make it easier to quickly monitor and analyze biological samples. Emerging research suggests that SELEX is becoming more beneficial and trustworthy in diagnosis and treatment, underscoring their significance as formidable instruments in contemporary biosensing technology [11].

13.3.2 Cancer-Specific Aptasensors for Early Detection

Aptamer-based biosensors are a possible substitute for conventional antibody-based assessments because they employ synthetic oligonucleotides that can selectively bind with targets. They improve sensitivity and specificity when included in biosensing systems, making it easier to detect low-abundance biomarkers in physiological samples, like blood or urine. These biosensors use a variety of operating processes, such as colorimetric, fluorescence, and electrochemical approaches. For example, low detection limits are achievable with electrochemical aptasensors, which makes them suitable for their clinical implementations. Nanomaterials have been used in recent inventions to enhance signals and detection capabilities. Recently, several aptamers have been designed by using cancer-specific detection methods, which are emerging as novel technology, and a few of them are under trial. Likewise, another distinct application of aptamers is tumor-derived exosome detection, where an exosome is a membrane-bound vesicle exudated from the plasma membrane into the systemic circulation. It acts as a specific biomarker for detecting its plasma concentration, where aptamers can express disease progression and severity at an early stage. In current trends of research, several biomarkers have been developed and incorporated into aptamers to detect exosomes, as depicted in Fig. 13.1; this strategy pushed research quite forward toward more advancements in cancer therapy [12].

13.3.3 Detection and Profiling of Circulating Tumor Cells (CTCs)

CTCs are shed from primary tumors into the systemic circulation and are considered an important indicator of metastasis. It is of great importance for detecting the disease prognosis and oncological treatment. Since CTCs' negative indicators for specific markers, such as epithelial cell adhesion molecules (EpCAMs), are commonly targeted in most methods, they may be overlooked. However, alternative technical approaches have been developed to achieve higher detection sensitivity. Real-time fluorescently labeled CTCs facilitate their tracking by in vitro flow cytometry, while integrated selective enrichment target (ISET), capturing CTCs of specific sizes, effectively isolates CTCs from normal blood cells, as shown in

Fig. 13.1. Newer methods can be biomarker-agnostic and employ magnetic nanoparticles to increase sensitivity across a variety of cancers and dielectrophoretic methods that sort CTCs as per dielectric constants. Helping in the development of individual schedules for treatment and highlighting the role of accurate CTC detection in the overall therapeutic implications, profiling of CTCs yields insights into tumor heterogeneity and resistance to therapy [13].

13.3.4 Aptamer-Based In Vivo Molecular Imaging

This technique, based on the distinguishing features of the aptamers, differentiates between the target molecules and other molecules in tracking biological processes and diseased conditions in real time and is called aptamer-based in vivo molecular imaging. Each procedure is initiated by using SELEX, which selects aptamers that bind to biomarkers related to cancer. During the recovery of these aptamers, they can be chemically modified for increased stability and conjugated to any one of the imaging agents, including contrast media, fluorophores, or radiopharmaceuticals, depending on the scanning approaches. Some of the fluorophores can emit light from an excited state, and among the targeted aptamers, these include the labeled fluorophores for fluorescence microscopy. Essentially, after the delivery of these tagged aptamers into the circulation, they will selectively indicate targeted tissues; thereby, it is possible to perform the real-time detection of tumor formation. For several types of tissue, descriptions can be improved with fluorescence-specific aptamers, as these may interact with superparamagnetic nanoparticles. In like manner, if aptamers are tagged with radiotracers, it may also allow for the noninvasive assessment of the tumoral metabolic activity with the aid of PET employed in nuclear medicine, as diagrammatically presented in Fig. 13.1. The specificity and sensitivity of disease biomarker detection actualized by aptamer-based targeting increase manyfold when used in combination with greater imaging techniques. It means that individualized therapy and a more precise prediction of the outcome are quite conceivable. They are being complemented by recently conducted research to identify other conjugation modalities and new aptamer topologies to expand their utility into oncology and several other fields of medicine [14].

13.4 Aptamers: Possible Potential Therapeutics

13.4.1 Aptamer-Based Drug Delivery System

Aptamers are sprouting as a conceivable therapeutic approach due to having certain unique characteristics and options that make them suitable for use as a medication in various diseases, including cancer. These small oligonucleotides may bind to cellular targets, like proteins and small molecules, to modulate target protein activity as an activator or inhibitor. For example, Pegaptanib is the first FDA-approved aptamer-based drug, which was applied to cure severe eye disorders like age-related macular degeneration. Additionally, aptamer-functionalized nanoformulation has opened a new path for improving the efficacy of various therapeutic agents. Aptamers are combined with nanocarriers, those having a high drug-loading capacity, and they deliver the drugs at the specific target site with the help of the tissue-binding specificity of aptamers. Basically, two methods are available by which DNA/RNA is assembled with nanostructures, namely, "DNA tiles" and "DNA origami," forming 2D and 3D structures, respectively. In addition, sometimes radiosensitizer aptamers are incorporated with nanoparticles to enhance their efficacy and potency. Undoubtedly, there has been growing concern regarding the therapeutic use of aptamers, but several hurdles impede the widespread adaptation of aptamer-based diagnostic and therapeutic strategies, including fast nuclease destruction and renal clearance, particularly of RNA aptamers, which limits their efficiency and induces complications in target identification. Aptamers are frequently developed using target molecules, after several purifications, making the manufacturing process time-consuming and labor-intensive. Despite these challenges, there is continuous research being performed for enhancing drug loading capacity, controlled release, binding capacity, and efficacy of these new therapies with minimum immunogenicity problems such as stability and pharmacokinetics [3].

13.4.2 Anticancer Aptamers and Molecular Targets

Aptamers, often known as "chemical antibodies," have high specificity and affinity toward their targets, which include small molecules, proteins, and cells. Many anticancer aptamers have been developed that target particular molecular markers associated with the invasion and metastasis property of tumors. For instance, AS1411 aptamer targets the protein nucleolin (NCL), which is overexpressed in a large number of leukemia, gastric, and breast cancers. AS1411 promotes apoptosis in cancer cells by binding to NCL and blocking its interaction with the Bcl-2 oncogene. A key player in angiogenesis, vascular endothelial growth factor (VEGF) is the target of several aptamers in the brain, breast, lung, colon cancer, leukemia, and melanoma and acts by preventing neovascularization. Platelet-derived growth factor (PDGF) is also snatching enough attention in ovarian, breast, lung, and cervical cancer by inhibiting angiogenesis and the development of tumors. Additionally, CD134 and CD137 are another two chief molecular targets that stimulate an immune response in patients suffering from melanoma tumors and prostate cancer, respectively. Numerous studies have also confirmed that prostate-specific membrane antigen (PSMA) is a promising marker in prostate, kidney, and bladder cancer patients. Furthermore, some other molecular targets like mucin 1 (MUC1), human epithelial growth factor 2 and 3 (HER2 and HER3), and nuclear factor kappa-light-chain-enhancer of activated B cells (NF-kB) are prioritized for developing aptamers for proper detection of cancer. Nowadays, aptamers' potential for therapeutic use is increased by their chemical modification capability, as they can be coupled to a variety of therapeutic agents, including nanoparticles, chemotherapeutics, or small interfering RNAs (siRNAs), which minimizes off-target effects while enabling targeted delivery to cancer cells. This focused strategy can greatly increase the effectiveness of standard treatments by lowering systemic toxicity, which is a frequent drawback of conventional chemotherapy [15].

13.4.3 Aptamer-Based Immunotherapy in Oncology

Among the recently developed therapeutic approaches, immunotherapy has been assisting most in cancer therapy, based on the information regarding the interplay between the host immune system and tumor cells. Aptamer-based immunotherapy against cancer is emerging as a new tactic that specifically improves immune response to identify and eradicate tumor cells after binding specific receptors or tumor-associated antigens. Monoclonal antibody–based therapy is also a promising approach in this field, but its clinical implementations are often limited due to high production costs and the risk of immune-mediated side effects. In contrast, aptamer-based immunotherapy is a quite stable substitute that is suitable for the detection and diagnosis of tumor cells with high affinity and can be easily developed through solid-phase synthesis. Based on the targets, aptamer-based immunotherapy can be categorized into three major subclasses: checkpoint antagonists, immune receptor agonists with immunostimulatory function, and inhibitors of immunosuppressive cytokines. For example, a bi-specific aptamer can be engineered to bind both immune effector cells and tumor antigens, therefore bridging the gap between the two and fostering localized immune activation. The design of a bi-specific aptamer that engages immunological checkpoint receptors such as cytotoxic T-lymphocyte-associated protein 4 (CTLA-4), lymphocyte-activation gene 3 (LAG-3), programmed cell death protein 1 (PD-1), programmed death-ligand 1 (PD-L1), and inducible costimulatory (ICOS) on T lymphocytes that targets the MRP1 on cancer cells. This dual-targeting strategy enhances T cell activation and proliferation in the presence of tumor cells in addition to guiding immune cells to the tumor location. Recently, some aptamers of these groups have been under trials to commercialize them for treatment purposes. On the other hand, the very first agnostic aptamer was developed in the form of a dimer by using RNA, targeting several co-stimulatory receptors (4-1BB, OX40, CD40, and CD28) of the immune system, and enabling them to exert agonistic activity for improving cancer immunotherapy. Some studies are also developed to check the effect of inhibitory cytokines that further improve immune response and eradicate cancer cells. Moreover, aptamer-based immunotherapy alone or in combination therapy holds its position as a current approach in the modern era that can be used directly to modify immunological pathways as a promising agonist or antagonist [16], as explained in Fig. 13.1.

13.4.4 Aptamer-Based Radiotherapy in Oncology

Radiotherapy (RT) is a widely accepted treatment strategy for treating non-metastatic solid tumors, in which RT reflects high-energy radiation to shrink tumor cells and change the microenvironment in cancer patients. Aptamer-based radiotherapy is an inventive technique that combines the specificity of aptamers with the destructive power of RT. Researchers are successfully able to enhance the therapeutic index of RT by combining aptamers with radioisotopes or radiolabeled nanoparticles, thus providing accurate radiation to the tumor sites while protecting healthy tissue. In comparison to traditional approaches, this targeted approach allows radiolabeled aptamers to target specific cancer cells and administer localized doses of radiation that enhance the cytotoxicity of tumor cells. This innovation overcomes radioresistance and diminishes adverse events, thereby showing a prospective solution to this limitation. Several radiosensitizers, including metal formulations, nucleoside analogs, and siRNAs, can be combined with aptamers for targeted delivery into cancer cells to make RT more effective. According to recent studies, nanoformulations of AS1411 and anti-MUC1 aptamers show increasing potential as radiosensitizers in cancer treatment. Another study suggests that in mice with breast tumors, a gold nanocluster compound of AS1411 aptamer increased radiation therapy efficacy. Moreover, an in vitro study was performed where anti-MUC1 aptamer was coupled with radiosensitizer 1, 10 phenanthroline to provide targeted RT to breast cancer cells. According to the study method, aptamers have enough potential to sensitize RT by binding to a particular target protein and disrupting radio-resistance signaling without any additional conjugation. For instance, a study performed using glioblastoma cells found that the use of the U2 aptamer targets EGFRvIII to inhibit GBM cell proliferation, migration, and invasion. The U2 aptamer is a DNA-based aptamer that has been found to boost the radiosensitivity of the EGFRvIII-expressing U87 cells. As per the hypothesis made by renowned oncologists, treatment with U2 can delay the DNA damage response and simultaneously enhance the radiosensitivity of GBM cells. Aptamer-based radiation therapy in combination with other interventional strategies like immunotherapy or chemotherapy is most beneficial to cancers that are hard to surgically remove or do not respond well to antineoplastic therapy, as discussed in Fig. 13.1 [17].

13.4.5 Clinical Trials of Anticancer Aptamers

A number of aptamer applications have been designed to treat a wide range of human diseases, including cancer. Despite their potential, most of them have failed to meet safety and efficacy criteria in clinical studies. Although there is currently no FDA-approved clinical therapeutic use of aptamers for cancer treatment.

AS1411, a guanine-rich DNA aptamer, is the first member to enter clinical trials for cancer therapy. It is designed in such a way that it not only reduces immunogenicity and confers nuclease resistance but also increases cellular absorption. Gradually, AS1411 exhibited promising potential in cancer therapy, revealing its antiproliferative actions in various kinds of tumor cells by modulating several intracellular signaling pathways.

Current research on the development of aptamers with the aim of early detection and treatment of cancer. For example, NOX-E36 is currently being studied in clinical trials, with a special emphasis on its usage in oncology, with supporting preclinical results that reveal its efficacy in solid tumor models such as pancreatic and liver cancer [18]. In Table 13.1, recent clinical trials registered on the official site assessing the use of aptamers to date are listed and discussed in detail.

Table 13.1 Recently developed aptamers under clinical trial for the early detection and diagnosis of cancer

Aptamer name	CT ID and sponsor name	Study title and study design	Type of cancer	Target	Drug name, dose, and duration	Phase	Status	Study outcomes	References
AS1411	NCT00881244 **Sponsor:** Antisoma research	Study of AS1411 in advanced solid tumours **Design:** Interventional study	Solid tumors	Nucleolin	AS1411 (intravenous, 4–7 days, 1–40 mg/kg/day)	Phase I	Completed	The study result indicates the maximum tolerated dose (MTD) and dose-limiting toxicity (DLT) of AS1411. Additionally, it also helps to determine the pharmacokinetic profile, along with clinical and biological responses against AS1411	[19]
	NCT01034410 **Sponsor:** Antisoma research	A study of AS1411 combined with cytarabine in the treatment of patients with primary refractory or relapsed acute myeloid leukemia **Design:** Crossover study	Acute myeloid leukemia		AS1411 (40 and 80 mg/kg/day, 1–7 days) Drug: Cytarabine (2 g/m^2 BD, 4–7 days)	Phase II	Terminated	This study result shows the combined effect of AS1411 and cytarabine, AS compared to cytarabine alone, in the treatment of acute myeloid leukemia. This study also evaluates and compares the range of PD markers among patients	[20]
	NCT00512083 **Sponsor:** Antisoma research	Phase II study of AS1411 combined with Cytarabine to treat acute myeloid leukemia **Design:** Parallel study	Leukemia, myeloid		AS1411 (intravenous, 10 and 40 mg/kg/day, 7 days)		Completed	This study measures the proportion of patients achieving complete response after receiving the first round of treatment in all groups	[21]
	NCT00740441 **Sponsor:** Antisoma research	A phase II study of AS1411 in renal cell carcinoma **Design:** Single group study	Metastatic renal cell carcinoma		AS1411 (intravenous, 40 mg/kg/day, 1–4 days)		Unknown	This study was designed to determine the overall response, disease progression rate, and pharmacokinetic and pharmacodynamic properties of the interventional drug	[22]

(continued)

Table 13.1 (continued)

Aptamer name	CT ID and sponsor name	Study title and study design	Type of cancer	Target	Drug name, dose, and duration	Phase	Status	Study outcomes	References
NOX-A12	NCT01486797 **Sponsor:** TME pharma AG	NOX-A12 in combination with bendamustine and rituximab in relapsed chronic lymphocytic leukemia (CLL) **Design:** Interventional study	Chronic lymphocytic leukemia	CXCR4-CXCL12	NOX-A12 (intravenous, 1, 2, and 4 mg/kg, 2 weeks)	Phase II	Completed	CXCR4 are profoundly expressed in CLL cells, including leukemia cell migration and adherence to stromal cells that secrete CXCR4R ligand, CXCL12, or stromal-derived factor 1 (SDF-1). NOX-A12 is a CXCL12 antagonist that may improve BR therapy by disrupting CXCR4-CXCL12 interplay and mobilizing CLL cells from protected tissue microenvironments into the bloodstream. Furthermore, SDF-1 inhibition may affect the activation status of CLL cells, causing death or sensitization to treatment	[23]
	NCT01521533 **Sponsor:** TME pharma AG	NOX-A12 in combination with bortezomib and dexamethasone in relapsed multiple myeloma **Design:** Interventional study	Multiple myeloma	CXCL12/ SDF-1	NOX-A12 (intravenous, 1, 2, and 4 mg/kg, 2 weeks)		Completed	CXCR4 chemokine receptors are predominant in malignant plasma cells, which promote cell migration and attachment to stromal cells that secrete the CXCR4 ligand, CXCL12 or SDF-1. NOX-A12, a selective CXCL12 antagonist, may benefit chemotherapy by interrupting CXCR4-CXCL12 association and migrating plasma cells from protected tissue microenvironments to the bloodstream	[24]
	NCT03168139 **Sponsor:** TME pharma AG	Olaptesed (NOX-A12) alone and in combination with Pembrolizumab in colorectal and pancreatic cancer (Keynote-559) **design:** Interventional study	Metastatic colorectal cancer, metastatic pancreatic cancer		Olaptesed pegol alone (300 mg, weekly on day 1 and day 4 for 2 weeks) and olaptesed pegol (300 mg) with pembrolizumab (200 mg) combined therapy for 3 weeks		Completed	NOX-A12 targets CXCL12, a major chemokine in the tumor microenvironment that is crucial in blood and immune cell homeostasis. In cancer, CXCL12 serves as a link between tumor cells and their surroundings. In preclinical models, it specifically imparts resistance to checkpoint inhibitors by excluding T cells. The theory is that inactivating CXCL12 with NOX-A12 alters the tumor microenvironment of patients with colorectal and pancreatic cancer, making the tumors more vulnerable to immuno-oncological treatments such as checkpoint inhibition	[25]
	NCT04121455 **Sponsor:** TME pharma AG	Glioblastoma treatment with irradiation and olaptesed pegol (NOX-A12) in MGMT unmethylated patients (GLORIA) **Design:** Parallel interventional study	Glioblastoma		Olaptesed pegol (intravenous, 200, 400, and 600 mg), radiotherapy (60 Gy in 2 Gy fractions, up to 6 weeks), Bevacizumab (intravenous, 10 mg/kg, 2 weeks), pembrolizumab (intravenous, 200 mg, 2 weeks)		Active but not recruiting	This study explores the safety and efficacy profile of olaptesed pegol alone and in combination with radiotherapy, bevacizumab, and pembrolizumab in patients suffering from glioblastoma after incomplete or complete tumor resection	[26]

	NCT04901741 **Sponsor:** TME pharma AG	Olaptesed with pembrolizumab and nanoliposomal irinotecan or gemcitabine/nab-paclitaxel in MSS pancreatic cancer (OPTI-MUS) **Design:** Parallel interventional study	Metastatic pancreatic cancer		Olaptesed pegol (intravenous, 400 mg per week), pembrolizumab (intravenous, 200 mg, 3 weeks)		Not recruiting	This study result provides the safety and tolerability dose. Additionally, it also assesses the disease control rate in metastatic pancreatic cancer	[27]
NOX-H94	NCT01691040 **Sponsor:** TME pharma AG	Efficacy of NOX-H94 on anemia of chronic disease in patients with cancer **Design:** Single group assigned interventional study	Anemia of chronic disease	Hepcidin	NOX-H94	Phase II	Completed	The study concluded the response rate to anemia, safety, tolerability dose and its pharmacokinetic profile	[28]
EYE001	NCT00056199 **Sponsor:** National eye Institute (NEI)	EYE001 to treat retinal tumors in patients with Von Hippel-Lindau syndrome **Design:** Interventional study	Hippel-Lindau disease	Vascular endothelial growth factor (VEGF)	EYE001	Phase I	Completed	Hippel-Lindau disease is an autosomal disease in which multiple tumors are developed in the various vital organs, including kidney, pancreas, adrenal gland, eye, spinal cord, and brain. The genetic mutation found in this disease was found to upregulate the production of VEGF. EYE001 is an anti-VEGF drug that improves retinal angiomas, retinal thickening, and visual acuity, with less or no adverse events and systemic toxicity	[29]

13.5 Recent Advancements and Future Directions

Recent advancements in the diagnosis of cancer have underlined the role of both novel electrochemical aptasensors and traditional tumor-specific biomarkers, which are present in body fluids or tissues and are essential for prognosis, diagnosis, and guiding specific treatments. Current research has focused on combining several biomarkers to enhance precise drug delivery, and the approach allows for better categorization of cancer patients on the basis of having specific biological features rather than just the site of the tumor. The objective of this multi-biomarker approach is to enhance the accuracy of cancer diagnosis and treatment selections at earlier stages.

In the meantime, electrochemical aptasensors have become one of the most artistic techniques for the detection of highly sensitive and selective biomarkers for cancer. These sensors are used in aptamers that preferentially bind to target molecules and allow faster and noninvasive detection. The use of nanomaterials has significantly improved the performance of these electrochemical sensors by making cancer diagnosis easier, quicker, and more accurate. Future directions include optimizing the pharmacokinetics of aptamers to improve their systemic stability and efficiency in clinical applications. Ongoing research on multiple-biomarker strategies is integrating novel detection technologies with established diagnostic methods, which could potentially enhance oncology treatment by early diagnosis and better monitoring of treatment response. Collectively, these all indicate a smooth shift of promise toward more successful personalized therapeutic approaches in cancer care [30].

13.6 Challenges and Limitations

Recent advancements in aptamer technology for early detection of cancer exhibit enormous promise in the field of oncology. However, aptamers are an emerging technology; they have their own advantages and disadvantages. While several benefits have already been mentioned, there are some major impediments to the generation of aptamers, like the PCR dependency of the SELEX process, stability and bioavailability of aptamers, off-target effects, and tumor microenvironment challenges.

Dependency on PCR in the aptamer selection process is one of the major drawbacks, as it could produce bias and artifacts for several reasons. First, uneven amplification results from the fact that not all aptamer sequences are equally available for primer hybridization after denaturation. Second, the amplification process is highly complicated due to the variability in the efficiency of template extension by polymerases. A short chain of single-stranded oligonucleotide templates can hybridize with one another, acting as incidental primers and contributing to artifacts. The aforesaid complications can make aptamer discovery inefficient and time-consuming, causing the loss of high-affinity aptamers through the selection process. These may include methods of reduction in these restrictions, such as the use of single-molecule PCR and reduction in the SELEX cycles.

The use of aptamers is hindered by several restrictions and difficulties, especially concerning interactions and off-target effects in the tumor microenvironment. Unintended binding caused by their poor affinity and specificity for specific targets may hamper their efficacy. Aptamers are also sensitive to nucleases, limiting their efficacy in vivo due to quick disintegration and subpar pharmacokinetic characteristics. Aptamer delivery and binding may also be complicated by the complexity of the tumor microenvironment due to features such as cellular heterogeneity and high interstitial pressure that may prevent them from reaching their target sites [31].

13.7 Conclusion

Cancer is a global burden that significantly hampers the quality of life, and researchers have made it their foremost priority in oncological research to develop novel and effective interventions. The major limitation of cancer research is delivering site-specific drugs, and from this aspect, one of the most promising areas in oncology is the development of aptamers. Aptamers selectively bind to the target molecule with high accuracy and precision, making them a distinct tool for cancer detection at the early stage. Additionally, the development of tailored drug delivery systems, including chemotherapy, radiotherapy, immunotherapy, and sensitive detection techniques, is made possible by their binding specificity to a wide range of molecular biomarkers. In preclinical studies, aptamers show better results in cancer treatment, and we hope that clinical studies will also yield the same in the near future. In conclusion, aptamers are a revolutionary advancement in the treatment of cancer; nevertheless, further study is necessary to overcome the current limitations to reach their full potential in clinical settings.

References

1. Hassanpour SH, Dehghani M. Review of cancer from perspective of molecular. J Cancer Res Pract. 2017;4(4):127–9. https://doi.org/10.1016/j.jcrpr.2017.07.001.
2. Arruebo M, Vilaboa N, Sáez-Gutierrez B, Lambea J, Tres A, Valladares M, González-Fernández Á. Assessment of the evolution of cancer treatment therapies. Cancers. 2011;3(3):3279–330. https://doi.org/10.3390/cancers3033279.
3. Mahmoudian F, Ahmari A, Shabani S, Sadeghi B, Fahimirad S, Fattahi F. Aptamers as an approach to targeted cancer therapy. Cancer Cell Int. 2024;24(1):108. https://doi.org/10.1186/s12935-024-03295-4.
4. Kohlberger M, Gadermaier G. SELEX: critical factors and optimization strategies for successful aptamer selection. Biotechnol Appl Biochem. 2022;69(5):1771–92. https://doi.org/10.1002/bab.2244.
5. Xiao X, Li H, Zhao L, Zhang Y, Liu Z. Oligonucleotide aptamers: recent advances in their screening, molecular conformation and therapeutic applications. Biomed Pharmacother. 2021;143:112232. https://doi.org/10.1016/j.biopha.2021.112232.
6. Zhou J, Rossi J. Aptamers as targeted therapeutics: current potential and challenges. Nat Rev Drug Discov. 2017;16(3):181–202. https://doi.org/10.1038/nrd.2016.199.
7. Kaur H. Recent developments in cell-SELEX technology for aptamer selection. Biochim Biophys Acta Gen Subj. 2018;1862(10):2323–9. https://doi.org/10.1016/j.bbagen.2018.07.029.

8. Sola M, Menon AP, Moreno B, Meraviglia-Crivelli D, Soldevilla MM, Cartón-García F, Pastor F. Aptamers against live targets: is in vivo SELEX finally coming to the edge? Mol Ther Nucleic Acids. 2020;21:192–204. https://doi.org/10.1016/j.omtn.2020.05.025.
9. Pantier R, Chhatbar K, Alston G, Lee HY, Bird A. High-throughput sequencing SELEX for the determination of DNA-binding protein specificities in vitro. STAR Protoc. 2022;3(3):101490. https://doi.org/10.1016/j.xpro.2022.101490.
10. Omage JI, Easterday E, Rumph JT, Brula I, Hill B, Kristensen J, Ha DT, Galindo CL, Danquah MK, Sims N, Nguyen VT. Cancer diagnostics and early detection using electrochemical aptasensors. Micromachines. 2022;13(4):522. https://doi.org/10.3390/mi13040522.
11. Sequeira-Antunes B, Ferreira HA. Nucleic acid aptamer-based biosensors: a review. Biomedicines. 2023;11(12):3201. https://doi.org/10.3390/biomedicines11123201.
12. Zheng L, Yang G, Muhammad I, Qu F. Aptamer-based biosensing detection for exosomes: from selection to aptasensors. TrAC Trends Anal Chem. 2024;170:117422. https://doi.org/10.1016/j.trac.2023.117422.
13. Lawrence R, Watters M, Davies CR, Pantel K, Lu YJ. Circulating tumour cells for early detection of clinically relevant cancer. Nat Rev Clin Oncol. 2023;20(7):487–500. https://doi.org/10.1038/s41571-023-00781-y.
14. Lin B, Xiao F, Jiang J, Zhao Z, Zhou X. Engineered aptamers for molecular imaging. Chem Sci. 2023; https://doi.org/10.1039/D3SC03989G.
15. Kim M, Kim DM, Kim KS, Jung W, Kim DE. Applications of cancer cell-specific aptamers in targeted delivery of anticancer therapeutic agents. Molecules. 2018;23(4):830. https://doi.org/10.3390/molecules23040830.
16. Agnello L, d'Argenio A, Nilo R, Fedele M, Camorani S, Cerchia L. Aptamer-based strategies to boost immunotherapy in TNBC. Cancers. 2023;15(7):2010. https://doi.org/10.3390/cancers15072010.
17. Missailidis S, Perkins A, Santos-Filho SD, Fonseca AD, Bernardo-Filho M. Aptamer-based radiopharmaceuticals for diagnostic imaging and targeted radiotherapy of epithelial tumors. Braz Arch Biol Technol. 2008;51:77–82. https://doi.org/10.1590/S1516-89132008000700013.
18. Bates PJ, Laber DA, Miller DM, Thomas SD, Trent JO. Discovery and development of the G-rich oligonucleotide AS1411 as a novel treatment for cancer. Exp Mol Pathol. 2009;86(3):151–64. https://doi.org/10.1016/j.yexmp.2009.01.004.
19. Van den Avont A, Sharma-Walia N. Anti-nucleolin aptamer AS1411: an advancing therapeutic. Front Mol Biosci. 2023;10:1217769. https://doi.org/10.3389/fmolb.2023.1217769.
20. Stuart RK, Stockerl-Goldstein K, Cooper M, Devetten M, Herzig R, Medeiros B, Schiller G, Wei A, Acton G, Rizzieri D. Randomized phase II trial of the nucleolin targeting aptamer AS1411 combined with high-dose cytarabine in relapsed/refractory acute myeloid leukemia (AML). J Clin Oncol. 2009;27(15 suppl):7019. https://doi.org/10.1200/jco.2009.27.15_suppl.7019.
21. Jabbour E, Short NJ, Ravandi F, Huang X, Xiao L, Garcia-Manero G, Plunkett W, Gandhi V, Sasaki K, Pemmaraju N, Daver NG. A randomized phase 2 study of idarubicin and cytarabine with clofarabine or fludarabine in patients with newly diagnosed acute myeloid leukemia. Cancer. 2017;123(22):4430–9. https://doi.org/10.1002/cncr.30883.
22. Rosenberg JE, Bambury RM, Van Allen EM, Drabkin HA, Lara PN, Harzstark AL, Wagle N, Figlin RA, Smith GW, Garraway LA, Choueiri T. A phase II trial of AS1411 (a novel nucleolin-targeted DNA aptamer) in metastatic renal cell carcinoma. Investig New Drugs. 2014;32:178–87. https://doi.org/10.1007/s10637-013-0045-6.
23. Steurer M, Montillo M, Scarfò L, Mauro FR, Andel J, Wildner S, Trentin L, Janssens A, Burgstaller S, Frömming A, Dümmler T. Olaptesed pegol (NOX-A12) with bendamustine and rituximab: a phase IIa study in patients with relapsed/refractory chronic lymphocytic leukemia. Haematologica. 2019;104(10):2053. https://doi.org/10.3324/haematol.2018.205930.
24. Ludwig H, Weisel K, Engelhardt M, Greil R, Cafro AM, Petrucci MT, Dümmler T, Zöllner S, Zeitler S, Riecke K, Kruschinski A. Anti-CXCL12/SDF-1 Spiegelmer® Nox-A12 alone and in combination with bortezomib and dexamethasone in patients with relapsed multiple myeloma: results from a phase IIa study. Blood. 2013;122(21):1951. https://doi.org/10.1182/blood.V122.21.1951.1951.

25. Suarez-Carmona M, Williams A, Schreiber J, Hohmann N, Pruefer U, Krauss J, Jäger D, Frömming A, Beyer D, Eulberg D, Jungelius JU. Combined inhibition of CXCL12 and PD-1 in MSS colorectal and pancreatic cancer: modulation of the microenvironment and clinical effects. J Immunother Cancer. 2021;9(10) https://doi.org/10.1136/jitc-2021-002505.
26. Giordano FA, Layer JP, Leonardelli S, Friker LL, Seidel C, Schaub C, Turiello R, Sperk E, Grau F, Paech D, Link B. Radiotherapy and olaptesed pegol (NOX-A12) in partially resected or biopsy-only MGMT-unmethylated glioblastoma: interim data from the German multicenter phase 1/2 GLORIA trial. https://doi.org/10.1200/JCO.2022.40.16_suppl.2050.
27. Tran LC, Özdemir BC, Berger MD. The role of immune checkpoint inhibitors in metastatic pancreatic cancer: current state and outlook. Pharmaceuticals. 2023;16(10):1411. https://doi.org/10.3390/ph16101411.
28. Park EJ, Choi J, Lee KC, Na DH. Emerging PEGylated non-biologic drugs. Expert Opin Emerg Drugs. 2019;24(2):107–19. https://doi.org/10.1080/14728214.2019.1604684.
29. Choyke PL, Glenn GM, Walther MM, Patronas NJ, Linehan WM, Zbar B. von Hippel-Lindau disease: genetic, clinical, and imaging features. Radiology. 1995;194(3):629–42. https://doi.org/10.1148/radiology.194.3.7862955.
30. Bhardwaj H, Noumani A, Himanshu JK, Chakravorty S, Solanki PR. Recent advancement in the detection of potential cancer biomarkers using the nanomaterial integrated electrochemical sensing technique: a detailed review. Mater Adv. 2024; https://doi.org/10.1039/D3MA00621B.
31. Shigdar S, Schrand B, Giangrande PH, de Franciscis V. Aptamers: cutting edge of cancer therapies. Mol Ther. 2021;29(8):2396–411. https://doi.org/10.1016/j.ymthe.2021.06.010.

Regulatory Frameworks and Intellectual Property Rights (IPR) for Aptamer-Based Cancer Diagnosis and Therapy

14

Praveen Halagali, Shreya R. Naik, Vamshi Krishna Tippavajhala, Mahalaxmi Rathnanand, Rashmi Pathak, Himanshu Sharma, Javed Iqbal, and Shriyansh Srivastava

Abbreviations

IPR	Intellectual Property Rights
IP	Intellectual Property
SELEX	Systematic Evolution of Ligands by Exponential Enrichment
PSMA	Anti-prostate-Specific Membrane Antigen
PTK7	Anti-protein Tyrosine Kinase 7
CTCs	Circulating Tumor Cells
PET	Positron Emission Tomography
MRI	Magnetic Resonance Imaging
CT	Computed Tomography
SPECT	Single-Photon Emission Computed Tomography
VEGFR2	Vascular Endothelial Growth Factor Receptor 2

P. Halagali · V. K. Tippavajhala · M. Rathnanand
Department of Pharmaceutics, Manipal College of Pharmaceutical Sciences, Manipal Academy of Higher Education, Manipal, Karnataka, India
e-mail: praveen.mcopsmpl2023@learner.manipal.edu; vamshi.krishna@manipal.edu; mahalaxmi.r@manipal.edu

S. R. Naik
Department of Pharmacology, Rani Chennamma College of Pharmacy, Belagavi, Karnataka, India

R. Pathak
Department of Pharmacy, Invertis University, Bareilly, UP, India

H. Sharma (✉)
Teerthanker Mahaveer College of Pharmacy, Teerthanker Mahaveer University, Moradabad, UP, India

S. Srivastava et al. (eds.), *Biosensors and Aptamers*,
https://doi.org/10.1007/978-981-96-8387-1_14

EpCAM	Epidermal Adhesion Molecule
HER2	Human Epidermal Growth Factor Receptor 2
FRET	Fluorescence Resonance Energy Transfer
CSCs	Cancer Stem Cells
HCV	Hepatitis C Virus
FDA	Food and Drug Administration
GMP	Good Manufacturing Standards
EMA	European Medicines Agency
HPLC	High-Performance Liquid Chromatography

14.1 Introduction

Aptamers are, however, short single-stranded DNA transfusions or single strands of oligonucleotides with molecular weights in the range of 6–30 kDa and nucleotide counts ranging from 20 to 80 that can fold into 3D conformations. Aptamers have similar conformational recognition to complex formation and antibody-antigen recognition, using high specificity as well as affinity. Aptamers bind to their targets via electrostatic interactions, hydrogen bonds, van der Waals forces, shape complementarity, and the arrangement of flat moieties, having dissociation constant (Kd) normally varying from pico- to nanomolar. Therefore, aptamers, sometimes known as "chemical antibodies," can operate as targeted ligands, agonists, or antagonists. [17]. The formation of an aptamer-target complex by aptamer conformational recognition of targets is graphically represented in Fig. 14.1.

Aptamers are magnificent substitutes/additives for monoclonal antibodies, which are affected by high production costs and immunogenicity. Aptamers provide unequivocal benefits due to their nucleic acid properties and microscopic size, which increase their value and therapeutic relevance for industrialization when compared to antibodies. In a variety of ways, aptamers are more clinically applicable than antibodies: (i) Aptamers are effectively nontoxic and non-immunogenic in vivo. The primary reason behind this is that the immune system does not recognize oligonucleotide aptamers directly. Unlike antibodies, aptamers lack redundant Fc regions to which Fc receptors can be bound, leading to unanticipated adverse effects. (ii) Aptamers have a strong ability to cross tissue barriers

J. Iqbal
Nursing Department Communicable Disease Center-Hamad Medical Corporation, Doha, Qatar
e-mail: jiqbal3@hamad.qa

S. Srivastava
Department of Pharmacy, School of Medical and Allied Sciences, Galgotias University, Greater Noida, Uttar Pradesh, India

Department of Pharmacology, Delhi Pharmaceutical Sciences and Research University (DPSRU), New Delhi, India

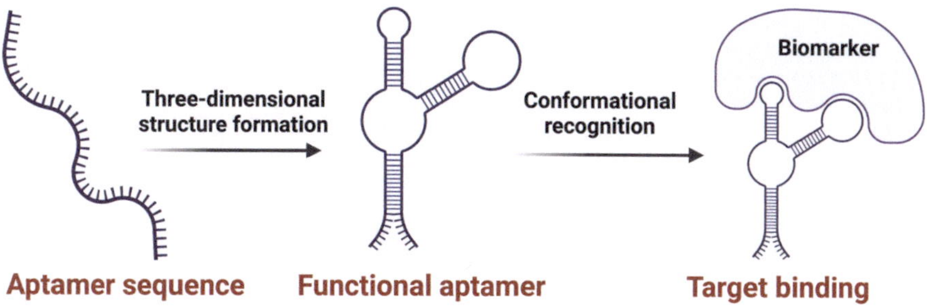

Fig. 14.1 A graphical representation of the formation of an aptamer-target complex by aptamer conformational recognition of targets

and are readily incorporated by their target cells due to their smaller size, therefore raising their therapeutic indices and optimizing the ratios of tumor to normal tissue and tumor to blood. (iii) A limitless variety of targets may be used for developing aptamers. The range of aptamer applications has been significantly increased by the successful development of specialized aptamers against a variety of targets to date, including tiny inorganic ions, medications, proteins, organic peptides, and even complex organisms or tissues. Additionally, aptamers have significant characteristics that make their industrialization easier. (iv) Aptamers can be stored and transported feasibly due to their thermally stable nature. (v) A specific aptamer can be altered and manufactured on a greater scale in a short amount of time with minimal batch-to-batch variance by using well-modification technologies and well-established chemical synthesis technologies. The benefits of aptamers over antibodies in terms of industrialization and clinical applicability are depicted in Fig. 14.2 [17].

Since the 1980s, researchers have been interested in RNA enzymes, which are nucleic acids that can fold into complicated formats and catalyze processes. These enzymes are the prerequisites of aptamers. Tuerk and Gold initiated Systematic Evolution of Ligands by Exponential Enrichment (SELEX) in 1990 after three different research teams separately disclosed iterative in vitro selection techniques for RNA enzymes. Building on earlier research, Ellington and Szostak dubbed the nucleic acids produced by selections "aptamers." The Latin word "apta" comes from "aptus," which means "fitting." The development of aptamers saw several additional significant turning points in rapid succession. The first two types of DNA aptamers were identified in 1992: thrombin-binding aptamer and specialized dye-binding aptamer. The parasite *Trypanosoma brucei* was bound by the first version of the aptamer that cell SELEX isolated, which was published in the year 1999. Macugen, the FDA's first aptamer therapeutic medication, was authorized in 2004 and was used in the treatment of macular degeneration. Technical improvements in DNA sequencing and manipulation, along with fresh approaches to selection, have simplified the selection process and reduced the entrance barrier over time. Nonetheless, SELEX's fundamental concept has not altered in more than three decades [20]. SELEX, or Systematic Evolution of Ligands by Exponential

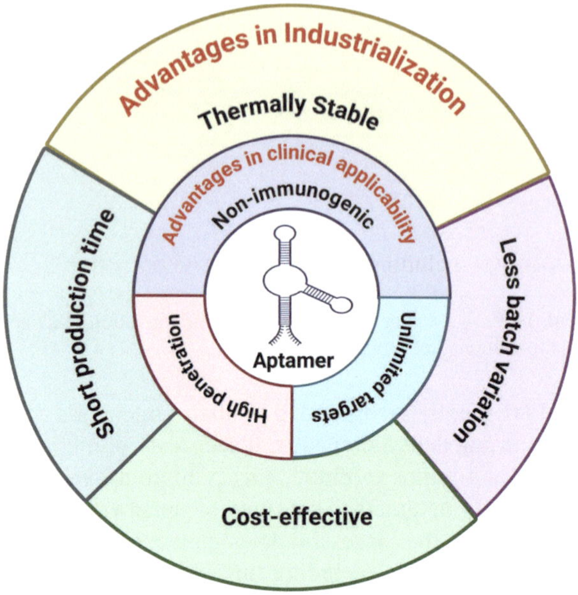

Fig. 14.2 Significant benefits of aptamers over antibodies in terms of industrialization and clinical applicability

Enrichment, is another name for in vitro selection. It is a Darwinian evolution process that generates aptamers by amplifying and selecting sequences that can carry out a specific function, like target binding or catalysis, through iterative rounds [2].

14.2 Importance in Cancer Diagnosis and Therapy

In clinical therapy, the majority of conventional antitumor medications have generated severe toxic side effects and are not selective. Aptamers are tiny nucleic acid ligands that have a high selectivity and precision for their targets. Via conjugation with medications, siRNA, nanoparticles, and other substances, aptamers are biomarkers that are closely associated with the development of cancer and can be employed as targets for screening and can be used as standalone medications. They also function as a method of targeted medication delivery capable of focusing on certain tumor cells, reducing toxicity to healthy cells, lowering the dosage required for the treatment, and improving therapeutic potential. AS1411, EpCAM, anti-nucleoli, anti-prostate-specific membrane antigen (PSMA), Sgc8, anti-protein tyrosine kinase 7 (PTK7), MUC1, anti-mucin1 aptamer, EpCAM, anti-epithelial adhesion of cells molecule, A10, and other tumor cell-targeting aptamers have all been screened by SELEX. Additionally, a variety of drug delivery techniques have been developed to target and treat specific tumor cells using these aptamers [6].

Cancer is the second leading cause of death in the world. Early accurate technologies for tumor diagnosis can allow physicians to monitor for the recurrence of tumors and metastasis, give estimates on prognosis, interpret treatment effects, and recommend treatment regimes. Antibodies are currently, frequently utilized in clinical tumor diagnostic techniques such as immunohistochemistry, in vivo imaging, flow cytometry, and tumor biomarker recognition. Moreover, the therapeutic uses of the antibodies have been somewhat restricted due to their drawbacks, which include restricted production methods, difficult chemical modification, high immunogenicity, low stability, and expensive manufacture. Aptamers offer clear benefits over antibodies in terms of stability, chemical modification, and production cost. They can also bind to targets with a high degree of specificity and affinity. It has been extensively utilized in several tumor diagnosis domains, including in vivo imaging, immunohistochemical analysis, and the detection of circulating tumor cells (CTCs).

The diagnosis and prognosis of cancer are significantly influenced by the sensitive detection of malignant cells. Certain tumor indicators, including CTCs, that are produced or released into the bloodstream by tumor cells at different phases of carcinogenesis and growth are suitable targets for liquid biopsies. Monitoring the state of the patient and the development of cancer will be greatly aided by the accurate and effective detection of CTCs when their intensity is low in the initial phases of the disease. However, since there are many fewer cancer cells in the blood than the vast majority of blood cells, the identification of CTCs is a very difficult task. Several aptamer-based analytic techniques have been used in recent years to identify CTCs by conjugating or combining several signal reporting technologies, including colorimetric, magnetic, electrochemical, and fluorescent technologies. Karnik et al., for instance, created a technology that uses a DNA network made up of repeated sticky aptamer domains to separate and collect CTCs. An electrochemical method for detecting liver cancer using CTCs was developed by Kashefi Kheyrabadi et al. A gold planar electrode coupled to a HepG2 cell-specific aptamer. Fan et al. created a technology that connects microfluidic devices with multivalent DNA aptamer nanoparticles to separate cancerous cells from the blood. Additionally, nanostructures functionalized with aptamers have been developed for cell capture and separation. By VEGF aptamer conjugation using magnetic beads to capture and concentrate CTCs, Wang et al. created a high-sensitivity CTC detection technology that targets dual aptamers. Pt-Au nanoparticles coupled with MUC1 aptamer were then used. Concentrated CTCs were used to incubate the nanoparticles. The colorimetric process was accelerated, and a sensitive signal was sent by Pt-Au nanoparticles in a mixture of hydrogen peroxide (H_2O_2) with TMB (3′, 3′, 5′, 5′-tetramethylbenzidine). The system has a threshold for detection of 10 cells/mL and a linear range of 10 to 105 cells/mL.

Molecular imaging concerns itself with the prognosis, monitoring, and detection of the disease. In this spectrum, aptamers are by far the major types of diagnostic agents in current cancer research, as these compounds are tagged to fluorescent compounds, radionuclides, or other imaging agents. Some of these in vivo imaging modalities for tumor imaging include positron emission tomography (PET), magnetic resonance imaging (MRI), computerized tomography (CT), luminescence imaging, and single-photon emission computed tomography (SPECT). Aptamer-conjugated targeting blood-brain barrier peptide IRD800CW-conjugated CD30 aptamer is used in vivo in imaging of lymphomas; Cy5-labeled pancreatic cancer-specific aptamer serves in vivo imaging of pancreatic cancer; glioma aptamer is used in vivo imaging of gliomas. They exhibit all desired characteristics—an adequate pharmacokinetic profile, favorable signal-to-noise ratio, rapid targeting, and accuracy specificity. MRI can be improved by conjugating aptamers to magnetic beads along with fluorescent molecular imaging. For example, glioma MRI imaging uses the aptamer of the vascular endothelial growth factor receptor 2 (VEGFR2) coupled with magnetic nanomaterials. Magnetic nanomaterials coupled with an epidermal adhesion molecule (EpCAM) aptamer for stomach cancer MRI imaging, etc. All of them greatly increase the sensitivity, biocompatibility, and tumor-targeted imaging capabilities while lowering cytotoxicity, which increases MRI's potential for clinical use [6].

14.3 Aptamers in Cancer Diagnosis and Therapy

14.3.1 Mechanism and Advantages of Cancer Detection Using Aptamers

14.3.1.1 Aptasensors

Early detection of cancer is important for preventing disease and its cure. For the diagnosis of cancer-related proteins, cancer cells, and small molecules, many kinds of sensors have been built. Although a maximum of them are dependent on antigen-antibody target proteins, they are recorded and seen using binding assays, which typically need a sandwich system to find their targets. There are two different types of antibodies in a sandwich system for the identification of a target. The affinities of antibodies differ from batch to batch, which is the major reason for the major incompatibilities raised during the evolution of diagnostics of dependable sensors. To reduce the above difficulties, aptamers were tested as a cancer diagnostic tool because of their specificity and higher binding forces for cells related to cancer and molecules. Aptamers can detect the difference between cancerous and noncancerous cells due to their ability to distinguish between proteins with similar structures. In contrast to antibodies, when aptamers attach to their targets, they undergo a conformational shift. The shift in the conformation helps to create distinctive, flexible aptasensors, which is not possible with antibodies. Thus, for the signal switch unit and identification unit in the creation of aptasensors for biomarkers linked to cancer, aptamers are used [19].

Optical Aptasensors

Due to its great sensitivity, fluorescence was used as the output signal while assembling biosensors with aptamers for the detection of cancer-related biomarkers and cancer cells. Fluorescent aptasensors served as the measure to identify cancer early using cancer-related biomarkers. For example, Freeman et al. developed a range of various VEGF detection techniques based on optical aptasensors. Cho et al. prepared VEGF165 as the target of a single-step surface-enhanced aptasensor, a common indicator of cancer angiogenesis.

Electrochemical Aptasensors

Apart from fluorescent aptasensors, electrochemical sensors were used because of their great sensitivity for accurate identification of cancer cells and biomarkers, their inexpensive cost, and their potential for therapeutic use. Generally, there were two approaches to the production of electrochemical aptasensors. The first method was the sandwich structure, which was the same as that of the antibody target antibody used to identify the cells and biomarkers of cancer. The next method relied on conformational changes of the aptamers after binding to the respective target. This conformational shift caused the electrochemically active molecules to move closer or farther away from the electrode, creating "signal-on" or "signal-off" aptasensors. A sandwich electrochemical sensor was created by Zhu et al. to identify breast cancer cells that overexpress human epidermal growth factor receptor 2 (HER2). First, the outermost layer of gold nanoparticles that had been altered on the electrode was conjugated with a HER2 nanoantibody (znti-HER2).

Other Aptasensors

Other than the abovementioned aptasensors, aptasensors of several types were developed to detect cancer cells and biomarkers associated with the disease [19]. Chemiluminescence, a sophisticated and versatile tool for detecting cancer cells is the one that does not interfere with autofluorescence, which is caused by photoexcitation in a chemiluminescence reaction. Cancer cells were detected using other signals like radiology, MRI, and ultrasound. Although most of these concentrate on in vitro *and* in vivo imaging.

14.3.2 Advantages of Using Aptamers

Production of aptamers is done chemically by a scalable process. Due to chemical production, aptamers are free from bacterial or viral contamination. They are not immunogenic, and aptamers are smaller. Therefore, they can efficiently access biological compartments, they have the capability to differentiate between specific as well as nonspecific targets, and they can also choose in contradiction to targets on the cell surface [10]. An aptamer's phosphodiester bond is chemically stable and can be reversibly denatured. Conjugation chemistries are orthogonal and simple to incorporate during synthesis to attach dyes or functional groups. Aptamers are suitably stable for long-term storage, and they can easily be transported at room temperature [15].

14.3.3 Current Applications

Analogously, aptamers and monoclonal antibodies can identify and attach to their targets. Thus, by their isolation, aptamers can be employed to recognize their targets molecularly. Aptamers have numerous therapeutic and diagnostic uses like target inhibitors and biosensors [21].

14.3.3.1 Aptamers for Diagnosis

Due to aptamers having high specificity and high affinity, they are the best agents and can replace traditional antibodies in food safety environmental protection, and clinical diagnosis. Aptamers can also be preferred for molecular identification of their targets, like that of monoclonal antibodies. Aptamers, being easy to develop, can be modified easily and have great stability; they are being used in many fields like molecular biology, biomedicine, and biotechnology.

Pathogen Recognition

The purpose of fluorescence resonance energy transfer (FRET) aptamers was to screen for *Escherichia coli* outer membrane proteins in a high-throughput manner to find surface enterotoxaemia *E. coli.* Aptamers are also being used for the identification of surfaces of *Campylobacter jejuni*. Aptamers can even diagnose multiple infections at once, showing their versatility and efficiency in diagnostic settings. Aptamer technology has recently advanced toward competing methods that can identify diverse diseases.

Wide-ranging pathogen identification: Indeed, aptamers have found broad applications in pathogen identification across different biological kingdoms, such as bacteria, viruses, and fungi. For instance, aptamers were created using SELEX to target *Leptospira interrogans*; these aptamers showed sensitivity and specificity for the identification of this pathogen in contaminated water samples. a) Enhanced sensitivity: By amplifying detection signals with PCR and similar methods, it is possible to increase aptamer-based detection sensitivity, which becomes particularly relevant when detecting low-abundance pathogens in complex samples. b) Point-of-care testing: Since they are fast and cheap, aptamer-based diagnostics can fundamentally fulfill these demands in resource-limited areas for rapid diagnosis at the point of care.

Cancer Recognition

Aptamers for cancer diagnosis and prognosis are developed for accurate and rapid diagnosis and prognosis assessments of cancer. They have been developed for the detection of various cancer indicators; tumor-associated proteins such as MUC1, HER2, and estrogen receptors were found in the cancer cell. Their targeting can be subjected to aptamers that are specific to the proteins implicated in various malignancies. Examples could include MUC-1-targeting aptamers that have been effectively used in the extremely sensitive quantitative detection of ovarian cancer biomarkers. Likewise, cancer diagnostics related to colorectal cancer have also identified aptamers such as SYL3C that bind specifically to EpCAM. Aptamer-nanoparticle systems: The ability of aptamers for detection is increased upon conjugation with nanoparticles. Examples include aptamer-gold nanoparticle (Apt-AuNP) systems, which improve the sensitivity and specificity of cancer cell identification in complex biological fluids like blood. Thus, these enable diagnosis to be made with greater precision by capturing cancer cells with their cages. In vivo imaging: Aptamers are tagged with imaging agents to diagnose cancers by noninvasive means. The use of aptamers in fluorescence and PET imaging is significant in the detection of cancers in living animal models. This feature allows for determining the tumor growth and response to different treatments, and this exhibits a real-time manner in operation.

Stem Cell Recognition

The development processes of the aptamers have proved ineffective against stem cells. There are only a listable number of aptamers against the stem cell markers such as cancer surface biomarkers, the epithelial cell adhesion molecule, CD44, CD133, CD117, and cancer stem cells (CSCs). Human pluripotent stem cells (hPSCs) can now be precisely labeled with aptamers. For example, alkaline phosphatase (ALPL), a marker that is highly expressed on the surface of PSCs, can be bound by the well-characterized DNA aptamer Apt19.

Monitoring Environmental Contamination

Aptamers can control and reduce the contaminants in the environment and the illness resulting from it. Antibiotics have heavy metals, pathogens, and toxins, which can be harmful to the human system. Antibiotics prepared from farm animals may get concentrated in human tissues. To overcome these issues, aptamers are developed against some antibiotics like tetracycline and chloramphenicol. Aptamers are also developed against various pesticides like fungicide carbendazim, acetamiprid atrazine, etc.

14.3.3.2 Aptamers Used in Biosensors

To simplify what aptamer configurations can be prepared, aptamers have a variety of uses in biosensors because of their combined capacity to attach to certain targets by creating stable tertiary structures. The purpose of aptamer-based biosensors is to detect illness biomarkers, such as platelet-derived growth factor, a protein linked to cancer, to ease the real diagnosis of cancer and the development of cancer prognosis. The activity of the biosensor can be enhanced by the use of different nanomaterials. For example, a graphene-based biosensor that targets β-globulin for the discovery of the human epidermal growth factor receptor 2 biosensor and for the detection of milk allergies.

14.3.3.3 Aptamers as Therapeutics

Aptamers having the capacity to inhibit targets of small molecules and protein ligands are regarded as good therapeutics. Target receptor function can be activated by aptamers or can also serve as transporters for delivering the medications to the target areas or cells. For example, aptamers can act as antiviral agents. HIV-1 can be neutralized by using RNA aptamers against a synthetic gp120 variant. RNA aptamers that target RIG-I can prevent the reproduction of influenza, vesicular stomatitis, and Newcastle disease viruses. Targeting the NS3 helicase domain of the hepatitis C virus (HCV), RNA aptamers that effectively block protease and helicase activities were created to suppress HCV.

14.4 Regulatory Frameworks for Aptamer-Based Products

A regulatory framework for aptamer-based products is developing as the effective method in therapeutics and diagnosis becomes recognized. The US Food and Drug Administration (FDA) has established particular requirements for diagnostic tests that aptamer-based assays must meet. One noteworthy instance is a small molecule aptamer-based test that was created to track the chemotherapy drug imatinib and satisfies FDA requirements for ligand-binding assays. This test showed:

- Accuracy and Precision: The test met FDA requirements for clinical diagnostics with an accuracy range of 97.1% to 101.8% and a precision range of 1.3% to 5.2%.
- Regulatory Compliance: To ensure adherence to safety and efficacy regulations, the aptamer was chosen to be target-specific and not interact with other medications.
- Manufacturing Standards: To guarantee uniformity and quality across batches and reduce performance variability, aptamer manufacturers should follow Good Manufacturing Practices (GMP).
- Clinical Trials: Before being approved, aptamers must pass stringent clinical testing to prove their efficacy and safety.
- Stability and Modification: To improve stability and lower renal clearance, therapeutic aptamers frequently need to be modified (e.g., PEGylated), which needs to be recorded throughout the approval procedure.

14.4.1 Overview

14.4.1.1 Approval Process

Aptamer-based product approval, especially in the therapeutic and diagnostics setting, includes several crucial steps that comply with regulatory standards established by organizations like the European Medicines Agency (EMA) and the US Food and Drug Administration (FDA). An outline of the crucial processes in this procedure is provided below:

- After being found, promising aptamers are thoroughly characterized to evaluate their stability, specificity, and binding affinity. This could consist of:

  Chemical changes: Modifications like 2′-O-methylation or PEGylation14 may be added to improve pharmacokinetic characteristics and stability against nucleases. Aptamers must undergo these changes to continue functioning in biological systems.
- Preclinical research on efficacy and safety is done prior to clinical trials.
- Efficacy shows in target biological models the ability of an aptamer to bind its target efficiently. Safety is conducted in order to ensure that the aptamer has no negative effects; hence, toxicological evaluations are undertaken.

- Aptamer-based products should undergo clinical trials that are much more extensive in order to demonstrate their safety and effectiveness in humans. That usually works out to be a series of three phases:
  Phase I Trials: These look into dose and safety aspects.
  Phase II Trials: These determine the effectiveness and the possible side effects.
  Phase III Trials: In these, the new treatment is used for comparison and contrast in larger populations alongside conventional therapies.
- On completion of clinical trials, the process moves to the formal regulatory filings that comprise:
  Data Compilation: Engaging all preclinical and clinical study data with manufacturing data all mixed into one body would make the filing of a New Drug Application (NDA) or Biologics License Application (BLA) an easier task.
  Review Procedure: The application is reviewed by the FDA or other relevant regulatory agencies to ensure that it meets the efficacy and safety standards.
- After this approval, continuing observations are to be made so as to ensure the safety and efficacy of the common public. This entails:
  Adverse Event Reporting: The manufacturers will need to report any adverse events known to be associated with the aptamer-based product.
  Periodic Review: The safety data will be reviewed at periodic times, as directed by the regulatory authorities, as more prescriptions are written for the product.

14.4.1.2 Manufacturing Conditions

Aptamers must adhere to all GMP guidelines to ensure the quality and consistency of products [9]. The manufacture of aptamer-based products entails several crucial procedures and conditions that guarantee the final product's effectiveness, stability, and quality. The process of aptamer manufacture has several main parts.

1. Chemical: The combination of phosphoramidite solid-phase chemistry for the production of aptamers is now the main method practiced since it is an established technology for producing oligonucleotides. Important characteristics are:
   (a) Scalability: The easy scalability of the whole procedure makes it possible for the production of very large batches ranging from grams to kilograms, thus rendering it suitable for both commercial and research purposes.
   (b) Automation: Automating modern synthesis lowers labor costs and allows for consistent manufacture.
2. Control Quality: In order for the aptamers to be in compliance with certification memberships for them to be used, the factor of quality control is extremely imperative at any stage in the general production process:
   (a) Purity: The purity and identity of aptamers can be confirmed by methods such as HPLC and mass spectrometry.
   (b) Functional Testing: Functional assays are performed on aptamers to indicate their binding affinity and selectivity toward their target molecules, ensuring that they operate appropriately in prospective application fields such as diagnosis or treatment.

3. Conditions for Folding: There are several prescribed conditions for the proper folding of aptamers:
   (a) Denaturation and Renaturation: In order for aptamers to fold nicely into an active morph, they undergo denaturation at high temperatures (about 94 °C for about 8 min) and are then cooled. Standardization of conditions such as these is generally considered vital since variation in them could impact binding efficiency.
   (b) Buffer: The buffer used for folding might negatively influence the stability and binding properties with which the aptamer is folded. Slight changes in the buffer composition or ionic strength should be closely monitored in order to maintain consistent performance.
4. Stability Features: In the biological environment, aptamers are required to resist degradation, especially by nucleases.
   (a) Chemicals: The aptamer may be made more stable by using phosphorothioate linkages or by utilizing nonnatural nucleotides; this would lead to resistance toward enzymatic degradation.
   (b) Storage Conditions: Aptamers may be lyophilized, which enables long-term storage without refrigeration, thereby simplifying logistics and reducing cold chain management costs.
5. Good Manufacturing Practices: Manufacturing processes must comply with GMP to ensure a safe and effective product:
   (a) Non-immunogenicity: Aptamer drugs, unlike protein-based therapies such as antibodies, are mostly non-immunogenic, which makes the regulatory processes even easier.
   (b) Documentation: All records on the synthesis procedure, QA processes, and stability studies must be kept well for regulatory submissions.

14.4.2 Clinical Trial Studies

Pegaptanib is the first and only medicinal aptamer that was authorized by the US FDA in 2004 to treat neovascular macular degeneration associated with aging as an antiangiogenic drug. Other than this, there have been several phases of clinical studies on pegaptanib for various diseases like AMD, proliferative diabetic retinopathy, and diabetic macular edema. It is presently approved in the United States, Europe, Brazil, Canada, and Australia. A pegylated 29-nucleotide DNA aptamer called E10030 was produced in response to platelet-derived growth factor B. E10030 binds to PDGF with sub-nanomolar affinity and interrupts the interaction of PDGF with the beta subunits of its receptors. When compared to ranibizumab, E10030 showed 62% more therapeutic effect in a randomized phase 2 trial that involved 449 participants with neovascular age-related macular degeneration. In phase 3 clinical trials, the use of the E10030 aptamer in conjunction with Lucentis was contrasted with Lucentis monotherapy in individuals with acute macular degeneration. There is no more data available as the study was stopped. ARC1905 is a pegylated 38-nucleotide RNA aptamer. It attaches to the human complement's C5 component and prevents its expression, which has a major role in innate immunity and inflammatory diseases. Clinical trials for AMD, idiopathic polypoidal choroidal vasculopathy, and geographic atrophy disorders have been conducted on ARC1905. AA1411 is a 26v base oligonucleotide rich in guanine with an unaltered DNA backbone. This aptamer is the first to be used in human cancer therapy clinical studies. Moreover, it is clinically evaluated for renal cell cancer in metastases and acute myeloid leukemia with advanced solid cancers exhibiting positive results with a lesser amount of side effects. Prolonged phase 1 trials were carried out in both non-small cell lung carcinoma and renal cell carcinoma patients and showed a nonsignificant result. Spiegelmer, also called NOX-A12, is a pegylated 45-nucleotide L-form RNA aptamer. These are single-stranded RNA oligonucleotides comprising a 40 kDa PEG branch. They target CXCL12/SDF-1, a major chemokine protein that has an active contribution to the proliferation of tumors and promotes the development of new blood vessels and metastases. The first medication used in human clinical research was given IV in 48 health patients in the age range of 18 to 60 years. This aptamer was determined to be safe and well tolerated by patients and demonstrated encouraging and sustained CXCL12 inhibition. In a phase 2a trial, 28 patients with relapsed or refractory multiple myeloma received NOX-A12 either alone or in combination with bortezomib/dexamethasone. The aptamer exhibited no toxicity, and also, its tolerability was found to be good. The US FDA has designated NOX-A12 as an orphan medication for the treatment of glioblastoma in conjunction with radiation therapy [22]. Notable clinical trials using aptamers for cancer detection and treatment are given in Table 14.1.

14.4.3 Challenges in Regulatory Compliance

(a) Developmental problems: Many steps of SELEX require PCR amplification for generating reaction mixtures. This amplification of the aptamer library may lead to artificial products, and bias of some nucleotide sequences is observed, which hinders the aptamer selection procedure. This may also lead to more time consumption and can also become a tedious process. Only a few aptamer-oriented commercial incubators have been established, like SomaLogic, Noxon, and Apta Biosciences. (b) Chemical problems: Aptamers can be highly modified when they bind to their respective targets. This modification may lead to nuclease degradation. (c) Approval issues: Only a single therapeutic aptamer has been approved to date. The introduction of aptamers in the market has not been an easy task. Even though a fine number of aptamers are being tested in different clinical trials, their development is facing skepticism, and investors are trading cautiously. A reversible adverse effect was observed in a phase III clinical trial of REG1 aptamer, which may hinder the progression of the emerging aptamers and make it yet more difficult to build a business around aptamers [14]. (d) Pharmacokinetic properties and other aptamer systemic characteristics are inconsistent and frequently unpredictable. (e) Unmodified aptamers have a higher

Table 14.1 Notable clinical trials using aptamers for cancer detection and treatment

Aptamer name	Type	Target	Targeted disease	Clinical status	References
Pegaptanib (VEGF165)	RNA	VEGF165	Diabetic retinopathy and age-related macular degeneration	Approved (marketed)	[8]
AS1411	DNA	Nucleolin	Renal cell carcinoma with metastases and acute myeloid leukemia	Phase II (NCT01034410, NCT00740441), phase I (NCT00881244)	[8, 12]
NOX-A12	RNA	CXCL-12	Various cancers (inhibits proliferation and metastasis)	Phase I/II ongoing	[12]
AGRO100	DNA	Nucleolin	Various tumors (anti-proliferation effects)	Phase I completed, safety established	[12]
68Ga-Sgc8	DNA	PTK7/CCk-4	Colorectal cancer	Early phase 1 (NCT03385148)	[8]
PNDA-3	DNA	Periostin	Breast cancer (metastasis inhibition)	Preclinical studies ongoing	[12]

chance of serum degradation. (f) Aptamer technologies are present to a great extent, enclosed by a single portfolio of intellectual property. (g) An aptamer's half-life is shorter because it is smaller in size, which makes it prone to renal filtration. (f) Aptamers have low drug loading capacity, and they are made using costly multistep procedures for design and synthesis. This may affect the commercialization of aptamer-based products. (g) Market competition: Aptamers face significant competition from established antibody therapies, which dominate the market due to their proven efficacy and safety records. This competitive landscape makes it challenging for new aptamer-based products to gain traction and funding for development. (h) Lack of standardization: The absence of standardized protocols for aptamer selection and production can lead to variability in clinical trial outcomes. Regulatory agencies require consistent methodologies to evaluate safety and efficacy, which is currently a challenge due to the diverse approaches in aptamer development [11].

14.5 Intellectual Property Rights for Aptamer Technologies

14.5.1 Patents on Aptamer Technologies

Sullenger et al. published the primary study suggesting that in 1990, it was discovered that RNA ligands may be utilized to stop a pathogenic protein from acting.

They showed that the TAR decoy, which HIV evolved to get cellular and viral proteins to attach to viral transcripts, might be used to stop the virus from replicating [16]. Tuerk and Gold's groundbreaking work was then responsible for the arena's 1990 opening. Using SELEX, an in vitro iterative screening and enrichment technique (Systematic Evolution of Ligands by Exponential Enrichment) [18], they extracted sequences that bacteriophage T4 DNA polymerase binds to from an RNA pool. This process later proved to be the field's groundbreaking patent (EP0533838) [1]. Ellington and Szostak used a comparable in vitro technique and independently published another work on the discovery of RNA ligands capable of binding to tiny chemical dyes in the same year [3]. They called this type of RNA molecule aptamer, a combination of the Greek term meros, meaning "part" or region, and the Latin term aptus, meaning "to fit." They also revealed single-stranded DNA sequences were selected from a large number of random sequences two years later [4]. Nucleic acid ligands that are short and single-stranded (DNA or RNA) and have been selected to bind with high specificity and affinity to their target molecules, which are often proteins, are referred to as aptamers. Some researchers have expanded this term to include peptides that exhibit comparable interactions and protein target modulation. The area of aptamers has advanced quickly; as of June 2008, there were almost 1000 articles (based only on a Medline search), 726 patents published globally, and 276 patents filed with the USPTO. Aptamer patents may be roughly divided into two classes: one that reveals the development of techniques for isolating and altering them and the other that identifies the kind of use it has. We attempted to evaluate every significant patent about therapeutic aptamers and their production processes in this chapter. Many times during this assembly, we discovered many patents on aptamers for a certain protein. This may be because of differences in their sequences, a new modification that was added, or a different isozyme target. Even though we have made every effort to highlight the most pertinent patents in these situations, we may have overlooked some crucial ones. Therefore, we sincerely regret if we have overlooked any patents that have significantly advanced the development of aptamers and therapies. Partitioning the ligands that are bound and those that are not is one of the most important and challenging phases in SELEX since poor partitioning methods can result in selection errors and the amplification of undesirable ligands. The majority of the aptamer generation–related patents have been submitted in this field. Various selection techniques are employed based on the aim, potential future applications, and accessible options. Although nitrocellulose membranes are frequently used to select RNA aptamers, this approach is limited to small molecule targets. Another selection method is affinity surfaces, where the immobilized target is treated with the oligonucleotide library [1]. Patents on aptamer technologies are given in Table 14.2.

Table 14.2 Patents on aptamer technologies [7]

Sl no.	Application number	Application date	Title
1	11201803600P	25.10.2016	DNA aptamer binding to cancer cell
2	16,749,175	05.02.2016	An aptamer for DNA that can attach to non-small cell lung cancer cells (H1975)
3	202011384675.2	30.11.2020	Quick screening of rectal cancer aptamer-containing tissue samples and use of the aptamer to create detection preparation
4	1,020,110,035,378	15.04.2011	A novel RNA aptamer with anticancer properties and a medication to treat cancer
5	202010140426.2	03.03.2020	Colon cancer nucleic acid aptamer is produced by quickly screening tissue samples and using it to prepare for detection
6	202080031891.0	30.03.2020	Aptamer specifically binding to cancer stem cells and use thereof
7	2,013,148,623	17.07.2013	Particularly binding to mouse colon carcinoma colon26 is a nucleic acid
8	202011371855.7	30.11.2020	Application of the nucleic acid aptamer truncation body in human non-small cell lung cancer
9	1,020,130,002,513	09.01.2013	Aptamer that selectively binds itself to an ERBB2 receptor
10	18,251,185	25.11.2022	Nanocomposite and preparation method and use thereof
11	201110172522.6	23.06.2011	Gastric cancer cells' nucleic acid aptamer sequence and applications
12	1,020,110,061,939	24.06.2011	An aptamer that binds to the ERBB2 receptor specifically and a composition containing the same
13	202010139631.7	03.03.2020	The bladder cancer nucleic acid aptamer was produced by quickly screening a tissue sample and using it to prepare for detection
14	15,424,896	06.02.2017	Ovarian cancer-specific aptamer and ovarian cancer detection technique
15	201110201214.1	18.07.2011	Prostatic cancer targets gene oligonucleotide aptamer, delivery mechanism, delivery carrier, and preparation techniques
16	201810572286.9	06.06.2018	EpDT3 aptamer-modified prostate cancer-targeting drug delivery vector and delivery system, and preparation and applications thereof
17	201811546124.4	18.12.2018	A nucleic acid aptamer that can identify human colon cancer and be used to create detection preparations
18	201811340422.8	12.11.2018	Aptamer for identifying drug-resistant cell strains in liver cancer and its use
19	200,910,083,075. X	28.04.2009	Aptamer for typing several non-small cell lung cancer subtypes and screening techniques for the same

(continued)

Table 14.2 (continued)

Sl no.	Application number	Application date	Title
20	201910536200.1	20.06.2019	Nucleic acid aptamer for identifying intestinal cancer serum marker regarding the use of nucleic acid aptamers for screening
21	201,410,720,055. X	01.12.2014	Aptamer for recognizing adriamycin-resistant breast cancer cells as well as a screening method and application of aptamer
22	2,018,117,251	20.06.2018	Pharmaceutical composition for treating cancer containing rage aptamer

14.6 Navigating Challenges in Regulation and IPR

14.6.1 Key Challenges in Regulatory Approval

14.6.1.1 Limited Clinical Approval and Experience

Till now, there is only one approved therapeutic aptamer from the FDA, and that is pegaptanib for clinical treatment for age-related macular degeneration 13. Cancer therapies have not seen any therapeutic aptamers approved, though there have been several that have progressed to different levels of clinical trials. It indicates the lack of a regulatory milestone as not enough clinical data exists, creating gaps in clinical experience required to comprehensively judge safety and efficacy for regulators [12, 13, 22].

14.6.1.2 Safety and Efficacy Concerns

The shift from preclinical experiments to clinical trials has normally created concerns about safety as well as efficacy. Although numerous aptamers have exhibited inadequacy in preclinical models in terms of potency, which questions the drug potential of these aptamers, there is no precise information on how safe they are, and there are limited regulatory acceptances of these drugs [13, 22].

14.6.1.3 Production and Scalability Issues

Generally, the method known as Systematic Evolution of Ligands by Exponential Enrichment (SELEX) is used to create aptamers. Compared to the procedure for producing monoclonal antibodies, which is comparatively more costly and time-consuming [5, 22]. The high price tags associated with producing aptamers may deter pharmaceutical companies from pursuing their development. Additional problems related to scaling up with acceptable quality may also add to the existing issues related to regulatory proceedings.

14.6.1.4 Pharmacokinetics and Stability

Pharmacokinetics and metabolic stability are often hindrances to aptamers. Due to their small size, they can easily be filtered through the renal system out of the blood and therefore have short half-lives, which could potentially limit in vivo therapeutic applications. Chemical modification can increase stability and increase circulation time, but such modification needs to be considered as regards its detrimental effect on aptamer binding activity and hence on its function [12, 22].

14.6.1.5 Regulatory Framework Adaptation

The existing regulatory frameworks are essentially focused on more traditional biologics such as antibodies. Aptamers differ in characteristics as well as mechanisms of action and need to be placed within regulatory frameworks adapted appropriately for those characteristics [8, 13]. Regulatory authorities should thus provide clear directives that detail every aspect of aptamer drug development—design, testing processes, and post-market surveillance.

14.7 Conclusion

Globally, cancer ranks as the second leading cause of mortality. Physicians can monitor tumor recurrence and metastasis, estimate prognosis, evaluate therapy outcomes, and recommend treatment regimens early with the use of accurate tumor diagnosis technologies. Nowadays, antibodies are widely used in histochemistry, in vivo imaging, flow cytometry, tumor biomarker detection, and other clinical techniques of tumor diagnostics. Furthermore, the therapeutic use of antibodies has been somewhat restricted by their disadvantages, which include restricted modes of production, difficulty in chemical modification, high immunogenicity, low stability, and expensive manufacturing. Aptamers provide distinct advantages over antibodies with regard to stability, chemical modification, and production cost. Molecular imaging is important in prognosis, monitoring, and disease detection. Aptamers are increasingly important as cancer diagnostic tools, often conjugated with fluorescent compounds, radionuclides, or other imaging molecules. The development of aptamers for cancer diagnosis and treatment also enjoys substantial policy support through regulation and intellectual property. By defining and meeting the standards of safety and efficacy and keeping rigorous patent protection, stakeholders seek to facilitate the journey from the lab to the bedside for aptamer technologies and improve the outlook for further research and development. It creates a setting that encourages growth in aptamer therapeutics to lead to better diagnostics and personalized therapies for enhanced patient care. These structures will be crucial in resolving the commercialization issues as they develop and ensure that aptamer-based products can contribute substantially to advances in cancer detection and treatment. Aptamers typically show tremendous promise for cancer diagnosis and therapy, owing largely to their specificity and versatility, while many constraints must be considered to improve practical applications. Ongoing work in aptamer technology must focus attention on establishing the pathways for curing issues concerned with stability, cell penetration, serum clearance, cross-reactivity, manufacturing difficulties, intellectual property conflicts, and insufficient knowledge of binding interactions. Addressing these issues will be the key to unlocking the potential that aptamers hold in clinical settings for the future.

References

1. Dua P, Kim S, Lee DK. Patents on SELEX and therapeutic aptamers. Recent Patents DNA Gene Sequences. 2008;2(3):172–86. https://doi.org/10.2174/187221508786241710.
2. Dunn MR, Jimenez RM, Chaput JC. Analysis of aptamer discovery and technology. *Nature reviews*. Chemistry. 2017;1(10) https://doi.org/10.1038/S41570-017-0076.
3. Ellington AD, Szostak JW. In vitro selection of RNA molecules that bind specific ligands. Nature. 1990;346(6287):818–22. https://doi.org/10.1038/346818a0.
4. Ellington AD, Szostak JW. Selection in vitro of single-stranded DNA molecules that fold into specific ligand-binding structures. Nature. 1992;355(6363):850–2. https://doi.org/10.1038/355850a0.
5. Gao F, Yin J, Chen Y, Guo C, Hu H, Su J. Recent advances in aptamer-based targeted drug delivery systems for cancer therapy. Front Bioeng Biotechnol. 2022;10 https://doi.org/10.3389/fbioe.2022.972933.
6. Han J, Gao L, Wang J, Wang J. Application and development of aptamer in cancer: from clinical diagnosis to cancer therapy. J Cancer. 2020;11(23):6902–15. https://doi.org/10.7150/JCA.49532.
7. https://clinicaltrials.gov. (n.d.).
8. Hu X, Zhang D, Zeng Z, Huang L, Lin X, Hong S. Aptamer-based probes for cancer diagnostics and treatment. Life. 2022;12(11) https://doi.org/10.3390/life12111937.
9. Kaur H, Bruno JG, Kumar A, Sharma TK. Aptamers in the therapeutics and diagnostics pipelines. Theranostics. 2018;8(15):4016–32. https://doi.org/10.7150/thno.25958.
10. Keefe AD, Pai S, Ellington A. Aptamers as therapeutics. Nat Rev Drug Discov. 2010;9(8):660. https://doi.org/10.1038/nrd3249.
11. Lakhin AV, Tarantul VZ. (n.d.). Gening L. Aptamers: problems, solutions and prospects.
12. Li Z, Fu X, Huang J, Zeng P, Huang Y, Chen X, Liang C. Advances in screening and development of therapeutic Aptamers against cancer cells. Front Cell Develop Biol. 2021;9 https://doi.org/10.3389/fcell.2021.662791.
13. Nuzzo S, Roscigno G, Affinito A, Ingenito F, Quintavalle C, Condorelli G. Potential and challenges of aptamers as specific carriers of therapeutic oligonucleotides for precision medicine in cancer. Cancers. 2019;11(10) https://doi.org/10.3390/cancers11101521.
14. Rozenblum GT, Lopez VG, Vitullo AD, Radrizzani M. Aptamers: current challenges and future prospects. Expert Opin Drug Discov. 2016;11(2):127–35. https://doi.org/10.1517/17460441.2016.1126244.
15. Santarpia G, Carnes E. Therapeutic applications of Aptamers. Int J Mol Sci. 2024;25(12) https://doi.org/10.3390/ijms25126742.
16. Sullenger BA, Gallardo HF, Ungers GE, Gilboa E. Overexpression of TAR sequences renders cells resistant to human immunodeficiency virus replication. Cell. 1990;63(3):601–8. https://doi.org/10.1016/0092-8674(90)90455-N.
17. Sun H, Zu Y. A highlight of recent advances in aptamer technology and its application. Molecules. 2015;20(7):11959–80. https://doi.org/10.3390/molecules200711959.
18. Tuerk C, Gold L. Systematic evolution of ligands by exponential enrichment: RNA ligands to bacteriophage T4 DNA polymerase. Science. 1990;249(4968):505–10. https://doi.org/10.1126/science.2200121.

19. Wu X, Chen J, Wu M, Zhao JX. Aptamers: active targeting ligands for cancer diagnosis and therapy. Theranostics. 2015;5(4):322–44. https://doi.org/10.7150/thno.10257.
20. Yang LF, Ling M, Kacherovsky N, Pun SH. Aptamers 101: aptamer discovery and in vitro applications in biosensors and separations. Chem Sci. 2023;14:4961. https://doi.org/10.1039/d3sc00439b.
21. Zhang Y, Lai BS, Juhas M. Recent advances in aptamer discovery and applications. Molecules. 2019;24(5) https://doi.org/10.3390/molecules24050941.
22. Zhou J, Rossi J. Aptamers as targeted therapeutics: current potential and challenges. Nat Rev Drug Discov. 2017;16(3):181–202. https://doi.org/10.1038/nrd.2016.199.

Correction to: Biosensors and Aptamers

Shriyansh Srivastava, Sachin Kumar,
Sathvik Belagodu Sridhar, Malakapogu Ravindra Babu,
and Shaik Abdul Rahaman

Correction to:
S. Srivastava et al. (eds.), *Biosensors and Aptamers*,
https://doi.org/10.1007/978-981-96-8387-1

The original version of the book was inadvertently published with incorrect spelling of author's name in online version.

The correction chapters and the book have been updated with these changes.

The updated versions of these chapters can be found at
https://doi.org/10.1007/978-981-96-8387-1_5
https://doi.org/10.1007/978-981-96-8387-1_6

S. Srivastava et al. (eds.), *Biosensors and Aptamers*,
https://doi.org/10.1007/978-981-96-8387-1_15

MIX
Papier aus verantwortungsvollen Quellen
Paper from responsible sources
FSC® C105338
www.fsc.org

If you have any concerns about our products,
you can contact us on
ProductSafety@springernature.com

In case Publisher is established outside the EU,
the EU authorized representative is:
Springer Nature Customer Service Center GmbH
Europaplatz 3, 69115 Heidelberg, Germany

Printed by Libri Plureos GmbH
in Hamburg, Germany